Abortion and Options Counseling

A Comprehensive Reference

Anne Baker

Revised and Expanded Edition

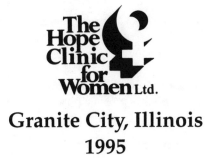

Granite City, Illinois
1995

Published by The Hope Clinic for Women, Ltd.
1602 21st Street
Granite City, Il 62040

Previously published in 1985 as: *The Complete Book of
Problem Pregnancy Counseling* by Anne Baker.

ISBN 0-9644777-0-X
Library of Congress Catalog Card Number: 95-75149

Printed in the U.S.A. by:
John S. Swift Co., Inc.
1248 Research Blvd.
St. Louis, Missouri 63132

Cataloging Data:

Baker, Anne, 1951–
        Abortion and options counseling: a comprehensive reference. — Rev.
and exp. ed.
        Previously published as: The complete book of problem pregnancy
counseling. 1985.
        Includes bibliographical references and index.
        ISBN 0-9644777-0-X
        1. Abortion counseling. 2. Pregnancy, Unwanted. 3. Counseling — Handbooks, manuals, etc.
II. Title. III. Baker, Anne, 1951– The complete book of problem pregnancy counseling.
IV. Hope Clinic for Women.
HQ767.4.B341995   LCCN: 95-75149

This book is dedicated to Sally Burgess-Griffin, the present Director of Hope Clinic, and to the memory of Laura Moody Zevallos, Executive Director of Hope Clinic from 1975 to 1992. To Sally, who champions a woman's right to quality health care, places a high value on learning, and who gave me the gift of time to record my experiences and share my knowledge here in this book. To Laura, who dedicated her life not only to a clinic and a cause but to people. Without Laura's and Sally's support this book could never have been written.

"The God who gave us life gave us liberty at the same time."
– Thomas Jefferson

Contents

Abortion and Options Counseling

Introduction

When I first entered the field of abortion counseling in 1976, little had been written on the subject. As I learned from trial and error and discussions of client cases with other counselors in the field, I vowed to record what I learned. My purpose was and is to share the information gleaned from experience.

The first edition of the <u>Problem Pregnancy Counseling Training Manual</u> was published in 1981. The Hope Clinic for Women, located in Granite City, Illinois, had been in operation for seven years and had been providing first trimester abortion services up to 14 weeks. The book continues to be geared for professional counselors and volunteers who want to learn how to increase their effectiveness in the field of abortion, pregnancy testing, and pregnancy options counseling.

In 1985 the revised edition was retitled <u>The Complete Book of Problem Pregnancy Counseling.</u> By 1985 Hope Clinic offered abortion services through 24 weeks and had survived a firebombing and other anti-abortion terrorism. The year 1985 also saw the completion of a joint study by Hope Clinic and Washington University researching women's decisions to tell or not to tell their male partners about their pregnancy. In 1988 we had a brief encounter with Operation Rescue anti-abortion terrorists; I finished research on women's emotional reactions and coping ability after an abortion; and our staff joined the 500,000 pro-choice demonstrators who marched on Washington, D.C. to protest the 1988 Supreme Court Decision in Webster v. RHS (allowing restrictions on abortion access). By 1994 I celebrated my 18th anniversary at Hope Clinic as Director of Counseling, and I am still learning about this multi-faceted field of counseling.

In this edition I have revised and expanded almost every chapter and have added many new chapters, some of which include Counseling the Abused Woman, Fetal Indications Abortion, How Women Cope After an Abortion and Implications for Pre-abortion Counseling, Interpreting Fetal Development: Is Abortion Killing a Baby?, and The Anti-Abortion Client.

This book can be thought of as two-in-one: a 50-page volume on pregnancy options counseling, and a 150-page volume on abortion counseling. Of course, many counseling issues are parallel in options counseling and abortion counseling, so some of the material in those sections is similar as well. I recommend going through the whole book at least once, and then using the Index when you need to find help with a difficult counseling situation.

No matter how long I remain in this field, it continues to captivate me. The expression, "I've seen it all!" does not apply to those of us in this field of counseling. There is always one more challenge just around the corner.

<u>Special Note About My Terminology</u>

You will notice that when I make a reference to a counselor I routinely use the female pronoun. This is simply because most abortion and pregnancy options counselors are female, and because the continual use of "he/she, him/her" is awkward. So if you are male, when you read "she," think "he."

When I refer to the person who performs an abortion, I use the term, "doctor" because at the time of this writing most abortion practitioners are physicians. However, I want to acknowledge the nurse practitioners, physician's assistants, and midwives who perform abortions and recognize that in the future the term "clinician" may be more appropriate.

History of Abortion

Abortion has been in existence since ancient times and practiced by women on every continent in the world (Gordon, 1976; Henshaw, 1986; Tietze & Henshaw, 1986; Tietze & Lewitt, 1977). Even when abortion is not legally or morally sanctioned by a society, the practice continues covertly and dangerously.

Women have resorted to many and various procedures and potions in order to induce a miscarriage when circumstances compelled them to do so (Gordon, 1976). In ancient times Japanese midwives inserted a type of seaweed into the cervix to interrupt the pregnancy. In Greenland, midwives used a thinly carved rib of the walrus in the same fashion. The people of the Torres Straits had a particularly frightening process in which the woman leaned against a tree while two people pressed a long pole into her abdomen. Ancient Indian practices involved grasping the uterus through the abdominal wall and twisting it until the fetus detached. A tenth century Persian physician recorded a process by which the root of the mallow plant was inserted into the uterus. In pre-industrial times, German, Tartan, and French women used the root of the worm fern in the form of a tea. Middle Eastern women used a potion concocted from the foam of a camel's mouth (Gordon, 1976).

It is sobering to realize that both birth control and abortion have not always been legal in the United States. The historical account in Linda Gordon's book, Woman's Body, Woman's Right, indicates that abortion and birth control methods were accessible only through word of mouth, catalogs, and midwives prior to the late 19th century. But from 1873 to 1938 birth control methods were illegal and labeled "legally obscene." In the early 20th century pioneers of family planning such as Margaret Sanger and Emma Goldman were thrown in prison for equipping married women with diaphragms in health clinics. From the 1860s to 1973 abortion was also illegal, and like birth control, went underground. There were some "therapeutic" abortions performed legally by doctors in hospitals when approved by two physicians, but most women had to rely on word of mouth for where to go.

ILLEGAL ABORTION

Women's desperation sometimes led them to self-proclaimed abortionists with no medical backgrounds. In the mid-twentieth century women sometimes paid hefty sums for having rubber catheters, knitting needles, umbrella ribs, coat hangers, or other objects inserted into the cervix in an attempt to cause an abortion. Women tried to self-abort using the same implements or douched with caustic solutions such as lye or ammonia, permanently damaging their bodies. They hoped to achieve an abortion but sometimes wound up dying in the process. So many women in so many different lands throughout time have willingly subjected themselves to any number of painful and dangerous practices to prevent an unwanted birth.

Some of the stories of illegal abortion experiences from the older women I have counseled and interviewed attest to this. Their descriptions of their humiliating, painful, and dangerous experiences make me wonder how they lived to tell the tale. The 1992 documentary, <u>When Abortion Was Illegal:</u> <u>Untold Stories</u>, by award-winner Dorothy Fadiman, is a poignant and powerful film that was nominated for an Academy Award. It can be purchased by writing to BullFrog Films, Iley, PA, 19547.

Desperation can be a powerful motivator. For those of you who have never talked to someone who has undergone an illegal abortion, here is an experience related to me by a woman I interviewed during my research. A 60-year-old woman I'll call Helen told me her abortion took place 35 years ago in a town in the Midwest. She explained, "I never told a soul since then until two years ago when a young co-worker was fretting about going to an abortion clinic for what she felt was a necessary abortion. I told her she didn't need to worry, now that REAL doctors perform the abortion in a REAL medical place. Worrying was for those of us back in the days before abortion was legal. We had no idea whether we'd come out dead or alive." Helen continued in a quiet, solemn voice. "I was 25 years old, married, and had two babies already - six months and two years old. I was married to a man who had been nice to me while we were dating, but after we married, he showed his true temper. He'd get mean over nothing. Once the babies started coming, he got worse. He'd hit me in the face and punch me in the stomach over things so small I didn't know what they were. I was always afraid he'd hurt my babies, and once he did threaten to throw the youngest at me from across the room. He told me he wouldn't have any more babies in his house! The look on his face told me if I had any more children, it would be the end of me - or them.

I had no family I could escape to. I had no job skills. He was the only way me and my boys were going to eat. Well, we didn't have birth control back then. You tried to use rhythm, but that didn't work. I had two rhythm babies to show for it. And, sure enough, I got pregnant again - the third time in three years. My only hope was an abortion.

My next door neighbor had three kids and we confided in each other. I broke down crying one afternoon in her kitchen and told her everything. She closed the door and told me about a lady she went to who did an abortion for her. She said it was scary, but she was OK afterwards. She gave me the number, and I made the arrangements. I was told to come alone at night. I had to go by bus. I had never been in that part of town before. A man met me at the bus stop and he said when I got in the car I had to be blindfolded - so I wouldn't know where we were. It was horrible, but it's what I had to do for me and my boys.

When the car stopped, I had to stay blindfolded till we got inside the house. When I opened my eyes I saw a tall, thin woman wearing glasses and a rubber apron. Her red hair was pulled tight into a bun on top of her head. She looked mean and gave me orders like a drill sargeant. I did as I was told. I handed her the $100 I had managed to scrape together with the help of my neighbor. That was a lot of money in those days! Then we walked up some dark stairs that led to the attic. That was the longest flight of steps I've ever climbed. The thought crossed my mind, 'What if I never come back down?' I felt horrible guilt, thinking if I died, then my boys would be left with their father. But this way, I at least had a chance to live. The other way... well, I hated to think of it!

When I reached the top, I was told to lie down on a board that was laid out on an old coil spring bed. She had a steaming basin of water and an orange rubber tube. I smelled some strong antiseptic, so I told myself at least she was trying to be clean. She told me to grip the sides of the board and not to scream. She stuck that tube up inside me and it hurt like hell. Then she told me to lay there for a while and she'd come back to check on me. When she returned, I was led back down the stairs and told I'd have some pain and bleeding and then I'd miscarry. I was ordered not to tell a soul, even if I had to go to the hospital. Then to make sure I had nothing to tell, the blindfold was tied back on, and out I went.

I was dropped off at the bus stop. I was in some pretty bad pain, but I guessed that was to be expected. By the time I was on the bus and halfway home, the blood started running down my leg. There was an old drunk half asleep on the seat across from me. I tried to mop up the blood with my handkerchief. I was never so glad when the bus arrived at my stop. I was also glad it was dark so nobody could see the lady with a blood-soaked dress hurrying down the street. I was praying like mad that my husband was still out with his buddies, and that my boys had behaved for my neighbor.

When I got there my neighbor cleaned me up and gave me some aspirin. It wasn't until the next day that I passed it. It hurt, and I passed a lot of blood. I felt real weak, but I still cleaned the house as good as I could and fixed his dinner when he came home, so he wouldn't be any the wiser.

After that experience, I really hated him. I vowed some day I'd get away from him. It wasn't easy, but eventually I made good on my promise to myself - and my boys.

Many a time I've said my prayers of thanks that I didn't wind up dead in that attic. I guess there were others who weren't as lucky. It's a world of difference between then and now - I mean the way abortions are done. When I hear people complaining about how terrible it is that abortion is legal, I think different. I think, 'Thank God!'"

Since abortion became legal in the United States in 1973, the abortion procedure has been transformed from a crude and dangerous practice to those that are sophisticated and safe. Now women not only receive safe medical care but emotional attention as well since most abortion providers offer some measure of psychological care.

Chapter One

Three Kinds of Pregnancy Counseling

There are three types of pregnancy counseling discussed in this book. They are:

• **Pregnancy Testing Counseling:** This occurs at the time the pregnancy test results are given.

• **Pregnancy Options Counseling:** This occurs some time after the woman knows she is pregnant.

• **Abortion Counseling:** This occurs at some point before the woman has an abortion and usually occurs on the day of her procedure.

The **content** of each of the counseling sessions can be quite similar, but the **focus** often varies because the woman's emotional and cognitive states can be different at these three points in time, and create different needs.

Pregnancy Test Counseling

When a woman receives a positive pregnancy test result, she is likely to react at a higher emotional level and a more confused thinking level than she would days after the confirmation of the pregnancy. The time of the pregnancy test is the moment of truth in which the counselor or nurse has confirmed the woman's suspicions. Her response may well be shock, alarm, panic, happi-

ness, fear, anger, or a mixture of these and other emotional reactions. The counselor's focus needs to be on helping the woman sort out her feelings about being pregnant. It is also appropriate to begin exploring her support system and what options she has already considered.

Options Counseling

When a woman seeks counseling days or weeks after receiving her test results, she has usually deliberated on her own and with significant others. What she needs is someone to listen intently and help her clarify what she thinks and feels about the alternatives and her ability to cope with each option. To help her reach a decision, she will need accurate information on adoption, abortion, and/or parenting.

Abortion Counseling

By the time a woman sees a counselor for the purpose of having an abortion, she is usually resolved in her decision. The counselor needs to focus on how the woman arrived at her decision, the degree of certainty she expresses about her decision, the level of emotional support she is receiving from significant others, her feelings and beliefs about abortion, her ability to cope post-abortion, and her fears and concerns about the medical procedure.

Pregnancy Options Counseling As Crisis Intervention

The characteristics of options counseling differentiate it from therapy and categorize it as crisis intervention counseling. Those characteristics include the following:

1. It is short-term counseling.

2. It involves an immediate problem and the immediate, usually intense emotions surrounding that problem.

In addition, an unplanned pregnancy may be a crisis that is further characterized by the following aspects:

1. It is a **major** life crisis, touching and seriously affecting more than the woman's life. Parents, family, children, and husband or boyfriend may be as deeply affected by the decision as the woman is.

2. Time is crucial. With pregnancy, indecision IS decision.

3. Finally, it is a physical as well as emotional crisis. Many times in early pregnancy the woman has constant nausea or vomiting, fatigue, severe appetite changes, breast swelling and tenderness, and she may be feeling generally "unwell." This often affects her daily life activities, including her job, school, and relationship with her children, male partner, and family. Pregnancy itself can dramatically change a woman's body in many ways, and it is a condition that is not easily concealed for very long.

Most of the time, pregnancy options counseling involves one session only. Depending on the facility, number of staff, and the woman's needs, this session can take anywhere from a few minutes to two hours, with the average time being one half hour to one hour.

Chapter Two

Exploring Our Attitudes as Options Counselors

Because of the highly emotional nature of the issues surrounding an unplanned pregnancy, it is imperative that each counselor in this field knows and faces her own attitudes toward abortion, adoption, teenage sex, sex outside marriage, birth control, risk-taking, teenage motherhood, fetal development, and single parenthood.

When a counselor fails to look at her own attitudes, how can she recognize her biases? If she fails to recognize her biases, how can she present a nonjudgmental approach to her clients? As in all counseling situations, the counselor's values and beliefs need to be kept separate from those of the client. Know whose values are whose! Since it takes self-awareness to know what triggers your own prejudices and cherished beliefs, start thinking...

ATTITUDES TOWARD ABORTION

1. What are your feelings about abortion in general? More specifically, under what instances do you believe abortion is OK? Not OK? Why?

2. At what gestational stage, if any, would you be against an elective abortion? A medically indicated abortion? For more in-depth exploration of this issue, refer to the section on fetal development and the chapter on second trimester abortion.

3. Should abortion be more restricted legally or less restricted in terms of cost, availability, gestational limits, and age of women? What about parental consent? Spousal consent? Why?

4. How would it affect **you** if abortion became illegal? How might it affect your female friends and family members?

5. Depending on circumstances, would you ever have an abortion yourself? If no, is it OK for someone else but not for you? Why?

6. Have you ever had an abortion? What was your experience? Positive? Negative? In what way? Do you still think it was a good decision? What were your feelings at the time, and how do you feel about it now? If you had or have any difficult feelings about your abortion, how have you coped?

7. How do you feel about a woman having an abortion who never used birth control?

8. How do you feel about a woman having more than one abortion?

9. How do you feel about a woman who is morally against abortion but insists upon having one?

10. How do you feel about an adolescent having

an abortion? A pre-adolescent? A teen having an abortion who has not told her parents about the pregnancy?

11. How do you feel about a married woman having an abortion?

12. How do you feel about a woman having more than one abortion using government funds to pay for the abortions?

ATTITUDES TOWARD ADOPTION

1. Do you believe the saying, "Adoption not abortion?" Why?

2. What exactly do you feel about a woman who places her baby for adoption?

3. What do you feel about a woman with children who carried to term and placed a baby for adoption?

4. Do you think, deep down, that adoption is preferable to or more noble than abortion?

5. Do you think, deep down, that adoption does harm to the adopted child, birth mother, adoptive parents, or all three? How?

6. How would you feel if you were pregnant, didn't have the financial means to raise a child, and didn't have abortion as an alternative?

7. Have you ever known or talked to an adopted child about the fact of his/her adoption? Think about that person's experiences, both positive and negative. Does this information color your outlook on adoption? How?

8. Are there any circumstances under which you would place a child of yours for adoption? How do you think you would feel?

9. Have you carried to term and placed a child for adoption? How have you coped with your feelings about it? Do you still feel it was a good decision?

10. Have you ever adopted a child? Have you ever wanted to adopt? How does that color your attitudes toward adoption as an alternative to an unplanned pregnancy?

ATTITUDES TOWARD PARENTHOOD

1. How do you feel about a 12- to 14-year-old girl who wants to keep her baby? A 15- to 17-year-old?

2. How do you feel about any woman who chooses to be a single parent?

3. How do you feel about a poor woman who wants to keep her baby?

4. Do you have any children of your own? Think about your experience as a parent. What are the joys? The hardships? What were some of the realities of parenting that surprised you?

5. What are some of your feelings about parenthood? For yourself? For others? For women in abusive relationships? For teens with abusive parents?

6. What do you feel about women who choose never to become mothers?

ATTITUDES TOWARD SEX

1. How did you view sex as a child? As a teenager? How have you changed?

2. What is your own sex life like presently? What would you like it to be if you're not presently satisfied?

3. What are your feelings and beliefs about virginity?

4. Do you believe sex outside marriage is wrong? For you or for others? Why?

ATTITUDES TOWARD PRE-ADOLESCENT AND ADOLESCENT SEXUALITY

1. What do you think about pre-teen girls having sex? What about pre-teen boys having sex? Why?

2. What do you think about adolescent girls having sex? What about adolescent boys? Why?

3. What were your sexual thoughts, feelings, activities, during your pre-teen and teenage years?

4. If you are a parent of a teenager, what are your hopes and fears for him or her regarding sexual activity? Why?

5. What kind of sex education and birth control information have you imparted to your children? What kind of sex education did you receive as a pre-teen? A teenager?

Why Adolescents Have Sex

Females

If female, she may:
1. Want to feel loved.

2. Want to express love to a special young man.

3. Want to feel desirable or sexy.

4. Want to experience pleasure.

5. Want to feel part of her peer group: "Everybody else is doing it. I must be abnormal if I'm not!" (This pressure is especially keen when a culture's media promotes and equates sex with success, desirability, and love).

6. Want to feel "adult."

7. Want to have a "relationship" with a young man.

8. Want to get back at her mother or father who harps on her clothing and behavior and who labels her "cheap" or "whorish."

9. Want to avoid saying no. (Females are still not conditioned to be assertive and get their own needs met).

10. Want to avoid displeasing, angering, or losing her boyfriend.

11. Want to cure boredom: "There's nothing else to do."

12. Want to have sex as a cure for loneliness. (Having sex is one way of fooling yourself into feeling close to someone).

13. Lose her inhibitions and good judgment while drinking alcohol or using drugs.

14. Feel pressured by the guy who pouts or uses "lines" to evoke guilt if she doesn't give in.

- "If you love me, you'll prove it."
- "If you arouse me and then leave me like this, I'll get sick and get blue balls!"
- "You know you want to, baby. Any real woman wants to ..."
- "You always put me off. Don't you love me?!"
- "You mean after paying for a whole evening's night out, I don't get anything in return? Is that any way to treat a guy?"
- "I can't help myself – you're driving me crazy, you're so sexy!"
- "If you don't want me like I want you, then we might as well break up. I can't go on like this."

15. Feel pressure from a boy's genuine love and sexual desire for her.

16. Want to satisfy curiosity.

17. Feel bodily tension from hormonal changes.

18. Lack sexual boundaries due to sexual abuse as a child or adolescent.

Males

If male, he may:
1. Want to experience pleasure.

2. Want to satisfy curiosity.

3. Want to "prove" manhood or adulthood.

4. Want to feel loved or to express love for a special girl.

5. Want to feel part of his peer group. He may feel left out if he thinks "everybody else is doing it."

6. Want to feel desirable and sexy.

7. Feel pressure from the media to be sexy and sexually active.

8. Feel pressure from the spoken or unspoken message from his father to "be a man – sow your wild oats." Some fathers derive satisfaction from thinking their sons are sexually active; some ridi-

cule their sons for not being sexually active.

9. Feel bodily tension from hormonal changes. He may be preoccupied with sexual sensations from unexpected, frequent erections.

10. Feel bored. "There's nothing to do."

11. Want a close relationship with a young woman.

12. Have sex as a cure for loneliness.

13. Lose inhibitions or become aggressive while drinking alcohol or using drugs.

14. Lack sexual boundaries due to sexual abuse as a child or adolescent.

15. Feel pressured by a particular situation or woman, thinking, "She'll think there's something wrong with me if I don't" or "she'll think there's something wrong with her if I don't want to."

There are by no means complete lists. Feel free to add thoughts of your own.

ATTITUDES TOWARD PEOPLE TAKING CONTRACEPTIVE RISKS

Have you ever felt critical of people who got pregnant while taking risks with birth control? Have you ever thought, "How irresponsible!?" Contracepting 100% consistently and 100% perfectly for all our reproductive years is a complex feat that few fertile human beings achieve. There are complex reasons why both men and women might fail to use their birth control methods at certain times. Take the time now to think about possible answers to these questions:

1. Why would a woman quit the Pill and either turn to a risky method of birth control or use none at all?

2. Why would a woman miss pills and not follow the instructions for missed pills?

3. Why would her partner also be willing to take these risks?

While you are thinking, imagine her in the context of a relationship with her male partner: What kind of man might she choose for a partner?

Why might she be having sex? What might their personalities be like? What emotional states might prompt a person to take risks? To gain a clearer understanding of why someone might take contraceptive risks, here are examples of reasons categorized by method.

Why A Woman May Take Risks With Birth Control Pills

1. She went through a period of time when she wasn't sexually involved with anyone but continued to take pills anyway. She fell into the habit of missing a pill now and then, thinking nothing of it, since she wasn't engaging in sex. When she then developed a sexual relationship, the habit of not attending to an occasional missed pill persisted.

2. When she and her male partner broke up and separated, she angrily threw her pills away, since they reminded her of what she no longer had or wanted in her life. Then, weeks later, her ex-partner returned, they reminisced about the good old times long into the night, and spontaneously plunged into a passionate reunion.

3. For years before she went on the Pill, she had not used any birth control with her first boyfriend, and no pregnancies resulted. They broke up. Her new partner insists she take the Pill. She agrees, but finds herself constantly nauseated. She figures it doesn't make sense to take something that makes her sick and so quits taking it. She relies on her presumed infertility. She does not know that different men have different levels of fertility, and that over time both men's and women's fertility can change.

4. Her boyfriend is very possessive and secretly wants her to get pregnant, thinking he'll trap her into marriage. He hides her pills, persuades her not to worry about missed pills, and coaxes her into having sex with him anyway. She allows herself to be swept away by his alleged passion.

5. Her religious upbringing creates a moral conflict between her desire for sexual intimacy and her belief that premarital sex is wrong. Being on the Pill engenders guilty feelings. Her unconscious compromise is to run out of her prescription, use rhythm, and wind up pregnant. The pregnancy and abortion are viewed as "teaching

her and her boyfriend a lesson" not to have sex again until married.

6. She was raised in a chaotic environment where consistency and doing things on time had no value. There were no "meal times," "time to do homework," "time to go to bed," etc. Sometimes meals were forgotten and she learned to ignore hunger. When she was sick her mother (or whoever was left in charge) would administer medicine only sporadically, if at all. Therefore, as an adult she did not internalize the ability to attend to time (take a pill every 24 hours, and remember to refill the prescription before it expires). Due to the chaos and neglect in her childhood, she also has not internalized self-worth or learned how to take care of herself.

7. Her parents are punitive and demand adherence to a strict moral code. Her greatest fear is her parents finding her birth control pills. In fact, one day her mother comes close to running across them, and instead of changing her hiding place, she throws them away, telling her boyfriend he'll have to use something. He acquiesces and uses condoms sometimes and withdrawal sometimes, and she winds up pregnant.

8. Her husband just died in an accident. He had long ago had a vasectomy, so she didn't need to think about birth control for many years. She and his best friend are crying and consoling each other late one night. Out of loneliness and sorrow, they unite in a spontaneous and desperate attempt to fill their sense of emptiness.

9. Her mother or father dies, and due to the disruption and confusion that accompanies grieving, she forgets pills. At the same time, she increases her sexual activity with her partner to maximize the feeling of closeness and relieve the feeling of aloneness.

10. She hears stories about women becoming infertile from being on the Pill for years. She fails to check out the facts and gets scared because she has been on the Pill for five years. She quits and unconsciously tests her fertility by not using another birth control method. Another variation on this theme is her doctor taking her off the Pill for a so-called "rest" from the Pill (even though she has had no problems on it). He/she instructs her to use "another method." She uses spermicides, or her partner uses condoms, but not in conjunc-

tion with each other and not consistently. They had been used to having sex spontaneously when she was on the Pill, and now they keep forgetting barrier methods require planning and preparation.

11. After one relationship ends she quits the Pill, thinking, "Why should I take a drug when I don't need it?" When she enters into a new relationship, neither she nor her partner discusses contraception before they become intimate. After a romantic evening of getting to know each other over a candlelight dinner, he asks her over to his place. There they start out on the couch, drinking wine and talking, and end up in the throes of passion. The thought of pregnancy fails to enter their minds until the next day. Or, she makes a hasty miscalculation of her possible ovulation time, convincing herself, "It's safe."

12. She has been abused emotionally and/or physically all her life. She is in an abusive relationship. She often behaves in ways that result in self-harm. Her self-destructive behavior is unconscious and habitual. She is angry with her boyfriend and, as usual, turns her anger in on herself. Her anger takes the form of having a one-night-stand shortly after running out of her prescription. When she finds out she is pregnant, she is terrified that her boyfriend might find out the baby is not his. She "accidentally" leaves the pregnancy test results semi-concealed, and he finds it.

13. A teenager has secretly been on the Pill, but her mother finds them. In a dramatic display of disapproval, her mother throws them away and declares that her daughter will not be having sex again! Daughter is angry, has sex anyway with no protection, and gets pregnant. Unconsciously she uses the pregnancy to punish Mom.

14. A woman in her late twenties lives with a man for several years. She wants to get married and have a family. He has an excuse every time she brings up the subject: "We need a stable income first; we need to buy a house first; we need a bigger savings account, etc." He asks her nearly every day if she has taken her pill on time. She runs out of her prescription and doesn't find the time to get it refilled. She gets pregnant, consciously or unconsciously, hoping to force a commitment.

15. She has had two abortions and years later reads anti-abortion literature that states women become sterile from several abortions. She "tests" her fertility by going off the Pill.

16. She has been on the Pill for years and assumes, "There's so much hormone in my system by now, I can miss pills without worrying." She disregards instructions for missing pills, thinking she's safe from years of use.

17. She is used to the convenience and spontaneity of the Pill, and has never felt a need to learn how to use spermicides or to keep a supply on hand. She feels awkward and embarrassed about buying and using them once the need arises. Instead she takes a risk, thinking, "Surely just this once won't hurt."

18. A teenager's parents are heading toward separation and possible divorce. She unconsciously starts to behave in ways that divert their attention from their own conflicts to her problem behavior. A responsible pill-taker in the past, she now starts missing pills. A teenage pregnancy creates a major family crisis and temporarily brings her parents closer together in their mutual concern for her.

19. Both she and her boyfriend fantasize about what a baby of theirs would look like and what they'd name their children. He gives her the message that if she got pregnant, they'd get married and have the baby. She "accidentally" misses pills.

20. She has tried several kinds of pills, continues to experience breakthrough bleeding, headaches, nausea, or weight gain. She talks to her doctor and he/she tells her "just keep on taking it." She gets frustrated and quits the Pill. She thinks the contraceptive effects of the Pill will linger in her body for several months after quitting them because a friend of hers went off the Pill and didn't get pregnant for six months.

21. She is experiencing financial hardship and finds the cost for the private doctor visits and pills too expensive. She has no knowledge of low-cost family planning clinics that are near her small town. She quits the Pill and relies on no-cost contraception: rhythm or withdrawal.

22. A senior in high school has been faithfully taking the Pill ever since her abortion when she was 16. She will soon graduate and both desires and fears going away to college in the fall. She accidentally misses one or two pills, and feels temporarily relieved when she finds out she is pregnant. Now maybe she can stay home, get married, and avoid separating from family, boyfriend, and friends.

23. She misuses the Pill because she doesn't know how the Pill works and how it doesn't work. Research has shown a substantial number of women who miss a period while on the placebo pills fail to start a new pack on time. They think they should wait till they have a period and then start a new pack. The research also shows a substantial percentage of women on the Pill wait to start a new pack if they are still bleeding past the last placebo (Williams-Deane & Potter, 1992). Or because they or friends of theirs did not get pregnant for several months after quitting the Pill in the past, they assume they can't get pregnant for several months after discontinuing the Pill. They assume it stays in their bloodstream. People also think because they did not get pregnant when they missed pills BEFORE, they won't get pregnant in the future when they miss pills.

Why People Take Risks With Condoms

A man might be sexually active and not use condoms because ...

1. He assumes the woman is on the Pill if she consents to have sex. He doesn't bother to ask or use a condom.

2. He assumes bad things happen to bad people, and thereby exempts himself from serious consequences, like sexually transmitted diseases or unwanted pregnancy.

3. He is afraid if he brings out a condom, the woman might reject him and think, "He premeditated the whole thing, that lecher!"

4. He is afraid to purchase condoms because he doesn't want to be seen buying them.

5. He doesn't like the feel of condoms or the interruption during sex play.

6. She doesn't like the feel of condoms or the interruption, and tells him so.

7. The condoms have broken or fallen off enough times for him to conclude, "They're no use anyway; why bother?!"

8. He is generally a risk-taker in his life and his approach to having sex is no different.

9. He wants to impregnate her, hoping she will then marry him (or stay bonded to him, if they are already married).

10. He feels that birth control is HER responsibility, and doesn't think about condoms as protection from disease.

11. He cares only about his own gratification, disregarding her welfare or the possibility of disease.

12. He has problems maintaining an erection when he tries to put the condom on.

13. He has experienced a condom failure in the past that has resulted in pregnancy and does not trust their effectiveness.

14. They both think they can skip the condom when she is at "the safe time of the month."

15. One or both are intoxicated by alcohol or drugs, and their judgment is impaired.

Why People Take Risks With Spermicides, Cervical Cap, Diaphragm And Sponge

1. She defers to him when he complains he can feel the diaphragm or sponge, and she discontinues use. She may have low self-esteem and believes his pleasure is more important than her welfare.

2. Either he or she (or both) has an allergic, burning sensation in reaction to the spermicide and finds it too painful to continue usage.

3. She continuously experiences yeast infections or vaginitis when using spermicides.

4. She has repeated bladder infections with the diaphragm.

5. They both think she can "skip it just this once" when she is at "the safe time of the month."

6. She hasn't become pregnant before when she skipped her method a couple of times, so she assumes she won't get pregnant the next time she takes a risk.

7. Either he or she (or both) hates the "mess" of spermicides.

8. One or both hates the interruption.

9. They don't have a place of privacy and have sex whenever and wherever there is an opportunity (a camping trip, a friend's empty apartment, etc.). They don't have a method with them when an opportunity arises.

10. They run out of supplies.

11. They alternate using spermicides and using withdrawal. The longer withdrawal works, the more they use it.

12. One or both are intoxicated using drugs or alcohol.

13. They have been separated or "broken up," have an unplanned reunion, and are carried away by emotion rather than thinking about consequences.

14. One or both are grieving a major loss (death in the family) and are not thinking clearly, needing closeness and intimacy, and unconsciously desiring "new life" to replace the life that was lost.

15. Their personalities and way of life could be generally categorized as "risk-taking" and spontaneous" rather than "organized" or "planning ahead" and their approach to having sex is no different.

16. She feels depressed and doesn't care what happens to her.

17. She generally behaves in ways that are self-destructive and leaves herself open for heartache and pain by skipping her method.

Why Women Take Risks With IUDs, Norplant And The Depo-Provera Shot

1. She dislikes touching herself and so does not check for the IUD string.

2. She fails to have it (either IUD or hormonal implants) removed at the designated time, thinking it will keep on working until she finds the time to go to the doctor.

3. Once it is removed, she isn't prepared to use another method. She is so used to the convenience of the device, the need for another method slips her mind, and she has unprotected intercourse.

4. She fails to keep her appointment for the next shot, and she thinks she is still protected.

5. She can't tolerate the breakthrough bleeding, discontinues the shot or Norplant, and both she and her partner fail to use another reliable method.

ATTITUDES TOWARD REPEATED ABORTIONS

When asked the question, "What are your feelings when you discover your client has had more than one abortion?" a counselor's response might include: "I feel...

- angry
- powerless (to help her change)
- weary ("What more can I do for her?")
- disgusted
- exasperated
- disappointed
- confused ("Why would anyone put herself at risk again?")
- sad
- a sense of failure as a counselor
- a sense of futility about motivating her to use birth control.

Getting in touch with negative feelings toward a client is usually difficult for those of us in the helping profession, since we view ourselves as compassionate people. Recognizing and admitting our own feelings are the first steps to counseling the repeat abortion client effectively.

Once we have identified our own negative feelings, we need to specify which circumstances affect us more negatively than others. Specific examples might include:

"If the woman was using birth control and it failed her, then I don't feel angry; I can empathize with her own exasperation with methods." OR

"If she's back the third time in one year, impatience and a hopeless feeling sets in." OR "If she has become pregnant four times because of missing pills and still insists next time she'll remember, I don't believe her anymore and feel angry she's still playing games." OR "If she had a painful abortion before, is obsessed with fear of pain and seems to be playing the victim, expecting me to rescue her, THAT really bothers me!"

It is crucial to examine those values that trigger our emotional reactions to repeated abortion. Upon scrutiny, the issue underlying our emotional response may be CONTROL: self-control, birth control, control of reproduction, control of our own and our partner's sexual desires, control over emotions and control of our lives. When other people let things happen to them, or when we feel out of control ourselves, we may respond with disgust or disappointment.

If we have always valued and practiced control in our lives, we may assume everyone else does or should. In that case, it is helpful to realize that many men and women live their whole lives (not just their sexual lives) presuming they have no control. These individuals may generally feel impotent to influence, direct, or alter the course of their lives, letting Mom or Dad, friend or spouse, teacher or priest make decisions for them because that's the way it has always been. Making decisions for themselves about anything is probably quite alien to them. And making a conscious decision about having sex and preventing pregnancy may be even more alien.

Throughout our lives we may have been given the encouragement and the opportunity to make decisions for ourselves until it seems second nature. "Think for yourself and plan ahead" may be a message some of us have readily adopted and strongly believe. "Be spontaneous, take chances" is another message some people have been taught to value. Everyone takes chances from time to time and plans ahead to some degree; still, some of us would characterize ourselves as "planners" and others as "risk-takers." Planners may think risk-takers are irresponsible. Risk-takers may think planners are boring. In the realm of contraception and sex, a counselor may feel irritated with a contraceptor's failure because the counselor herself has gone through the hassle of taking steps to prevent pregnancy. In fact, the counselor may have foregone some pleasurable moments because of her value of self-discipline. Planning ahead is certainly a discipline, sometimes requiring self-restraint. In regard to sex, haven't we heard people express disgust toward a couple who they thought "just couldn't restrain themselves! Why couldn't they have waited until after the trip to the doctor or drug store?" And yet we all have times when we let our need for immediate gratification overtake our better judgment in some areas of our lives. Is there anything we've gone ahead and done, knowing the possible consequences? For example, eating like there's no tomorrow after painstakingly dieting off five miserable pounds; going out with an ex-boyfriend or ex-husband after struggling so hard to stay strong and sever ties with him completely; putting off some project for tomorrow and then goading yourself to meet the deadline; smoking a cigarette after having quit for good (!) for the third time in two years; undergoing a second dental nightmare after you had sworn you'd brush and floss faithfully after the first root canal; OR taking "just one more drink" at a party, knowing you'll pay dearly with a hangover the next day. It seems that at times everyone feels the immediate pay-off of doing something NOW outweighs the possible bad consequences LATER.

After we've thought about a past instance in our own lives where immediate gratification prevailed over prevention, what about our own birth control background? Have we had it easy with methods? Used the Pill with never a side effect? Good memory, routines come easy? Have we used the IUD or Norplant with never a problem? Found the diaphragm a cinch? Easily incorporated the condoms and spermicides into lovemaking? If so, we might lose sight of the fact that contraception is a genuine ordeal for some people.

If we have struggled with contraception and through conscientious effort prevented unwanted pregnancies, our conclusion might be "If I can do it, so can they!" Unfortunately, there is no method of birth control at this time that is everything to all people. What method is 100% side-effect free, 100% safe, 100% effective, 100% available, and 100% convenient to use? Even abstinence is ruled out in the last category.

With the birth control methods now available, controlling fertility often means choosing security from unwanted pregnancy over spontaneity and freedom from hassle or health hazards. When people realize they can have one or the other but not both, they may feel a twinge of resentment or envy toward the person who has chosen the other value. This dynamic even applies outside the realm of birth control. For example, the ulcer-ridden but successful businessman may sound off on "those lazy-good-for-nothing kids who run around having fun and not making anything of their lives!"

"But how can anyone gamble when the stakes are so high?" someone may protest. "Another pregnancy and another abortion are pretty high stakes!" The risks might indeed be great, but that probably means that the immediate gain loomed even larger, even more important. Because "having sex" may mean "feeling close, feeling wanted, or feeling loved," those human needs might outweigh all risks at some point in a person's life. A powerful need can blind a person to possible consequences. People may not even be aware that a value-weighing process is taking place. Deliberating takes thinking and reflecting, and for the grand majority of both men and women, sex is simply not an intellectual act as much as it is a feeling act. How often have we counselors been astounded to hear a pregnant client remark, "Well, I really didn't think about birth control at the time..." When it comes to sex, most people FEEL - love, pleasure, closeness, disappointment, pain, or loneliness. If they're thinking at all, it might be something like, "I wonder what he (or she) thinks of me?" People do not necessarily think, "Now I will have intercourse. I do not want a pregnancy to occur. Therefore, I need birth control." The thought process might well be more complex than that. After concluding, "I need birth control," the next thought might be: "How do I bring up the subject without breaking the mood? Do I really want him to know I intend to keep on having sex with him? Do I really want to have sex with him again?" Sex is not a cognitive activity for many people. Perhaps it should be, but we all have to deal with what is.

It seems that women seeking another abortion thoroughly admonished themselves the first time they got pregnant and had an abortion, and swore it would never happen again. It is common for a counselor in the post-abortion session to hear a woman declare, "You'll never see ME again! I'm going to use my birth control forever after!" Directly after any stressful event in our lives, we of course vow never to let the same thing happen again, and we mean it. Then the farther away in time we get from the event, the more likely it is that we lapse back into old habits. We conveniently forget just how bad we felt last time.

While the memory of the last abortion may fade, the ongoing hassle of birth control may be accentuated with time. A comfortable rationalization may then take over: "Surely it's not likely that I'll get caught again! People only go through that kind of crisis once in a blue moon!" And then condoms are left in the drawer, or a pill prescription runs out, or the diaphragm is forgotten "just this once." And for each pregnancy there were two people who took that chance...a man and a woman...and both are responsible.

All too often the blame for a repeated abortion is directed toward the woman, even though she certainly didn't impregnate herself. Perhaps this is because the client we see is almost always the female, without her male partner. For a myriad of reasons, not all of which are his fault, the partner in the pregnancy usually remains the "invisible man." Since we often do not see him or speak directly to him, our focus is on the woman. She is the one in our office, and therefore she is the one to whom we react.

The blame might also be directed toward the woman because she has more to lose, so "she should be more motivated to take care of herself!" The belief that every woman should take care of herself is derived from the fundamental value of self-worth and self-reliance. Before a woman takes the step to protect herself from harm, she must feel that she is worth protecting. In addition, she must take the initiative to protect herself instead of waiting for a man to do it. Unfortunately, our culture has taught women to be dependent upon men for their protection. For years in the area of reproduction, women depended upon men to either abstain from sex or use condoms to prevent pregnancy. Even outside the realm of sexuality, years of conditioning and social sanction have directed women toward the role of passivity and dependence, NOT self-reliance.

The Women's Movement of the 1960s and 1970s fought to reverse this conditioning and expectation of female behavior. In the 200+ years of American history, it has only been since the 1960s

that female-oriented contraception (the Pill, IUD, etc.) has become the expected method of preventing pregnancy. Women are faced with the awesome responsibility of controlling reproduction. Although there have always been women who have defied society's norms and embraced self-reliance, many more conformed and then reinforced the value of passivity as a female trait in their daughter's behavior. Is it any wonder counselors see so many women whose life pattern is LETTING things happen to them instead of MAKING things happen? How often we have heard a client explain, "My doctor said I might want more children later, so he wouldn't give me a tubal sterilization." OR "My husband said he doesn't like condoms, so we did without." And that was that.

Many women wouldn't dream of pressing a man on the issue of using condoms, or questioning their doctor's reasoning, or defying their partner's warning not to take "those dangerous pills." Perhaps in such cases, a counselor's anger may find its source in an underlying frustration with this woman's passivity. This may be especially maddening to those who have struggled with their own conditioning. In this case, the old adage, "We despise in others that which we despise in ourselves," certainly holds true.

Whether or not we are dealing with the client's passivity, loss of control, low self-worth, or feelings of failure, the key to effective counseling is to recognize and understand specific issues that trigger our emotions. One of these issues is what we believe about abortion. Some pro-choice counselors are still unsure about their moral beliefs about abortion. What does it mean when a counselor states, "Oh, I believe abortion should be the woman's choice - whatever she wants to do is OK - but I myself would never have an abortion"? Why is it OK for someone else but not for me? Perhaps this counselor tends to believe that abortion is taking a life. We all need to ask ourselves,

1. What are the stages of fetal development?

2. How do I interpret that information?

3. Up to what stage do I think abortion is OK? Why?

4. Do I think a fetus is a person?

20

5. What do I think constitutes personhood?

If a counselor maintains that abortion is taking a life and yet is pro-choice, then she may view one abortion as excusable, but find repeated abortions unacceptable. That counselor will inevitably convey a message of disapproval to the client, if not in words, then by a gesture, a look, a sigh. Anyone who tries to shame others into more "acceptable behavior" will be disappointed with the results. The vast majority of people relate to verbal or nonverbal reproaches by clamming up and shutting off communication. Therefore, the client who perceives censure from her counselor will probably feel shame or resentment and respond by withdrawing. Once the communication has been cut off, it is unlikely the counselor can be of much help. Thus, the counselor has alienated the client and has rendered herself ineffective.

Many women I've counseled who are seeking another abortion are already criticizing themselves, sometimes fearing that "God won't forgive me this time..." They often feel embarrassed to face us again, thinking, "What will those people think of me?" We counselors need to be aware of our judgmental attitudes and free ourselves so we can help the client with her own attitudes and help her problem-solve. How can we free ourselves?

1. By believing and conveying to our client that failing to control her fertility does not make her a bad person.

2. By focusing on our purpose: helping her cut through her self-criticism and accept herself, and helping her get back in control of her fertility by exploring the problem and generating possible solutions.

3. By using thought-substitution, we can transform our thoughts of criticism to those of empathy. For instance,

• If the woman wasn't using birth control and we start thinking, "How irresponsible!" we could instead switch our thoughts to "Have I ever taken any risks with my well-being? Am I so superior?"

• If the woman appears passive ("It just happened"), and her passivity frustrates you ("Why doesn't she wake up and take care of herself!"), think: Were you always the magnificently asser-tive creature you are today? Can you relate to her lack of assertiveness?

• If the woman has had multiple abortions, and you start feeling frustrated, stop and think: a woman who starts ovulating at age 13 and goes through menopause at age 50 has 37 years in which she could get pregnant. Although it is not likely, she could have 20 children in her lifetime and miscarriages besides. And if we imagine all the combinations of children, miscarriages, and abortions a woman COULD have, the number of each can be staggering. In that light, even five abortions is a tiny number. Remember: if not repeated abortions, then repeated unwanted babies!

• If you feel YOU must be the failure, ("I was the one who counseled her last time. Where did I go wrong?"), think: it isn't fair to judge ourselves by our client's behavior. If the woman or the couple is not ready to face the fertility problem at the time of a second or third abortion, we cannot go home with her and put pills in her mouth or suddenly materialize in time to slip a condom on her partner. In addition, the crux of the fertility problem may be quite complex, something which would take a good deal of time to uncover. How much can we expect to accomplish in one or two counseling sessions? We can only suggest the client pursue counseling if that seems appropriate. We can't force her. We also cannot make others change their behavior when they are not ready to do so. We need to be realistic with what we can and cannot do in a short-term counseling session, and then LET GO of what we can't do. No matter how much we want to help people change and avoid additional crises, it is their life to live, mistakes and all.

Summary

Negative attitudes toward the repeated abortion client spring from our value system and interpretation of what abortion means. It is never the events themselves that cause distress; it's what we think about those events that causes negative feelings. If we view the event of repeated abortion as:

1. a reflection of our own failure

2. a moral infraction

3. an issue of women's passivity

4. an act of irresponsibility

negative attitudes result. When we harbor negative attitudes, we alienate the client and render our counseling ineffective. To be an effective counselor, we need to identify the source of our negative attitude, be willing to alter the way we view repeated abortion, and adopt an attitude of understanding and acceptance.

ATTITUDES TOWARD SECOND TRIMESTER ABORTION

Some people believe first trimester abortion is morally acceptable, but second trimester is not. They feel increasingly uncomfortable with abortion as the fetus grows in size and becomes more developed. The issue of when a fetus becomes a baby rises to the surface when people think about second trimester abortion. Even those who come to the conclusion they don't know when personhood begins may feel uncomfortable because of their uncertainty.

If you feel uncomfortable with second trimester abortion, you may find yourself needing "good reasons" to justify it. It may be difficult to avoid feeling disdain for the woman who says she knew about the pregnancy three months earlier but kept postponing the abortion because she was afraid. One of the ways caregivers can increase their comfort level with second trimester abortion is to keep their focus on the client - the woman. Understanding why delays occur may engender an accepting attitude. Reasons for the time delay are many and varied, but essentially the woman who seeks an abortion in the second trimester was unable emotionally, intellectually, or financially to seek an abortion sooner. Basically any woman in her second trimester who wants an abortion feels she cannot carry to term without considerable emotional or physical distress.

On the other hand, you may believe second trimester abortion is as acceptable and morally good as first trimester abortion. Some people believe a second trimester fetus is not the moral, physical, emotional, or intellectual equivalent of a person. They conclude that second trimester abortion is therefore not the same as killing a person. Even though they may believe fetal life

has some value, they may not believe it has the same value as the life of the woman or possesses the same rights as the woman. Therefore, her decision to keep or end her pregnancy is paramount. In addition, they may believe forcing a woman to carry to term is a form of slavery, and forced parenthood can lead to tragedy for both mother and child. In this light they view second trimester abortion as a moral good.

There are no right or wrong answers to the question, "When does personhood begin?" Those who believe it exists in the second trimester may never feel comfortable or **want** to feel comfortable with second trimester abortion. It is my belief that those staff members with accepting attitudes need to be the ones who administer to the emotional and physical needs of second trimester clients.

Chapter Three

Fetal Development

As a pregnancy options counselor, you'll need a working knowledge of fetal development to confront your own feelings about abortion at different stages of fetal development, and to convey fetal development information at the patient's request and help her interpret the information.

When learning about fetal development, keep in mind two questions:

1. What are the facts?
2. How do you interpret those facts?

Reader Beware!

In gathering the facts from books on fetal development, reader beware! Reading about fetal development can be confusing because each author will use the term "weeks" but rarely explain whether they are weeks from conception (gestational age) or weeks LMP (from last menstrual period). It is vital to know whether the author is referring to gestational age or LMP age because there is a difference of two weeks between the two. So, if a woman states she is eight weeks from conception, she is 10 weeks LMP (add two weeks to the gestational age), and the description of a 10 week LMP fetus will be the accurate description. Two weeks does not sound like a lot until you examine the development of one stage and then look at how much the development has progressed

two weeks later. For example, a human embryo at six weeks LMP cannot be distinguished in its appearance from a rabbit or turtle embryo. Two weeks later it is distinguishable as a human fetus. It is not until eight weeks LMP that its sex organs have begun to appear. I have found that most (but not all) authors of fetal development books are referring to LMP weeks.

DESCRIPTION OF FETAL DEVELOPMENT

Conception: Fertilization is a process in time. The "moment of conception" is actually a vague term. Biologically there are seven distinguishable events that comprise "conception" or "fertilization:"

1. contact of the sperm with the egg surface
2. activation of the egg's outer layer
3. formation of the fertilization core
4. entry of the sperm into the egg cytoplasm
5. completion of meiosis and final maturation of the egg nucleus
6. formation of the sperm and egg pronuclei
7. fusion of the pronuclei

These seven steps occur over a number of hours and culminate in the division of the zygote to form two cells (Grobstein, 1988).

The following information was taken from two sources: Before We Are Born by Keith Moore (1989) and A Child is Born by Mirjam Furuhjelm, Axel Ingelman-Sundberg and Claes Wirsen (1976).

One week LMP: The fertilized egg travels to the uterus and implants in the lining. Beginnings of yolk sac and amniotic sac are apparent.

Two weeks LMP: A flat, three-layered embryonic disc is formed. Inner cells will become the internal organs and the outer cells will form the skin, skeleton, and central nervous system.

Week 3 LMP: Neural tube formation occurs and the flat disc begins to fold and elongate. Body segments appear. Early blood vessel formation occurs. Chorionic villi burrow deep into the uterine wall, later to become the placenta.

Week 4 LMP (1/6 inch): Internal organ systems begin to differentiate.

Week 5 LMP (1/4 to 2/5 inch): It is now called an "embryo" due to cell differences. The heart begins rhythmic pulsing, but no blood is formed yet. Paddle-like limb buds appear. The spinal column is forming and looks like a long tail. Brain cells are beginning to differentiate, but there is no capability for consciousness or sensation of pain.

Week 6 LMP (1/2 inch): The tail is still present. Limb buds are lengthening. Eyes and ears are beginning. The heart is pulsing on the outside of the body. The human embryo at this stage cannot be visually differentiated by appearance from a pig, rabbit, chick, or elephant.

Week 7 LMP (3/4 inch): Skeletal and muscular development has begun. The tail is still apparent. Notches appear for fingers and toes. The heart becomes internal.

Week 8 LMP (one inch): The tail begins to disappear. Fingers and toes are present. External sex organs appear. Cartilage and skeletal growth occurs. Eyelids are fused closed. Still no blood is pumping through the beating heart. Its weight is less than an aspirin tablet. It is now called a "fetus."

Week 9 LMP (1.5 inches): The tail is gone. Its head is almost half the length of the whole fetus. Its heart tones may be audible by ultrasound. The

limbs are nearly complete. Weight: 1/15 ounce.

Week 10 LMP (1.75 inches): Its eyes move from the side to the front of its head but are still shut. The scrotum appears in a male. Lower body development begins to accelerate, but the head is still almost as large as body. Blood and bone cells form. Blood is now pumping through the heart. Early reflex movements are not perceptible to the mother. The fetus now has lips, tongue, and a thin skin. It swallows amniotic fluid, and its digestive system is working. It responds to touch with reflex movement but has no capacity for perception of pain.

Week 11 LMP (two inches): The internal organs begin to function. Urine is produced and excreted into the amniotic fluid. The sex organs are not distinguishable.

Week 12 LMP (three inches): The formation of arms, legs, hands, feet, fingers, toes, ears, and sex organs are completed. Reflexive rather than purposeful movements occur in the face and limbs, such as sucking thumb. All movement is reflexive from spinal cord.

Weeks 13 LMP (3.5 inches)
Week 14 LMP (four-five inches)
Week 15 LMP (five-six inches)
Week 16 LMP (six-eight inches)

Between 13 to 16 weeks there is rapid body growth. The skeleton is visible by X-ray. By four months movements can be felt by the mother. The fetal heart can be heard with a stethoscope. Fine hair covers the body. Formerly transparent skin becomes pink. Eyebrows and eyelashes appear. Survival outside the uterus is impossible. Weight: six ounces.

Week 17 - 20 LMP (eight - 12 inches from head to toe if straightened out from a curved shape). An oily substance called "vernix" covers and protects the skin from drying out. Fat begins to form. Myelinization of the spinal cord begins which forms insulation for the nerve cells. However, the ability to feel pain is highly improbable until the third trimester when both the cerebral cortex and neural connections are adequately formed (Grobstein, 1988).

Weeks 21 - 25 LMP (12-14 inches) The fetus is covered with a cheeselike secretion. The skin is wrinkled and eyes are open. The fetus continues to add fat and length but still has a skinny appearance. Proportions of the head and body are becoming more balanced. Capillaries are now visible in the skin. Hair appears. Fingernails present but not fully formed.

VIABILITY: If the fetus is between 22 - 24 weeks LMP and weighs at least 500 grams, it is said to have reached viability (Amon, 1988, Hovick, 1989, Kilbride et al., 1990, Moore, 1989, Reiter et al., 1991). According to the 1990 Stedman's Medical Dictionary, "viability" is defined as the capability of living outside the uterus. Until alveolar cells in the lungs begin to produce surfactant, the lungs will collapse instead of filling with air (Kantrowitz, 1990).

While there are accounts of some fetuses less than 24 weeks LMP surviving at birth, they can not do so without high technological intervention. Even with advanced intervention, survival is not guaranteed. Some hospitals have the most advanced equipment, and others are poorly lacking. A review of the literature indicates that neonatal weight is a better predictor of survival than gestational age (Hovick, 1989). Hovick found that even with technological intervention, weight less than 500 grams (one pound) has resulted in a 0% survival rate, and weights between 500 - 600 grams have a survival rate of 43%. Once the fetus reaches 1000 grams or 2.2 pounds, it has an 85% chance of survival. A weight of 1000 grams usually corresponds to a gestational age of 27 weeks (approximately seven months).

28 weeks (16 inches) Weight: two-three pounds. Because of immature lung development, the fetus cannot breathe on its own until seven months. At that time lungs are developed sufficiently for survival, but if born prematurely there are risks of cerebral palsy, mental retardation, blindness, hearing impairment, heart, respiratory, and circulation problems (Rosenblith, 1992).

32 weeks or eight months (18 inches) Weight: five pounds.
Until the fetus reaches roughly 30 weeks, there are no regular electrical patterns in the brain that resemble adult human brainwaves (Grobstein, 1988).

40 weeks or nine months: Length and weight varies, as with all stages of the pregnancy.

INTERPRETING THE FACTS: IS ABORTION KILLING A BABY?

It is important to note what **meaning** you attribute to the various stages of fetal development. Your **interpretation** of what the stages of development **signify** will result in forming your opinion to the question, "Is abortion killing a baby?" When asking the question, you are seeking to establish whether an embryo or fetus at some point in its development is the **same entity** with the **same capacities** as a born baby. **If it is the same,** then abortion is the same as infanticide. **If it is not the same,** then abortion is not "killing a baby." Remember, there is no consensus from scientists, doctors, philosophers, or theologians. Your conclusion is simply your opinion based on your interpretations. Your opinion may also be held by many others, but it is strictly an opinion.

Consider these questions: 1). Is the fetus in the uterus the same entity it will be once it is born? If so, at what point in its development is it the same? Why? If not, why not? 2). Is aborting a fetus the same thing as giving birth and then killing the baby after it's born? Why? Why not? In considering these questions and exploring your criteria for the answers, notice what IS NOT present at each stage of development as well as what IS present. Why is this approach helpful? Is a bowl of cold water mixed with raw carrots and onions and a raw soup bone soup? It has all the ingredients and the potential for soup, but what's missing? When deciding **if** and **when** a fetus becomes the equivalent of a born person, look at the "ingredients" that are there, and those that are missing. It will give you a more complete perspective. The following are some of the most common stages of development at which people declare a fetus becomes "a baby" and the criteria they use to support their answers. Included are reasons why some people disagree with each set of criteria.

Possible Criteria For Determining When A Fetus Becomes A Baby

1. When conception takes place. Conception is the time at which the egg and sperm unite in a seven-step process (Grobstein, 1988). Some people believe that the fertilized egg (zygote) is itself a person because the entire genetic code of what the person may become is present. Other people see a marked distinction between a fertilized egg and a

person, and point out a similar distinction between an acorn and an oak tree, between a hen egg and a chicken, or blueprints and a house. One has the potential to become something in the future, and the other is the end result in the here and now.

Some faiths teach that a soul is infused at conception ("ensoulment"). They teach that the zygote is fully human because it has a soul, period. Other faiths teach a soul is not infused until birth has occurred and the first breath is taken. The belief in a soul is a matter of faith, just as the belief of when ensoulment occurs is a matter of faith.

Some people choose conception as their criterion because the two reproductive cells, sperm and ovum, from which the embryo develops are living cells and originate from the human species. Therefore, they conclude the zygote is "a human life" because it is both living and human. Others say while it may be a form of human life, it is not the same kind of life as a fully developed nine-month baby and therefore does not have the same value.

2. When the embryo has a heartbeat (four-five weeks LMP). Some people believe that the beginning of a person's life is when the heart starts to beat because the end of a person's life comes when the heart stops beating. However, others say that at four weeks the heart might be beating, but the embryo was **living** before the heart started pulsing. And some people say the heart might be beating at four weeks, but there's no blood yet pumping through the heart until 10 weeks LMP. And no human being can be alive without blood pumping through his or her veins.

3. When the fetus has identifiable body parts (eight weeks). This is the time at which arms and legs, hands and feet, and fingers and toes have been formed. Some people believe when they can identify human body parts, then it's a baby. Others believe it takes more than arms and legs for a fetus to be the equivalent of a baby because a baby has and is much more than its arms and legs. For instance, a baby can breathe air, and an eight-week fetus can not.

4. When the fetus resembles a baby. The time at which people think a fetus looks like a baby varies widely.
Some people might look at an enlarged photo of an eight-week fetus and say it looks like a baby, and others will say not until late second trimester when its head and body are more proportionate, its skin has some fat underneath, it's bigger, and they can see a face. Some people believe if it looks like a baby, then it is a baby. Again, others believe it takes more than visual resemblance to constitute the equivalent of a born baby.

5. When there is quickening (16th to 20th week and beyond). This is when the fetal movements can be felt by the woman. Some people say once they can **feel** life moving around inside them, then it's a baby. Others say the fetus has been moving around long before the woman can feel it, and the only difference is that the fetus is large enough to cause sensations in the woman.

6. When the fetus is viable. There are two definitions of viability: 1). When a fetus will probably be able to sustain life outside the woman's body WITH the intervention of present day technology (approximately 22-24 weeks LMP). As technology becomes more sophisticated, earlier fetuses may fit into this definition. 2). When a fetus will probably be able to sustain life outside the woman's body WITHOUT technological intervention (approximately 28 weeks or seven months).

Viability is the time at which the fetus has enough lung development to be able to breathe. It has the capability to live apart from the woman's body, and some people view this as the first time the fetus is a totally separate life. However, some premature births at seven months may result in sustained life but one with blindness, mental retardation, heart and respiratory problems, and other serious impairment due to its underdevelopment. Because of this, some people do not view the seven-month fetus as the equivalent of the same fetus carried to full term and born healthy.

7. When the fetus has the same or similar brain and central nervous system development to that of a newborn. The exact timing is unknown, but the part of the brain and neural interconnections necessary for human thought and consciousness does not develop until the third trimester, and it is still incomplete at the time of birth (Francoeur, 1989, Bennett, 1989, Flower, 1989). In fact, brain cells are still reproducing up to two years after birth (Stratton, 1982). Dr. Dominick Purpura, neurologist, neuroscientist, and dean of the Albert Einstein Medical School states, "The things that

seem to be very important are a certain minimum number of nerve cells in the cerebral cortex, a certain minimum number of synaptic connections. Which says then, that if you don't have that number of neurons, or that amount of connections, you're not going to be able to produce the qualities of humanness, personhood." (Jaworski, 1989). Using this criteria, the minimal time for the beginning of personhood is at the middle of the third trimester, since organized brain waves similar to a newborn's are not present until 31 weeks.

8. When the act of birth takes place. Those who designate birth - whether by C-section or by natural birth - maintain that the fetus is not living on its own outside the woman's uterus until birth and is not interacting with its parents and family in the same way as a born baby does, and therefore until birth it is still a different entity.

This list contains the most common points of demarcation people use to determine when, if ever, a fetus becomes a baby before birth. It is by no means a complete, exhaustive list. For an in-depth examination of "personhood" from philosophical, theological, and Biblical viewpoints, I recommend reading the following: Simmons, Paul, (1990). Personhood, the Bible, and the Abortion Debate.

Donovan, Patricia, (1983). "When Does Personhood Begin?" Family Planning Perspectives, Volume 15, Number 1, January/February.

Knight, J. and Callahan, J. (1989). "Elective Abortion: The Moral Debate," Preventing Birth: Contemporary Methods and Related Moral Controversies.

For an anti-abortion stance from a professor of philosophy, read "The Unborn as Person" in Restoring the Right to Life (Bopp, Jr., 1984).

Values Clarification Exercise

Here is a beneficial exercise to help staff clarify their values and feelings about the morality of first and second trimester abortion. It also helps them discover if their values would permit them to l). refer for an abortion, both first and second trimester, 2). be present in the procedure room, and 3). choose an abortion herself - both first and second trimester. The group facilitator makes five cards, each one bearing one of these descriptions:

STRONGLY AGREE, SOMEWHAT AGREE, DON'T KNOW, SOMEWHAT DISAGREE, AND STRONGLY DISAGREE.

Place each card on an imaginary line on the floor in a continuum. Ask the group members to move to the card that best describes their feelings after each one of the following sentences is read. After they have moved to the appropriate spot on the imaginary line, ask the participants why they agree or disagree. Make the statement that there are no right or wrong answers. The purpose is to provoke thought and clarify beliefs about fetal life in relation to abortion and in relation to the woman choosing abortion.

1. Abortion is destroying living tissue.

2. Abortion is ending the potential for life.

3. Abortion is ending a human life.

4. Abortion is ending some form of human life.

5. Abortion is killing a human being.

6. In an abortion, removing a first trimester fetus from the uterus is the same as smothering a newborn.

7. In a second trimester abortion, removing the fetus from the uterus is the same as smothering a newborn.

8. I could and would refer a woman for an abortion if she was 24 weeks.

9. I could and would refer a woman for an abortion if she was 26 weeks.

10. I would be willing to assist a woman through a 24-week abortion procedure.

11. I would be willing to assist the doctor during a 24-week abortion.

12. If I were 46-years-old, divorced, suffering financial hardship, and my partner left me in my 24th week, I'd probably have an abortion.

13. I can think of a situation in which I would probably have an abortion in the first trimester.

14. I can think of a situation in which I would

choose to have an abortion in the second trimester.

15. Whether it is an eight-week or 24-week abortion, a woman should have the legal right to terminate her pregnancy.

16. Whether it is an eight-week or 24-week abortion, my feelings about it are the same.

This exercise can be modified by reading off each of the nine criteria for deciding when personhood begins, or make up criteria of your own.

Does Third Trimester Abortion Exist?

The reason I have mentioned only first and second trimester abortion is because third trimester abortion is extremely rare. The National Abortion Federation is aware of extremely few physicians who are willing and able to provide an abortion in the third trimester. A third trimester abortion is performed only in cases of severe fetal abnormality or if the woman's life or health is in imminent danger. (Grimes, 1984). Those of us who have been in the field of abortion since its legalization in 1973 know of no physicians who will perform an abortion on a healthy fetus "the day before full term delivery," as the anti-abortion propagandists allege.

Chapter Four

Pregnancy Test Counseling

O nce a counselor has examined her attitudes, she is ready to learn the specifics of pregnancy options counseling. A logical place to start is to learn pregnancy test counseling.

POSITIVE RESULTS

The first thing to realize when giving a positive result is that not every woman is going to be unhappy with the results. Usually women who come to a family planning clinic are interested in contraception, NOT pregnancy. Many positive pregnancy test results are met with disappointment and long faces. Fortunately, some women do welcome the news. As an undergraduate practicum student at Planned Parenthood years ago, I recall having one hand on the Kleenex box every time I gave a positive result because of the number who became upset and cried. One day a woman burst into tears at the news, and as I passed her a tissue I thought, "Oh, this poor soul is surely in anguish!" To my surprise and delight she smiled through her tears, shook my hand, and said, "This is the happiest day of my life! Here I thought I was sterile!" So I learned not to assume.

Reactions And Feelings

Every woman should be given the opportunity to express her feelings and explore her situation in private. One of the first questions you need to ask is, "How do you feel about the results?"

If She Is Crying

Receiving a positive pregnancy test result can confirm a person's worst fears and often triggers an outpouring of tears. If she starts to cry, silence is an appropriate response, as is the gentle statement, "It's OK to cry." Some women start to talk, revealing the source of their tears before you even ask. Other women may chide themselves, stating, "I told myself I wasn't going to cry!" You may make any number of responses that conveys understanding and permission to cry…"Sometimes tears are a good thing," or "We all need to cry sometimes when we don't want ourselves to." She may let herself cry or she may steel herself against any display of emotion. Whatever her inclination, let it be and follow her lead.

If She Appears Uncomfortable

If she seems upset and uncomfortable, not knowing quite what to say or where to begin, you could comment, "From your reaction it seems a bad time for you to be pregnant." She will confirm your hunch or express confusion and ambivalence. Ask her if she would give you an idea of her situation. As she unravels the bits and pieces of her situation, reflect back to her both the feeling and content of her statements. This is the time to employ your active listening skills. After you have helped her clarify and define the problem, you can both begin to examine the options.

If She Seems Stunned And Is Unresponsive

If she sits silently staring into space and is not responding to your statements or questions even after periods of silence, she is probably **unable** to communicate at this time. It is fruitless to continue asking questions and prodding for answers. Attempts at problem-solving are pointless. Gently let her know that she probably needs time to soak in the information. Would she like to be alone with the person who came with her? Tell her she is welcome to talk to you later when she has collected her thoughts. If there is an office she and her friend can occupy for awhile, then she can ask you for appropriate information before she leaves. This is especially helpful if she has come a long distance to your facility. If time and space do not permit this course of action, suggest she and her friend call or come back later if she needs to ask any questions and receive information. You may give her written information on all her options and encourage her to call you back soon.

Content of the Pregnancy Test Counseling Session

The following is a mental outline of the flow of events that usually takes place in a pregnancy test counseling session. Every session does not follow precisely in this order or even cover everything in these suggested 11 steps. The outline is simply a way to structure your thoughts when delivering a positive result.

1. Allow her to express her feelings.

2. Reflect back to her what you see and hear her telling you.

3. Evaluate her ability to respond. Does she appear shocked?

4. If she is responsive, ask if she has already thought about what she would do if her results were positive.

5. If she is responsive, help her to list all her options: carry to term and raise the child, carry to term and place the child for adoption, or have an abortion.

6. Ask who she would want to talk to before making her decision.

7. Let her know she is not expected to make a decision right now.

8. Calculate an approximate length of pregnancy based on her last menstrual period and inform her she needs a pelvic exam or sonogram to evaluate it more accurately.

9. Explain the time element when deciding what to do: 1). Early prenatal care is a wise idea if she is carrying to term, 2). After 14 weeks an abortion becomes a two-day process that costs more than a first trimester abortion, and she may have to travel out-of-state to a second trimester provider.

10. Offer to answer any questions and give her appropriate referrals and reading material.

11. Invite her to call back if she wants to talk further.

NEGATIVE RESULTS

Reactions and Feelings

When giving a negative pregnancy test, it is helpful to ask, "How do you feel about the results?" Is she relieved or disappointed? Sometimes, of course, you don't have to ask, depending on her visible reactions. Often the woman is confused, wondering why the pregnancy test is negative when she has been missing periods. Although there are reasons why a woman can miss periods and not be pregnant, it is also true that pregnancy tests are not always accurate. I have seen more than one woman having a second trimester abortion because all the pregnancy tests in her first trimester were negative. Possible reasons why she may not be pregnant and still miss periods include problems with ovaries, pituitary gland, or central nervous system, menopause, birth control pills, hormonal implants, and Depo Provera shots, to list a few.

Determining If Results Are Accurate

Since pregnancy tests taken from urine are not as accurate as blood tests, she may want a serum pregnancy test for greater accuracy. However, there are questions you can ask that may help determine whether the test is probably right or wrong.

1. "When was your last NORMAL period?" She needs to be at least 14 days late for her period before most urine tests are accurate. Always have a calendar handy. If she is too early in the pregnancy, the results could show negative. She needs to wait until she is at least seven weeks from the last period to maximize the probablility that another pregnancy test or pelvic exam will be accurate.

2. "Have you had any symptoms of pregnancy, such as breast soreness or swelling, nausea, appetite changes, bloating, tiredness, sleeping more than usual, frequent urination or dizziness? If she does have symptoms, then it is likely the negative results are in error. Some women who have been pregnant before KNOW when they're pregnant. Some women will even inform you, "Last time I was pregnant the test didn't show up positive until I was three months along." This is a definite cue to suggest a blood test or sonogram instead of having the urine test rerun.

3. "Are your periods usually regular or do you usually miss periods now and then?" Sometimes when a woman has an irregular menstrual cycle, she has difficulty knowing whether she is pregnant or whether she is just missing periods as usual. An irregular cycle might explain a negative test. Nevertheless, always encourage the woman to investigate further with a blood test or sonogram.

4. "Do you have the Norplant? Do you get the birth control shot?" Either of these can cause missed periods, but then again neither method is 100%.

5. "Have you been on birth control pills? Did you miss any? Did you go off them recently?" Sometimes missing pills or quitting them can cause a temporary cessation of periods. On the other hand, a woman can get pregnant by missing or quitting them. Even if all clues point to the accuracy of the negative test, suggest she make an appointment with her doctor to determine why she is missing periods.

6. "Were you wanting to get pregnant?" If she does not want to become pregnant, she must understand she needs to start using a method of birth control right away. Most people will need spermicides and condoms until they see their doctors and receive their contraceptive of their choice. The issue of contraception is an especially important one to bring up with adolescents. Some teens who experience a pregnancy scare may breathe a sigh of relief when given the negative test. They sometimes conclude, "I've learned my lesson, and I'll never have sex again!" But a few weeks later they are having sex again. In this case there are ways to explore the reality of their intention to abstain. (See the chapter on abstinence). She may conclude, "Everything's OK now. I can go back to having sex and not worry anymore." Asking her, "How would you have felt if the test had been positive?" may help her consider the issue of birth control. If her boyfriend is out in the waiting room, this is an excellent opportunity to talk about birth control and condom use with both partners. They are probably motivated, having just been faced with a scare. The counselor needs to demonstrate spermicides and condoms and explain where they can be purchased. Giving them a birth control guide for deciding on a future method and briefly demystifying the pelvic exam and pap smear may help pave the way for a trip to the doctor and conscientious contraception.

If She Is Disappointed With Negative Results

Some women have been trying to get pregnant. Instead of birth control, they may need a pamphlet or other resource on infertility. If she has been trying to get pregnant for over one year, and if she has already read about infertility, she and her partner need to talk to their doctor or be referred to an infertility specialist.

After the Pregnancy Test

After the pregnancy test counseling session, the woman will return home. If she hasn't done so already, she will come to grips with the fact that she is pregnant. At some point she will probably confide in someone or several people. After some time of deliberation, she usually comes to a decision. However, for those women who feel "stuck," an options counseling session might be useful.

Chapter Five

Options Counseling: Building Rapport

BUILDING RAPPORT

Building rapport is such a basic tenet of counseling that it merits discussion at this point. Building rapport means engaging trust and putting a person at ease. When you have rapport, the client feels comfortable enough to communicate feelings and thoughts with a minimum of inhibition. In therapy trust can be built gradually over the passage of weeks or months. However, in short term counseling the counselor usually has one chance, one short session in which to create that bond. Therefore, from the moment you greet the client to the moment the session ends, you need to do and say those things that will foster trust. Trust is necessary to open communication; without communication you are powerless to help that client in any way. Therefore, you need to send her nonverbal and verbal messages that it is safe to reveal herself.

Nonverbal And Verbal Elements Of Building Rapport

Some of the simple nonverbals that encourage trust include appropriate smiling, good eye contact, attentive body posture or mirroring the way the client is sitting, matching the client's speed or slowness in her speech, and facial expressions and gestures that indicate acceptance, interest, and empathy. Verbals that build rapport include explaining the purpose of the counseling session, using her name, sharing appropriate information about yourself, actively listening to her, and interjecting appropriate humor.

Simple nonverbals that inhibit or destroy trust include lack of facial expression or eye contact, and any gestures, noises, facial expressions or body posture that indicate disinterest, disapproval, annoyance, or extreme nervousness. Some of the verbals that damage rapport include any remarks or statements that are critical, chiding, preaching, blaming, shaming, discounting, or inappropriate smiling and laughing.

There are schools of thought as well as techniques designed to establish trust and rapport, such as Neuro Linguistic Programming (NLP), and hypnotherapist Milton Erickson's technique of "pacing." Frogs Into Princes by Richard Bandler and John Grinder, and The Magic of Rapport by Jerry Richardson are two excellent references on NLP's method of building rapport.

In The Magic of Rapport, Richardson explains that establishing rapport quickly and effectively requires getting into alignment with the client. He describes a number of ways you can align yourself with any client, and starts by explaining Milton Erickson's technique of pacing.

Pacing

You are pacing another person if you:

1. Speed up or slow down your rate of speech to match theirs.

2. Sit the way they are sitting, hold your hands as they are, and use some of their gestures.

3. Repeat some of the same phrases, images, and words they use.

4. Turn up or down the volume of your voice to match theirs.

5. Express shared beliefs and ways in which you agree.

Social scientists have discovered that these alignments occur naturally and unconsciously when two people are conversing harmoniously with each other. To an observer, each may even appear to be the mirror image of the other. Next time you find yourself thoroughly engaged in an agreeable conversation, notice how you are both sitting or standing.

This theory maintains that when you are pacing a client, she will feel more comfortable with you because she will feel you are truly "with" her. The more comfortable she is, the more apt she is to communicate freely. And the more freely she communicates, the more you will discover what her individual needs are and can tailor the session to meet those needs.

While some counselors perceive the techniques of N.L.P. as "manipulative," others view the techniques as strategies that help them establish rapport quickly.

Active Listening

This skill is fundamental to effective counseling and is also part of establishing rapport. Without it you are handicapped. When a person engages in active listening, she pays close attention to both the content of the message given and the feelings behind it. The listener then reflects back to the speaker both feelings and content of the message. For example, the client states, "My boyfriend wanted me to get an abortion but wouldn't even give me any money for it! I tried talking to him last night but he claims he still doesn't have the money. I'll get even, don't worry!" An active listening response would be, "Sounds like you're feeling angry because he's not willing to take any of the responsibility and has dumped the financial burden all on you! And you're not going to let him get by with it!" Clues to the person's emotions include her tone of voice, the way she sits, the look in her eyes, and other nonverbal behaviors that accompany what she says. Two people can make the same statement and convey different feelings by their nonverbals. The reasons why active listening is so helpful are:

1. It indicates to the speaker she has been heard and understood.

2. It promotes further communication.

3. It helps the speaker clarify her thoughts and feelings.

4. It helps the listener understand what the speaker is thinking and feeling.

5. It enables both listener and speaker to problem-solve.

When you are first learning active listening, you can use the format, "It sounds like you feel _____ because _____." Variations include "Let me know if I'm hearing you right. Did you say _____?" "Correct me if I'm wrong, but are you feeling ___ because ___?" "From what you said, it sounds like ___," "What I'm hearing is ___," "So you're saying that you're feeling ____ because ___?" Try to vary the format so you won't sound mechanical. Soon it will become second nature.

One last word about active listening. Don't be upset if your response is off-target. Whatever your response, the speaker will either agree and elaborate or disagree and correct the inaccuracy. This process will help her thoughts become clearer to herself as well as to you. People don't always know what they're feeling or why. Active listening can help them find out. For more information on active listening skills, read Leadership Effectiveness Training by Thomas Gordon, The Skilled Helper by G. Egan, and Short-Term Relationship Counseling by Terry Beresford.

Chapter Six

Decision-Making and Ambivalence

EXPLORING THE DECISION IN OPTIONS COUNSELING

1. Let her define the problem. Encourage her to talk and explain her entire situation to help you understand.

2. Reflect back her feelings and thoughts to help her clarify what the problem actually is. No one can really solve a problem until he or she can identify precisely what the problem is.

3. Find out the alternatives she has been considering.

4. Fill her in on ALL alternatives if she has left any out.

Helping the Ambivalent Client

1. What are the pros and cons of each alternative, in terms of consequences? It's helpful to make six lists, two for each option: parenthood, adoption, and abortion. The lists might read:

• Positive Consequences of Keeping and Parenting the Baby.

• Negative Consequences of Keeping and Parenting the Baby.

• Positive Consequences of Placing the Child for Adoption.

• Negative Consequences of Placing the Child for Adoption.

• Positive Consequences of Having an Abortion.

• Negative Consequences of Having an Abortion.

When making these lists, it is important she use the word "abortion" instead of "not keeping the baby," or other terminology because the only way to keep from carrying to term is through an abortion process. Denying the reality NOW can create regret LATER. This is the same reason to use the word, "parenting," along with "keeping the baby."

2. Ask how she would probably feel and how she would cope as time went by 1). after an abortion, 2). after she kept the baby, and 3). after she placed for adoption. This allows her to examine the pros and cons from the standpoint of emotional well-being now _and_ in the future.

3. Ask under what circumstances would she like to become a parent? How are her present circumstances different than what she wants? What would it take to get what she really wants?

How would she feel about taking that action? How would she cope?

4. What are her goals for the coming year? For the next three years? How important are her goals? How would each alternative help or hinder the achievement of her goals?

Life Losses And Gains

Sometimes it helps to reframe the consequences of each alternative in terms of life losses and life gains. List everything she can think of in answer to the questions, "What would you stand to lose in your life if you carried to term?" Do the same for the question, "What would you gain? How would carrying to term benefit your life?" Then repeat the questions for the adoption and abortion alternative. If she has children and expresses concerns about her children's welfare, ask, "What would your children stand to lose if you carried to term and kept the baby, placed it for adoption, or had an abortion? How would they benefit if you carried to term, placed for adoption, had an abortion?" Then summarize her answers and allow her to reflect on what she has said.

Conflicting Values And Priorities

Help her identify any conflicts between her values and each alternative. She may place a high value on motherhood and want children, but at this time in her life she places a high priority on getting her education. She views her education as the means by which she will be able to have a decent paying job some day and avoid a life of hardship and poverty for both her and her children.

She may not want to be pregnant at this time in her life for a number of compelling reasons, but the only way to "undo" the pregnancy is through an abortion. A conflict arises if her belief about abortion is that it's killing.

Exploring The Client's Belief About Abortion

"Is abortion killing a baby?" is one of the difficult questions most women think about when faced with the decision to carry to term or end a pregnancy. When you ask, "What did you used to believe about abortion before this became a personal issue?" you will find the replies usually fall in the following categories.

1. "I've always believed abortion should be the woman's choice, but only in certain cases." Rape, incest, and life endangerment are the usual exceptions many people have professed as "legitimate" reasons for having an abortion until they or a loved one are faced with an unplanned pregnancy. Then they discover other "legitimate" reasons for ending a pregnancy, or they may feel ashamed that their reasons don't measure up.

2. "I've always believed abortion was killing." For many people the saying, "abortion is killing" becomes an automatic response because they have seen and heard it so frequently on anti-abortion billboards, TV commercials, programs, and the media coverage of anti-abortion activists. After giving it more thought, some people discover they no longer believe or only half believe what they've said all along, while others believe it more strongly than before.

3. "I never thought abortion was wrong." Some people have never held the belief that abortion was killing or that only certain reasons were "legitimate."

4. "I never thought about it enough to know what I believed." They state that until it became a personal issue, they never gave it a thought. They may still not know what they believe.

The belief that abortion is "killing" or "not killing" is one of the main issues that creates extreme ambivalence for some women when considering abortion. For a thorough discussion of how to explore the client's belief, refer to the chapter on Guilt.

The woman in conflict may be trying to choose between what she considers the lesser of two evils: bringing a child into the world when she can't provide adequately for its basic needs, or "ending its life." She is trying to decide: 1). Which is MORE wrong? and 2). Which can she LIVE with for the rest of her life? When she feels they are equally wrong, the conflict is acute, and she usually resorts to making the choice that will more likely result in MANAGEABLE levels of guilt or sadness and less likelihood of deep regret, depression, shame, or trauma.

Reality Testing For Single Parenthood

If a client is unsure whether she will be able to raise a child on her own, or when a teenager assumes parenthood will be "a piece of cake," here is an approach to take.

Let her know parenthood can work out when a pregnancy occurs at a time that is not ideal as long as she finds workable solutions to the following questions:

1. Do you have a place to live before and after the baby is born? If you are planning to live with someone else, have you **asked** them and received a definite answer?

2. If you plan to live on your own, have you priced rent and utilities? Have you found an affordable apartment yet? Do you need to set aside time to start searching?

3. How will the doctor, pre-natal care, hospital, and pediatrician bills be paid for? Have you found out how much these bills will be?

4. Do you have medical insurance? Are you eligible for any government assistance? Have you contacted the Department of Public Aid in your state to check your eligibility?

5. If you already know exactly how much aid you will receive, have you added up your expenses to find out if this amount will cover everything?

6. If your expenses are more than the aid you'll receive, how will you cover the remaining expenses? Have you asked your parents how much they are willing to provide for you and the child?

7. Do you or your partner have a job? How much does it pay? Will this amount cover rent, utilities, food, transportation, clothing, laundry, babysitter, doctor, and other bare essentials for you, him, and the child?

8. Will you or your partner need to take a second job to cover costs? Will you need to continue working after the baby is born?

9. Do you know someone who will give or lend you baby clothes, maternity clothes, crib, blankets, car seat? Have you priced those articles yet?

10. Do you have a babysitter who will take care of the child if if you need to go to work or to school? Have you asked them, and have they given you a definite answer? How much will they charge for babysitting?

11. Do you want to continue your education? How will you accomplish this? Will you go to night school? Day school? Who will watch the baby while you're in school and when you need to study and do homework? Will you need to go to work as well as attend classes? Have you planned a schedule to see how this can work?

12. If you plan to attend college, who will pay for it?

13. How much time do you want to spend with your child? Will you have enough time to satisfy both you and the child? What will your daily schedule be like, including weekends, to allow time for all you need and want to do? Will it be OK if you don't have time for going out with friends? What kind of recreation and fun do you NOT want to give up? How can you schedule some of this recreation after the baby is born?

14. How will having the baby affect your family? How will it affect your relationship with each one? Have you talked to them? What do you want and need from them? What are they willing to give? What do they want and need from you? What are you willing to give?

15. If there is bitter conflict between you and your family over this decision, are you willing to live with that conflict? What is the probability of them reconciling differences with you or you with them?

16. If your parents want you to have an abortion, and you want to keep the baby, have you asked them and your boyfriend and his parents to come together for a family conference? Have you considered seeing a family counselor? Any Mental Health Department offers family counseling on a sliding fee scale based on what you can pay.

17. Will your decision to parent a child come the closest to giving you what you want in your life at this time over all the other alternatives?

The Need For Factual Information

Give her any other factual information she doesn't have that will help (such as the description of the abortion procedure, a referral to find out if she is eligible for state aid, or information on the adoption process). Sometimes fear of the unknown appears as indecision. For example, someone who is terrified of pain or believes infertility will result from abortion can appear undecided about what to do. Or the woman who is afraid she will never know what happened to her child once she has placed for adoption may be in a quandary. But once she has the facts, the obstacle creating indecision sometimes melts away dramatically.

Exploring How Her Decision May Affect Significant Others

When helping someone think through her decision, it is also beneficial to ask who else's life would be affected by the decision. People don't exist in a vacuum, and often women are concerned about how their decision will affect others in their lives. Who is important to her in her life and how would they react to the pregnancy and each alternative? Whom has she already told? What were their reactions to the pregnancy? Are there any other significant people in her life she would like to tell? How would they probably react? How would their reactions affect her? Does she need to find out for sure how they would react? For instance, if she says she really wants the baby, but isn't sure if her mother (or boyfriend) would help her, she needs to find out. The alternative may be having an abortion and then finding out **afterwards** her mother or partner would have been very willing to help her take care of the baby. The more facts she has on which to base her decision, the greater the potential for a sound decision.

Exploring How Significant Others Are Affecting Her Decision

Conflicts between what she wants and what her partner or parents want are another major cause of ambivalence for some women. The desire to keep the peace or please parents or partner may make it difficult for her to follow her own desires and meet her own needs. The more attachment she feels toward the person who op-

poses her own desires, the more painful it may be to make her decision. For example, the woman who states she is in love with her partner will probably have more difficulty than the woman who says she could care less what he thinks. The teenager whose survival depends upon her parents will probably be in a greater quandary than the woman who no longer needs her parents for her survival. If the woman lives with the person who opposes her decision, there is greater opportunity for on-going conflict than if she lives apart from them. In addition, the woman who generally looks outside herself for answers and approval will probably be more affected by her partner or parents than the woman with greater inner strength.

The Time Crunch

Many major life decisions must be made under time constraints. Although you can reassure her she doesn't have to make the decision right now, let her know approximately how long she has to make a decision about having an abortion. Check her last menstrual period or suggest a pelvic exam or sonogram for more accuracy. If she is even considering an abortion, she will need this information. Most women do not know the cost, safety factors, and accessibility of abortion at various points of gestation.

If she is considering carrying to term, finding a doctor and getting prenatal care as soon as possible is important.

Training Video For Options Counseling

The video, "No Single Answer," (1993) is an excellent training tool for options counselors. Terry Beresford and Joan Garrity demonstrate and discuss three different counseling scenarios at the time of the pregnancy test. This video can be purchased by writing to Planned Parenthood of Northern New England, 51 Talcott Road, Williston, VT 05495-8116.

Chapter Seven

Common Dilemmas

"I Want An Abortion, But I Can't Afford It."

Sometimes the cost of an abortion seems prohibitive, and that can create feelings of despair. The first reaction to the fee may be, "Oh, there's no way I can come up with that much money!" Even though the situation may seem hopeless at that moment, there still are options.

1. Whom has she told? Are there any friends or family members who could help, especially knowing her alternative would be to have a baby under her circumstances? If the client doesn't want family or friends to find out, the fact is they **will** find out if she has the baby. Admittedly, telling Mom or Aunt Gertie might be unpleasant, but the alternative of having an unwanted child may be more than unpleasant. If she can't think of anyone, here are some relations and acquaintances other women have found to be a help in need: a friend, cousin, sibling, aunt or uncle, a step-parent, grandparent, boyfriend's parent, a classmate or co-worker, a supervisor or boss. Some have even been surprised to find that one or both of their parents were very supportive once they knew the truth.

2. Is the client or male partner employed? When will they receive their next paycheck? How far along will she be in the pregnancy then?

3. Do they have any savings?

4. Do they know they could use a major credit card?

5. Is there anything she or her partner could sell?

The point is, how badly does she want the abortion? The more she wants it, the more options she'll be willing to try. There certainly will be times when the client truly has no financial resources. You need to know if the abortion provider will reduce or defer fees. Some can and some can't, depending on their own costs.

"I Want The Baby, But I Can't Afford It."

1. Explore ways of obtaining financial assistance, including her and her partner's relatives, charitable organizations, and government assistance.

2. How does she feel about raising a child on a very limited income? Has she known anyone who has relied on government assistance? I once saw a woman who told me, "I'm used to being poor. I was raised on welfare. I know what it's like wearing second hand clothes and eating beans all the time. But I'll be damned if I'll make somebody else live like that! I don't ever want a child of mine to have to poke around in someone else's trash for

their dried up, thrown- away Christmas tree like we did!" On the other hand, some women feel having a baby under any financial circumstances is preferable to having an abortion or placing their baby for adoption.

3. How would she like to be able to provide for a child? What goals does she have for her financial future? What does she need to do to achieve those goals?

4. How would she feel about receiving government aid or relying on her parents <u>temporarily</u> until she is able to get a job and provide for herself and her child?

"I Want The Baby, But My Boyfriend/ Husband Wants Me To Have An Abortion."

If the client makes this statement, here are some questions to ask.

1. "Tell me more about your desire to have this baby." Encourage her to talk about what she wants.

2. "Why does he want you to have an abortion? What do you think about those reasons?"

3. "What are you feeling about him? What do you think will happen to the relationship if you have the abortion? What will probably happen if you don't?"
 If she is thinking about agreeing to the abortion to hold onto the relationship, how will she probably feel if weeks or months later they break up anyway? How will she feel about her decision?

4. "How will you feel toward him afterwards if you have the abortion? How will you probably feel toward yourself?"

If her partner is available to talk to, it is helpful to talk to them both. You can then facilitate communication between the two, helping to remove communication blocks and misunderstandings. Most of the time they are not listening to the feelings behind each other's words, and that leads to frustration and anger. However, sometimes a breakup was on the way, and this pregnancy is "the last straw."

"I'm 30 Years Old And Don't Have Any Children, But I Don't Want To Struggle As A Single Parent."

This woman is feeling the pressure of the biological timeclock. As a single woman, she is faced with the dilemma of wanting children but wanting to be married before having children, and fearing that her time is running out for having both.

Sometimes she gets pregnant to test her partner's intentions. When he abruptly suggests an abortion or otherwise indicates he isn't interested in marriage or fathering a child, she may conclude, "I'm wasting my time with him." Often he feels content to continue the relationship after the abortion, but she feels rejected and disappointed, preferring to end the relationship. If they have been lovers for years, severing the ties may be very painful to her despite her anger. She is then dealing with two major decisions and two endings. Not only is she disappointed in her boyfriend, but her hopes for a future (marriage and motherhood) have been crushed.

It may be helpful to help her clarify her life goals.

1. What does she hope for in her 30s? 40s?

2. How strongly does she want to be a parent?

3. By what age does she want to have a baby? Is there a reason she does not want to be any older than that?

4. What does she need to be able to have a baby by that age?

5. Does she definitely want to be married before having a child?

6. Would she ever consider single parenthood as a viable option for herself? Under what circumstances? How could she plan and create those circumstances by the time of her cut-off age?

7. Would she rather never have a child (biologically) than be a single parent? How will she view this decision if at age 40 she is still single, has no children, and discovers she is going through menopause?

8. Has she thought of other ways to be significantly involved in a child's life other than being a biological parent? Would this option give her satisfaction?

If she states that taking a chance on never having children would be devastating to her, then she is gambling with very high stakes. Depending on the client, it may be wise to request that she have another counseling session before taking an action that cannot be undone. One 32-year-old client told me she wanted children but not if the child would have one parent. She was adamant about that stipulation. She stated she could accept a life without a child of her own better than she could accept all the consequences to her and the child if she struggled as a single parent. She added, "If I never have another opportunity to be a Mom, then I'll be the best Aunt I can be. I have two nieces and three nephews and can see them whenever I want." She chose to go through with the abortion.

Another 36-year-old client declared her life would be "unfulfilled" if she never became a mother. She told me throughout her ten-year marriage she had always longed to get pregnant, but it never happened. She had been divorced for three years when she became involved with another man. To her amazement she became pregnant. "I was so happy when I found out. It was a dream come true until he told me he already had grown kids and wasn't going to start over. He walked out, and now I'm alone." She said she worked at a low-paying job and couldn't support a child "the right way." The only person who might be able to help her raise the child was her 60-year-old mother, whom she had not told.

We talked about the abortion in terms of losses and gains, and it was clear the gains were small and the losses were great. I asked her to describe "the right way" to raise a child, and as she spoke, her perception changed. She started out describing a context of marriage, house, and money. But she ended up stating the right way could mean "just enough money to cover necessities and lots of love." She knew she had the latter ingredient, and with her mother's help might have the former as well. Upon my suggestion, she left to go home and talk to her mother. She never returned.

"At First I Was Happy, But Then My Situation Changed."

Health Risks

It is a common mistake to assume this client will feel justified in terminating the pregnancy because of her doctor's advice. Frequently this woman expresses guilt and a sense of powerlessness rather than moral justification. She may struggle with feelings of selfishness for taking care of her health at the expense of the potential life she's carrying. The lower her self-esteem and the stronger her desire for the baby, the harder the struggle.

Her family and friends and a caring partner are usually 100% supportive because they don't want anything to happen to her. But she is often plagued by the nagging doubt, "Am I really worth it?" This is true even for some of the women who were told their life would be in serious jeopardy if they carried to term.

Of course you are not going to change a person's self-esteem in one session. However, you can explore:

1. The level of confidence she has in her doctor's judgment.

2. Her reasons for not taking the risk of carrying to term.

3. How carrying to term and suffering the predicted consequences would affect significant others in her life.

4. Her support system.

5. Her feelings and how she expects to cope afterwards.

A 23-year-old insulin-dependent diabetic woman told me, "They almost lost me and the baby when I gave birth a year ago. My blood pressure went sky high, and I became unconscious. They had to do an emergency C-section at eight months. It was a while before we both got out of the hospital. My Mom and husband were frantic, and my doctor told me afterwards not to risk another pregnancy." She continued, "The only reason I'm here is because if I died, my little girl wouldn't have her mommy, and I couldn't do that to her. And if this baby lived, there'd be two

41

children without their mother. If only I knew everything would be OK, I'd try it." She started to cry and said, "I just feel so selfish. What right do I have to take a life?"

I reflected, "It feels selfish to protect your own life by having to end this potential life." She sobbed and shook her head yes. I ventured, "Sometimes caring for the self and others **equally** is hard to do." She blurted out, "Don't I know it! My mother's not a well woman and I'm an only child, so it's up to me to do what I can for her. I've got a baby to care for and a husband who needs attention, and on top of it all, I've got to make sure I eat the right foods and take my insulin!" She sobbed long and hard while I sat quietly with her. Then she blew her nose and said, "Whew! I've been under a lot of pressure, trying to keep it all under control. I know I'm making the right decision and the Good Lord understands. I'll probably feel relieved afterwards - and a little sad, naturally. I'm just grateful I have my daughter."

In our remaining time together we reframed the abortion in terms of 1). a loss to be grieved, and 2). an act of caring for the self in order to care for her daughter. We also discussed ways of coping with guilt, and she gratefully received a referral for spiritual counseling.

The Baby Fantasy

The woman in this situation is often a teenager. From the beginning of the pregnancy she has been thinking in terms of "the baby" and sometimes has already named it. She may have told her friends and boyfriend she is going to have a baby and has been looking at baby clothes in stores. Usually she has hidden it from her parents. As the pregnancy progresses, her mother suspects she's pregnant, confronts her, and paints a vivid picture of the realities of raising a child.

At the same time she is facing her parents' displeasure, her boyfriend may have started going out with other girls or generally exhibiting irresponsible behavior. What started out as the dream come true is now a dreadful nightmare. She realizes that getting married, moving out of the house, and getting out of school is not going to happen like she thought. She is faced with the prospect of battling with her parents the whole nine months while some other girl goes out with her boyfriend. Her choice may be between keep-

ing peace in the home and the status quo or having the baby and risking parental rejection. She may be torn between two thoughts: 1). Once the baby is born, her parents will relent and love her and the child and 2). They'll reject her and the baby, and she'll be miserable. If she is basing her decision on assumptions, you need to help her find the facts. What have they told her? If they are threatening to kick her out of the house, where else could she live? Would she consider a home for single mothers as a temporary option? How would she feel about that? She may be viewing her situation as "I have no choice but to have an abortion." You can reframe what you've heard by summarizing, "Sounds to me you'd rather keep the peace and live at home without a baby than to have the baby and risk losing your home." If her fantasy entailed moving out of the house and into a home with her boyfriend, her goal may have been one of adult independence. If so, you can help her plan other ways of achieving independence, such as finishing school, getting a job, going to college out of state, and acquiring financial independence. And by using a reliable method of birth control, she can be more in charge of when the next pregnancy will occur.

Financial Crisis

A financial crisis is another reason why a woman might change her mind about carrying to term. Losing everything in a fire, natural disaster, or going bankrupt can change her course of action dramatically. Sometimes she or her partner loses his or her job. If this is the case, has she considered how she will view this decision if in three months they find another job? Is she able to accept the decision based on limited knowlege of the future?

Extreme Nausea

Some pregnancies are terminated due to the debilitating condition of hyperemesis: the woman can't eat or drink anything without vomiting. She becomes weak and dehydrated, and requires hospitalization. Often she is in jeopardy of losing her job due to excessive absences. She may be neglecting her children and quarreling with her partner. A very pale and sick client explained, "All I do is lie in bed and throw up. I'm so weak, I can hardly stand up. Sometimes I just lie on the bathroom floor with my head hanging over the toilet. I can't take it anymore!" She could barely keep her head up and carried a plastic bowl with her "just in case." She had just been discharged from the hospital for dehydration and severe weight loss. "I went from a size 14 to a size five in one month," she said. "My doctor said I'd have to stay in the hospital until I could eat again. How am I going to pay for all that when I lose my job, and who's going to take care of my kids while I'm laid up in the hospital?" she stated. Most of these clients want the abortion over with as soon as possible and are looking forward to feeling "normal" again.

However, some of these pregnancies are planned and wanted, and the loss is deeply felt. Some women who had to choose between their own survival and that of the baby feel selfish, guilty, and defeated. One of my clients was a newlywed who had looked forward to her first child. She struggled long and hard to endure the debilitating effects of hyperemesis, but landed in the hospital several times. She hung on for 15 weeks, hoping the next day would be different and the severe vomiting would finally end. It continued to get worse. She stated she could no longer walk without help, her arms and legs shook spasmodically, and she was now severely depressed. Her husband told me, "I'm scared she is dying." She stated, "It has become a mental as well as physical sickness. I've lost all desire for everything except I want my life back. I never thought I'd say this, but I lost the desire for the baby, and when that happened, I lost everything keeping me alive. I just want to walk again and have a drink of water and well – **live.**" She and her husband were deeply grieved but determined the abortion was best. She said she felt like such a failure that she had told her husband, "If you want to divorce me, I'll understand." She said he replied, "I will never let you go!"

Partner Rejection

Sometimes the woman reports that her partner was happy when they discovered she was pregnant. They both agreed to keep the baby. She states her decision to carry to term was contingent upon his agreement to stay with her and help support the child. Then when she found out he was seeing other women or he told her outright he was no longer interested in helping her parent the child, she faced a new set of circumstances.

One 18-year-old broke into tears as she explained what happened. "For the past year he kept telling me he wanted to marry me and have a baby. He was constantly talking about what our baby would look like and what we would name it. When I told him I was pregnant, he was happy. We announced our engagement to everybody, sent out the invitations, and the wedding date was set. We even bought baby clothes. A week before the wedding, he called me to say he couldn't go through with any of it. I couldn't believe what I was hearing. He had thought it over, he said, and decided he wanted no part of it. I asked him, 'What am I supposed to do? I don't have any money to pay the hospital bill or support this child, and neither do my parents!' All he said was 'Give it away' and hung up. I haven't been able to reach him since."

A client in these circumstances needs to ask herself honestly if her decision to end the pregnancy is an act of anger aimed at her boyfriend. What exactly are her reasons for ending the pregnancy? Is the abortion going to benefit her life or simply serve as a retaliation against her ex-boyfriend? How does she expect to feel after the abortion, and how will she cope? How probable is it that they'll get back together? How will she feel about having had an abortion then? Does she expect to regret her decision? How strong is her support system, and how receptive is she to using her support system?

Diagnosis Of Severe Fetal Abnormality

When a woman has been happily expecting a baby and then is told the baby has a severe abnormality, she may feel as though her world has come to an end. The blow is enormous. Some women continue the pregnancy and prepare themselves for the consequences. Others choose not to put themselves, their families, or the child through the suffering. With either choice there is grief and loss.

Does she have enough information from her doctor upon which to make the decision? Which option does she feel she can cope with and live with better? Who will be there to support her emotionally?

An excellent booklet for assisting couples with the decision to end or continue an abnormal pregnancy is <u>A Time To Decide, A Time To Heal</u> (Minnick, Delp, & Ciotti, 1991). For extensive information on counseling couples who have chosen to end a pregnancy due to fetal indications, see the section, "Clients Who Choose Abortion Due To Fetal Indications," in Chapter 18.

Chapter Eight

The Adoption Alternative

Whenever a client is struggling with issues surrounding abortion but states vehemently she CANNOT have the baby, make sure you go over the adoption alternative. Having counseled thousands of women with an unplanned pregnancy, I have seen **few** who have opted for adoption, but that doesn't mean **every** client won't. Even those women who declare, "I don't believe in abortion" frequently don't believe in adoption either.

REASONS CLIENTS MAY REJECT ADOPTION

When a client is asked about adoption, the reasons for rejecting it are almost always the same: "If I went all the way through the nine months of pregnancy and the pain of labor and delivery, I would be too attached to the baby and wouldn't be able to part with it once it was born. Besides, I'd always wonder if it was **really** being cared for even if I knew where it was, and if the child ever wondered why its mother gave it away. No, I could never do that to a child, and I couldn't go through the ordeal myself!"

Single parenthood is more socially accepted in many communities now than in years gone by; consequently women seem to feel more comfortable keeping their baby than placing it for adoption. Therefore, the vast majority of women with

unplanned pregnancies are weighing the pros and cons of having the baby and keeping it versus terminating the pregnancy. It is still unwise to assume nobody wants to place for adoption. So, bring it up if the woman herself does not mention it. And if she simply states, "I could never do that," ask "What made you decide you could never place for adoption?" You will be helping her to explore the specific reasons for rejecting the adoption alternative. Listen for any misconceptions. For example, if the woman states, "I couldn't stand not knowing where my child was or if it was being taken care of," you need to inform her that in many areas the woman CAN know where her child has been placed and kept informed of the child's general well-being. However, it is true that she will not have **control** over how the child is parented or cared for.

It is not uncommon for a woman who insists she could never place her baby for adoption to lament, "I feel so selfish. Here I am having an abortion when all those couples want to adopt!" She needs to let go of a source of unnecessary guilt. To let go, it is important that she separate HER problem – unplanned pregnancy – from the problem of infertile couples – no pregnancies. The two problems have nothing to do with each other. The fertile women of the world have no obligation to furnish the infertile people of the world with babies. And if the infertile people believe otherwise, then isn't it selfish of them to expect such a sacrifice on their behalf! The question is, does she PREFER to place her baby over all other options?

PROS AND CONS OF PLACING FOR ADOPTION

Has she considered the pros and cons? Here are some of the positive aspects of this option:

1. The baby would probably be placed in a good home with loving parents. The social service agencies screen prospective parents thoroughly, and those people wait on lists that are years long.

2. Many agencies give the birth mother a voice in the placement of her child. She may be able to choose the couple's religion, educational background, age, etc.

3. In some states she has the option to keep the child's file "open" or "closed." If she wants the child to have access to her in the future, she can leave the file open. If she would prefer never having contact with that child, she can request the file be closed. You need to know what your state's adoption policies are. However, it is true that having a closed file does not guarantee that child will never be able to locate the birth mother. In addition, the trend at this time and for the future seems to be open files.

4. Many hospitals give her the choice of whether she'd like to see or hold the baby. Policies vary among hospitals. Many adoption agencies encourage the birth mother to have contact with the baby, partly to help her grieve the loss afterwards.

5. If she places the child for adoption and goes through the Department of Children and Family Services, medical expenses would be covered. She would not have to pay the cost herself.

6. Many (but not all) adoption agencies now offer on-going emotional support before, during and after the birth. There are ways of coping with any feelings of loss, sadness, and guilt after the adoption process. Some women have placed their babies and though they may think of it from time to time, they still feel satisfied with their decision.

7. Some women feel a deep sense of satisfaction that they gave such a precious gift to someone and made them so happy.

8. Some women feel good about themselves living up to their values and standards about giving life and avoiding abortion.

9. If she equates abortion with murder and hasn't the financial means to keep the child, adoption allows her to avoid both the moral dilemma of abortion and the financial dilemma of raising a child.

Some of the negative aspects of adoption include the following:

1. Some women are unable to detach themselves from the baby once it is born. The less emotional support she has from the outside, and the less inner resolve she has, the more likely it is that she will change her mind after the birth. How much support and resolve does she have?

2. Some women fear that the father of the child would claim it and not allow her to place it for adoption. He DOES have parental rights. Would her partner take the baby? Would she want him to?

3. Some women fear the adopted child would find her some day in the future and create a crisis at some later date. Despite "closed files" there ARE other ways a child could possibly locate her. There are no guarantees.

4. Some women fear they would feel guilty about giving their own child away. They fear they would be plagued by thoughts of where the child was, how the child was doing, did the child wonder why its mother gave him/her away, how old would the child be now, and does the child blame her? And whenever they'd hear of a child abuse case of an adopted child, they'd worry that it was their child.

5. Some women fear they would want the child back after it was too late.

6. In order to place a child for adoption, the woman must go through the nine months of pregnancy and childbirth. Many women do not want to continue months of nausea or fatigue or other potentially debilitating symptoms of pregnancy. Some would lose their jobs if they continued the absenteeism caused by the sickness.

7. Some would lose their jobs once they left to deliver the baby and recuperate. Some would have to drop out of school. Some women want to avoid all their co-workers, classmates, friends, or family members knowing about the pregnancy. Women cannot conceal a pregnancy forever. Eventually people would find out and then she would need to contend with their reactions.

8. Some women want to avoid their parents' reactions, especially when they strongly suspect rejection, censure, disappointment, or sorrow.

9. If the woman already has children, she often considers how they would react seeing their mother give their brother or sister away. And if the woman is single or divorced and has teenage children, she often considers what kind of example she is setting, having a baby out of wedlock and then "giving it away."

10. Some women who reject adoption are themselves adopted. They often say, "I have wonderful parents, but I know how it feels to be adopted, and I would never do that to anyone else."

11. Some women have already placed one child for adoption and swear they could never go through it again. Some express deep regret.

12. Although adoptive parents are screened for their desire and ability to provide a good, loving home for the child, there are no guarantees how the child would be parented, and the woman has no control over the situation. Legally, she would have no rights over the child and its care.

However, for the few who are considering adoption, all pregnancy options counselors should have basic knowledge of the current adoption practices in their area and adoption agency referrals.

CHANGING PRACTICES AND LAWS IN THE ADOPTION FIELD

The Hope Clinic counselors have an annual inservice on the changing adoption scene from the coordinator of a local Department of Children and Family Services or a Childrens Home and Aid Society. The following are some of the questions we ask to keep up-to-date:

1. What information is given to the adoptive parents about the biological parents? Do they know why she placed the baby for adoption?

2. Does the adopted child have legal access to her/his file?

3. What does your agency do for the adolescent who intends to place for adoption? Do you help make arrangements for continuing her education during the pregnancy? Do you offer family counseling if her parents are upset with her carrying to term? Can you arrange for a place to stay if her parents make her leave home?

4. Are all the woman's medical expenses paid if she places for adoption? What if she changes her mind and keeps the baby?

5. How long is the waiting list for adoptive parents-to-be?

6. What are the biological father's rights to the baby? What if he has been abusive to the woman?

7. What kind of ongoing counseling does the woman receive if she chooses to place her baby for adoption? How does this service vary from agency to agency?

8. How many women change their minds once the baby is born?

9. What is the legal process (briefly) for relinquishing parental rights?

10. What happens to the baby once it leaves the hospital? Who takes it before the adoption papers are signed?

11. How are prospective adoptive parents screened?

12. Does the biological mother receive information on the adoptive parents of her baby? What kind of information is available to her?

13. Does she have access to information on how the child is doing as time goes by?

14. What are some of the reasons a parent might place an older child for adoption?

15. What procedure does the woman go through

if she decides to place her baby for adoption - from her first visit with the agency to postpartum?

16. How many infants were placed for adoption last year?

17. How many older children were placed?

18. What constitutes "hard-to-place" children? What are the chances of adoption for babies with AIDS or who were born to drug-addicted mothers? Has there been any follow-up on these families as the child gets older?

The answers to these and other questions change from year to year and from area to area.

Chapter Nine

The Abortion Alternative

Once she has decided to end the pregnancy, the woman will make an appointment for the abortion. At this point, she continues to act upon this decision in very concrete ways. She will need to:

1. Get the money for the abortion fee.

2. Plan her transportation and possibly someone to accompany her to the clinic.

3. Figure out how to get there and how long the trip will take.

4. Arrange for a babysitter to watch her children, if necessary.

5. Fabricate alibis for the people she does not want to know where she is going.

6. Set her alarm clock the night before the abortion.

7. Remember to follow the clinic's instructions for the morning of the abortion (don't eat breakfast, do take a shower or bath, bring pregnancy test results or first morning urine sample, be on time, etc.)

8. Make the trip to the abortion clinic.

9. Walk through the door, possibly in the midst of protesters.

10. Fill out preliminary forms in her chart.

11. Walk into the counseling office and sit down.

Each of these actions, together with the initial decision-making process, requires thought and energy and serves to reinforce the major decision to have the abortion. Most women do seem sure of their decision on the day of their procedure, despite nervousness and fears. However, a counselor cannot assume this is the case, since some people do choose to change their mind.

PROFILE OF WOMEN CHOOSING ABORTION

According to the statistics gathered from the Alan Guttmacher Institute, most of the American women obtaining abortions are under 25 years of age, although ages range from nine into the 50s. Most are unmarried, but nearly one in five are married. Most are employed and one in three are earning less than $11,000 per year. Most (70%) are Caucasion; however, compared to the number of Caucasians in the American population who have abortions, Hispanic and African American women have disproportionately higher rates of unintended pregnancy and abortion. The vast majority (90%) of abortions are done in the first three months of pregnancy (less than 12 weeks), and less than 1% of abortions are performed after 20 weeks. Women who obtain abortions represent every religious faith. One out of six abortion patients state they are born-again or evangelical Christians. Almost one out of three are Catholic, and Catholic women have a higher rate of abortions in the United States than Protestant women. (Alan Guttmacher Institute, 1990, Cook, 1990, Henshaw, Forrest, & Van Vort, 1987, and Henshaw & Silverman, 1988).

Some people think there is a "type of woman" who chooses an abortion. In my experience of counseling thousands of women, I have found there is ONE and only ONE "type" of woman: pregnant. People having abortions include every imaginable occupation, economic bracket, race, and religion. Here are some of the women I've counseled:

1. Religious people who are active in their church: Catholics, Lutherans, Mormons, Pentecostals, Jews, Baptists, Christian Scientists, Jehovah's Witnesses, Muslims, Hindus, and any other denomination you can name.

2. "Pro-life" political activists, counselors from pro-life pregnancy testing centers, daughters and nieces of officials in "pro-life" organizations, and pro-lifers who marched on Washington, D.C.

3. Female ministers, male ministers' wives and daughters, Sunday school teachers, congresswomen, women in the Armed Forces, day care workers, dancers, teachers, therapists, lawyers, doctors and nurses, housewives with six children, models, and athletes chosen for the Olympics.

4. Grandmothers who got pregnant during the change of life.

Knowing about the men who impregnate these women and who support their decision to have an abortion is equally enlightening. Review the above list and instead of thinking "female," think "male." You can add priests, evangelist preachers, professional hockey and ball players, librarians, dentists, builders, physicists, plumbers, engineers, congressmen, TV and radio personalities, seminary students, mayors, and pediatricians to the list. What "type" of male supports a woman's

decision to have an abortion? Human. Period.

Some men agree with their partner's decision but provide no support of any kind. Some give the woman the money for the abortion, others provide transportation, and many provide emotional support and their presence at the clinic on the day of the abortion.

HOW MANY WOMEN CHOOSE ABORTION – AND WHY?

In the United States in the 1980s there were approximately 1.6 million women who chose to end their pregnancies each year (Tietze & Henshaw, 1986). Whenever the number of abortions being performed is cited, someone invariably proclaims, "There are too many abortions in this country!" Whenever I hear this pronouncement, I can't help but wonder, "What do they think is the RIGHT number?" And once an abortion provider reached its quota of abortions, who are all the people that will have to be sent away? Abortion isn't about numbers, it's about people. The question, "Why are there so many abortions?" can partially be answered by the simple fact of the laws of probability. No contraceptive is 100% effective. There are millions of men and women in their reproductive years whose imperfect contraceptives fail them, or who fail to use their contraceptive consistently and perfectly. Thus, numerous unintended pregnancies occur every year.

REASONS WHY PEOPLE CHOOSE ABORTION AS THE BEST ALTERNATIVE

Research shows most women base their decision to have an abortion on a number of reasons. Two of the most frequently cited reasons are lack of financial resources and emotional unreadiness for the responsibilities of parenthood (Torres & Forrest, 1988). Janet, a 19-year-old waitress, described her financial and emotional unreadiness for parenthood in this way: "I work part time and go to school full time with the help of financial aid. My boyfriend has a full scholarship and works part-time too. My mother lives on a modest income and couldn't help out even if she wanted to. I don't know where my father is. When I was growing up, we never had enough of anything. My mother did the best she could, but I refuse to put any child of mine through all that suffering.

I'm struggling to get an education so I can get a decent paying job some day. I work hard for my grades. I have a chance to make a better life for my children some day. If I had this baby, I'd be dragging us both down, and I don't know if there'd be a way back up. My mother and I had a lot of love between us, but you need more than love to provide for a child."

When women have one or more children they are raising by themselves, they state their first responsibility is providing for the children they already have. Bonnie, a 22-year-old mother of a two-year-old son, stated, "It's all I can do to pay my bills now. My son's father is unemployed and he's not always around. I can't count on him even when he has a job. I'm working two jobs to make ends meet. If my mother wasn't available to watch my son while I'm at work, I wouldn't have enough money to pay for day care. I'd have to take on a third job, and I don't think I'd ever see my son. Everything would fall apart if I had this baby. Already with this pregnancy I'm tired all the time and feeling sick. I can't afford to lose my energy. I've got to keep going. If I had this baby, I'd have twice what I have now. I'd probably wind up having to go on welfare, and my son would suffer and so would this one."

Many adolescents who choose abortion describe their emotional unpreparedness for parenthood in this way: "I'm still a kid. How can a kid take care of a kid? And I wouldn't want my Mom having to take care of my kid. Once I'm old enough and ready to have a child, I want to be the one who takes care of it. I want to be the mother, not some kind of sister."

Usually women under the age of 24 are still in school and feel their education is extremely important. Learning a job skill or earning a degree means the difference between a low paying job or any job at all and making an adequate living. Many women state they do not believe it's realistic to rely on a man to support them. They want to have what it takes to get a job that pays a living wage. Nancy stated, "I saw what happened to my sister once she dropped out of school and had her baby. She got married, but five months after the baby was born, she and her husband fought so much, he left. She went on welfare for awhile, then moved back home with our parents. She's 24 and they support her. She found a part time job, but she can't find a good job because she doesn't

even have a high school education, much less any advanced education or job skills. She's depressed most of the time and my parents really wish she would get out on her own. It's a mess, and I feel sorry for my nephew."

Women over 35 choose abortion largely because their children are almost grown. Neither the woman nor her partner feels able to "start all over again" and raise another child. When women are in their 40s, they and their partners also fear fetal abnormalities, such as Down's Syndrome. Sometimes she has received a diagnosis of severe fetal abnormalities, or she may have a health problem that will get worse if she carries to term.

Women may choose an abortion because the pregnancy is a result of rape or incest, and they fear carrying to term would intensify their trauma.

Many abused women who fear violent repercussions from their partner and who are trying to sever ties with him may choose abortion.

Those women whose pregnancy symptoms are so severe (eg. hyperemesis) they can no longer function normally may choose to end the pregnancy.

Women who are being treated for cancer or other life-threatening illness may seek an abortion when their doctor tells them their treatment must stop until after she has the baby to avoid fetal damage.

Women who need their medication to manage mental illness may also choose abortion when they learn they would have to quit their medication if they carried to term (to avoid fetal damage). They may also feel unable mentally to assume the responsibility of parenting a child.

There are as many reasons for choosing an abortion as there are individuals, and those I have listed above are some of the more common reasons. In general, women choose abortion because: 1). They feel their physical, emotional, financial, and/or mental well-being and that of their family will be threatened by going through nine months of pregnancy and having a/another child; and 2). They feel they are unable to provide adequately for the child. They choose abortion rather than adoption because 1). Carrying a pregnancy for nine months can present physical, emotional, and financial hardships for themselves and their families; 2). They consider parting with the child at the end of nine months too traumatic; and 3). They feel they can cope better after an abortion than after placing their child for adoption.

HOW WOMEN FEEL ON THE DAY OF THE ABORTION

The most common feelings women experience are anxiety and fear. The sources of the fear are many and varied. They may be afraid of the unknown or that someone they know will see them. Before they even arrive they may be afraid of protesters, or that the clinic will be dirty and the workers unprofessional. They also may fear needles, doctors, pelvic exams, pain, complications, and fear they'll feel sick or sore when they leave for home.

Other than fear, women may experience any or all of the following: tension, tiredness, sadness, shame, guilt, ambivalence, anger, or relief that the day has finally arrived. They may also feel foolish for being in the predicament in the first place. This is especially true for older women or women in the medical profession.

The women may also be preoccupied with any number of emotionally-charged issues, such as sexuality and contraception, parenthood, religion, the relationship with parents or partner. Finally, many women feel physically sick due to the pregnancy and stress. They experience nausea, weakness, dizziness, cramps, or fatigue. Since the woman will be going through a potentially uncomfortable medical procedure "awake," and since her emotional state has a direct effect on her physical experience, it is important to address her fears. For those few clinics who routinely offer general anesthesia, people can have plenty of fears about "being knocked out" despite their desire to BE "knocked out.".

With this as background, it becomes apparent why addressing each person's state of well-being in a pre-abortion counseling session is important.

Chapter Ten

Abortion Counseling

GOALS AND OBJECTIVES OF ABORTION COUNSELING

Since abortion is as much an emotional experience as it is a physical one, the goals of a pre-abortion counseling session should include the following:

1. Making sure the woman has considered all her alternatives and that she understands whatever decision she makes is HER choice.

2. Empathizing with her.

3. Assessing for signs of potential poor coping post-abortion (see Chapter 13, How Women Cope After Their Abortion).

To realize these first three goals, you need to:

- Help her clarify her beliefs about abortion.
- Explore and validate her feelings about her decision in light of her beliefs.
- Explore how she is expecting to feel afterwards and how she expects she will cope with her feelings.
- Reinforce her strengths and expectations for coping well.
- Teach constructive ways of coping, if appropriate.

- Assess her receptivity to using constructive strategies and resources for her well-being afterwards.
- Address any rejection of responsibility for the decision.
- Examine her support system and how she is affected by the people she has told.
- Assess her need for post-abortion counseling and give referrals if appropriate.

4. Calming the woman's fears and helping her relax. You can accomplish this by behaving in a professional, knowledgeable, and soothing manner, and by pinpointing her fears. Depending upon the nature of the fear, you can give appropriate information, help her problem-solve, or teach relaxation techniques. You can also let her know any questions she has are welcomed and will be answered.

5. Informing her of the abortion procedure and possible complications for her own information and so that she can sign an informed consent.

6. Helping her regain a sense of control over her fertility. You can achieve this by exploring the client's contraceptive history, finding out what problems she has had, giving her credit for the contraceptive efforts she has made in the past, and helping her decide on a future method of birth control suitable to both her and her partner.

This process will help give her a feeling of closure and preparedness for the future.

THE BARE MINIMUM APPROACH TO PRE-ABORTION COUNSELING

Some abortion providers believe only the basics are necessary in the pre-abortion counseling session:

1. Giving information about the procedure and possible complications.

2. Asking if the abortion is what the woman herself wants to do.

This certainly is better than no information and no questions asked, but there's a lot missing for both the woman and the legal protection of the clinic.

PHILOSOPHY AND METHOD

There are several different philosophies surrounding the number and kind of pre-abortion counseling sessions that are necessary for the client's welfare. In fact, these philosophies can be viewed on a continuum. One philosophy views counseling of any kind unnecessary and asserts informed consent is enough. On the other side of the spectrum is the double-counseling approach, where the woman receives two counseling sessions, once on a day prior to the procedure and again on the day of the procedure. Other approaches fall somewhere in between. Most abortion clinics seem to follow one of these four philosophies.

The One-Step Counseling Session

On the day of her abortion procedure, the woman receives an individual counseling session in which a trained, qualified counselor talks with her about her decision, feelings, and support system, and ensures she is informed about the procedure and possible complications before signing consent forms. The reasoning behind this approach includes:

1. The woman is given a private, one-to-one session to encourage her to reveal how she is feeling. An individual session allows the counselor to tailor the counseling session to fit her needs. One woman may be feeling confident, relaxed,

supported by one or more significant others, and ready to get on with the abortion. Her session may take no more than 15 minutes. Another woman may sit down, burst into tears and unravel a myriad of troubling issues. The counselor may spend an hour with her. The average time for counseling sessions of this nature is one-half hour.

2. Most, but not all, women have their minds made up by the time they arrive for their appointment at the abortion clinic. It is up to the counselor to ask that it IS her decision, both for her sake and for the legal protection of the clinic.

3. Many women have to travel long distances to get to the closest abortion clinic. Providing both the counseling and the procedure all on one day saves her additional problems, since transportation and time spent away from school, work, or home can be problematic for many people.

The Two-Step Counseling Approach

This belief maintains that women need two counseling sessions: options counseling and pre-abortion counseling. The former is done on a day preceding the abortion procedure and the latter is done on the day of the abortion. The first session is usually in-depth, exploring her decision, options, feelings, and support system. The second session focuses more on her understanding of the procedure, possible complications, aftercare, and a briefer discussion of her decision and feelings before signing consent forms. Reasons for this two-step process are:

1. To allow the client to discuss issues surrounding the pregnancy and then have time to go home and process what was discussed.

2. To have a more efficient patient flow on the day of the procedure when the doctors and nurses are there, since the second counseling session takes less time than the longer, first session.

Using Either One-Step Or Two-Step Approach, Depending On The Client

Some clinics employ the one-step approach for most clients, but will suggest going home and rescheduling the abortion if the woman expresses extreme ambivalence in the counseling session. Hope Clinic usually uses the one-step approach, but if a woman seems upset while making her appointment, she will be given the choice of talking to a counselor on the phone or coming in for an options counseling session. Hope Clinic counselors also will use the two-step approach in cases of extreme ambivalence or extraordinary distress on the day of the procedure.

Those clinics that usually use the two-step approach may accommodate a woman's special transportation or time needs by scheduling both her counseling and procedure all on one day.

The Informed Consent But No Counseling Approach

Some clinics hold the view that most women don't need or want any pre-abortion counseling. They provide just a description of the procedure and possible complications, and an acknowledgement that it is HER decision, so she can sign an informed consent. These information sessions often take place in a small group setting, and may require the clients to watch a standard film that thoroughly informs them of the procedure and possible complications. Reasons for this approach include:

1. They maintain a mandatory counseling session is an invasion of her privacy.

2. There is no need to hire qualified counselors, so it decreases clinic costs.

3. Informed consent takes far less staff time than counseling, so again it decreases clinic costs.

4. It decreases patients' waiting time in the waiting room.

5. They maintain that since most women have their minds made up, they don't need counseling prior to the abortion.

Some clinics using this approach will employ one counselor for times when a client appears extremely upset or requests counseling.

Using this approach takes the risk of not meeting the woman's individual needs, therefore there is potential for more anxiety and pain during the procedure (unless she is under general anesthesia) and in recovery. In addition, there is no assessment of her emotional well-being and ability to cope post-abortion. Omitting this may be a disservice to her and put the clinic in jeopardy. There is too much documented research on factors that enhance or hurt women's coping ability post-abortion to ignore. (See Chapter 13, How Women Cope After Their Abortion).

Since the 1980s, the intensity and sophistication of anti-abortion combat against abortion providers has steadily increased. "Pro-life" lawyers are volunteering their services to disgruntled women and their parents or male partners who "regret" the abortion. No longer are the lawsuits restricted to medical claims. Clinics have been sued by people claiming personal damages due to **lack of counseling** or inadequate counseling and subsequent emotional distress, so the no-counseling approach can leave a clinic unprotected legally.

Granted, even with the best of counseling, some people will still blame the abortion clinic for everything that goes wrong in their life from that day forward. But documentation that counseling took place is the ounce of prevention that could be worth a pound of cure.

GROUP OR INDIVIDUAL COUNSELING?

There has been a lot of debate among abortion counselors over the appropriateness of group pre-abortion counseling.

Group Counseling

Those who support group counseling cite the following reasons in its behalf:

1. Women may not feel so alone. They may develop a camaraderie with each other in a group, especially if they have repeated contact with each other, as in a three-to-four-day second trimester procedure. Therefore, they may feel supported by each other.

2. The clinic does not need to hire as many counselors, so costs are lowered.

3. Less staff time may be required since several people are seen at one time, so again costs are lowered.

Individual Counseling

On the other hand, proponents of individual counseling give the following reasons:

1. Pre-abortion counseling is by nature very short-term, usually one session. If it is only one session, there is neither enough time nor the repeated contact that is necessary to build the kind of trust and bonding that makes a group effective.

2. Many people do not feel comfortable revealing personal feelings in a group of strangers. Therefore, women may feel more anxious and fearful when seen together in a group rather than more comfortable and supported.

3. Since people are likely to feel more inhibited in a group of strangers, individual needs may not be met.

4. A woman may be more likely to feel she has been treated as an individual when seen individually, whereas if she was afraid she would be "herded through an abortion mill," group counseling may appear just that to her.

Group Information Session And Individual Counseling

Some clinics use the group approach only for informational purposes. For example, the procedure, possible complications, aftercare instructions, and sequence of events are explained in a small group setting. Then, after receiving information to help allay fears of the unknown, she receives an individual counseling session that covers exploration of the decision, her feelings, support system, birth control, and any special concerns she has.

Some clinics invite the significant others to join the women in their informational group. Others do not, thinking that those women without a supportive partner or parent would feel the lack more acutely by comparison.

Significant Others Groups

There are some clinics that hold additional information groups for the significant others accompanying the woman. This information group involves the woman's male partner, family mem-bers, or friends, and helps to calm their fears, dispel their misconceptions, and/or increase their awareness of the political issues of abortion.

We at Hope Clinic have tried all the above approaches and prefer holding group information sessions for the women followed by an individual counseling session. If we had the additional space to hold significant other groups, we would do so. Using the combination of group information and individual counseling helps prevent counselor burn-out (less repetition in giving instructions), promotes smooth patient flow, and yet retains the individual treatment for each patient.

TOPICS COVERED IN THE PRE-ABORTION COUNSELING SESSION

In the session preceding the abortion, the following topics should be included:

1. Description of the procedure, possible complications, and aftercare instructions (either in a group or individual session).

2. Her options.

3. Her decision: Why she has chosen abortion, and whether she feels certain about the decision.

4. Her support system: Whom she has told about the pregnancy and abortion and their reactions.

5. Her feelings about abortion and expectations for coping post-abortion.

6. Her choice of birth control method for the future, and discussion of any past problems with methods.

7. Her signature on the consent forms.

Chapter Eleven

Clients' Emotional Reactions In The Abortion Counseling Session

You will undoubtedly see many different reactions. Here are some of the most common:

1. Nervous

2. Calm - real or feigned

3. Tearful

4. Withdrawn

5. Angry

6. Talkative

7. Upset due to harassment from anti-abortion protesters

Nervous

Imagine yourself going to the doctor for a Pap smear or to the dentist for a checkup. Nervous? Now, imagine yourself going to a doctor you've never met, in a place you've never been, for an abortion which you know little or nothing about. It is no wonder the majority of our clients are nervous. Some have butterflies in their stomachs; others are terrified to the point of tears.

Let the client know nervousness is NORMAL before an abortion, and help her clarify what she

fears. Different people fear different things. Usually an explanation of the clinic process, abortion procedure, and complications relieves much of the anxiety.

Most people are fearful of pain - some more than others - and most people want to know, "Is it going to hurt?" Everyone can benefit from a discussion of relaxation tips unless they appear to be and state they are calm and relaxed (see chapter on Managing Pain and Fear of Pain). If she relates a past painful or unpleasant abortion experience, then you and she can strategize how this experience can be different. For instance, a 20-year-old client related an extremely painful and emotionally distressing abortion experience she had at age 16. What stood out in her mind was her parents' unwillingness to help her raise the child and her fear of the abortion. She remembered crying and getting sick in the recovery room. I asked her to tell me everything that was different this time.

"This time it's all my decision," she asserted. "My parents don't even know about it, and I'm here with my boyfriend." Her boyfriend was very supportive. "When I was 16 the guy dumped me, so I felt all alone." She continued, "I'm older now and I've had pelvic exams and one abortion, so I know what's going on. Back then I never had anything like that done." In addition, she said she had gone to a clinic where there was little or no counseling beforehand - just a brief explanation of the procedure. And, finally, she was glad to hear Hope offered a variety of pain management strategies, such as pain relievers and muscle relaxers. "All I had back then was a local anesthetic," she said woefully. We both agreed there were considerable differences between this experience and the one at age l6, and she appeared far more confident in her ability to handle the situation.

Calm

Sometimes the woman is genuinely calm and collected, which is much to her advantage. Perhaps a friend had an abortion and already calmed her fears, or maybe she had an abortion before with no problems and little pain. This genuinely calm demeanor is not that uncommon, especially for patients who have had an unproblematic previous abortion, or who are in their thirties and older. On the other hand, a calm exterior may be a defense or "front" for inner turmoil. It may be her way of numbing painful emotions and appearing composed in front of all the people in the waiting room. Some women are relieved to let it all out during the counseling session behind closed doors. Others will maintain the facade no matter what. It is often better to leave their defenses intact rather than break through them. This control may be their usual way of coping under severe stress, and it may help them get through a frightening experience. We all have our own ways of coping with stress.

Sometimes you can detect a discrepancy between her non-verbal and verbal messages. You might gently confront her by describing what you see: "You are telling me everything is OK and yet your leg is shaking. You look very nervous." If her response is defensive, don't push. You may uncover the source of her tension when discussing the male partner, parents, or attitude toward abortion. For example, one client seemed relaxed until I brought up the subject of her partner: "It doesn't make any difference what he thinks - it's my life!" she snapped. I concurred, "Regardless of what anyone else thinks, it's your life and your decision." Then she went on, "He told me I was murdering my baby if I had an abortion, and then I find out he's left for Alabama!" "How maddening! Adding insult to injury!" I remarked. She looked me squarely in the eyes and said, "He's a jerk and not worth talking about!" I added, "Yes.

We don't need to waste our breath on him!" She laughed and said, "And then there's my mother!" "What about your mother?" I inquired. "When I told my mother, she told me I was going to hell for killing my baby, and that I wasn't welcome in her house. My sister is the only one who thinks I'm doing the right thing, but she lives 200 miles away and the phone calls are expensive," she replied. We spent some time talking about her own beliefs about the morality of abortion, who else she could talk to, and how she would handle her mother's reactions to her abortion.

Sometimes the woman will appear calm throughout pre-abortion counseling. It may not be until she is in the recovery room that she lets go. She may cry or become angry and demanding. Before you start berating yourself for your failing to perceive her true feelings, do realize that some people are experts at hiding emotions. She may have had a lifetime of practice. Nonetheless, without burdening yourself with feelings of guilt or self-doubt, you could discuss the case with another counselor. Explore what (if anything) you might have detected. There will always be a next time.

Tearful

There may be any number of reasons why the woman is crying. Don't assume. It could be fear of the procedure, release of tension, sadness, frustration, guilt, or anger, to name a few. Whatever the cause, she is allowing the release of strong feelings. So give her time, let her cry, and let her know crying is OK. Some counselors feel drawn to touch the client in a consoling way. However, some people do NOT liked to be touched, especially by someone they just met, and will tense up or draw back. There are other effective and less intrusive ways of comforting and supporting someone in distress. Just being with her quietly as she cries, attending to her, and listening empathetically are all ways of showing you care. Crying can be cathartic, and often there is renewed strength after the tears have been wiped away.

Withdrawn And Uncommunicative

Sometimes the non-verbal client is naturally shy; sometimes she is preoccupied with disturbing thoughts and emotions she does not wish to disclose to anyone, including you. It may take time to engage this client's trust, and in the framework of a one-time counseling session, you may never gain it. However, you might start by getting in alignment with her: the way she is sitting and the softness of her voice. Communicating with withdrawn clients takes time, so tell yourself from the beginning to take your time, even if you have been going at a fast clip on a busy morning. Shift from high gear into low gear. Sometimes slowly retracing the steps she has taken from the time she suspected the pregnancy to the pregnancy test and up to the present day can help her tell you her story. Sometimes you will detect a glimmer of interest and increased energy when she is talking about something that does not directly relate to the abortion. When this happens, go ahead and digress a little to sustain the energy and forge a better bond.

Frequently the uncommunicative client is between the ages of 11 and 14. In addition to the above interventions, you may also try the following technique suggested by a junior high school social worker. Give her a list of feelings that are illustrated by cartoon faces and ask her to circle the ones that best describe how she's feeling right now. While she's looking over the paper, occupy yourself with something else, so she doesn't feel watched. Ask her to let you know when she's finished. You may also give her the written sentence, "What I want to do about the pregnancy is …" and ask her to circle her answer (have the baby and parent it, place the baby for adoption, and have an abortion). Sometimes answering a questionnaire is less threatening than answering an authority figure.

If after all your best efforts she remains unresponsive, and you do not have a clear sense the abortion is her decision, let her know you'd like another counselor to see her. You might explain, "I don't want to stand in the way of your receiving good care today. I understand that different people feel comfortable with different counselors. You wait here while I find another counselor so you'll feel more comfortable." By leaving her alone for a few minutes, she may feel a release of tension. Sometimes the second counselor has more success with the client because of a dynamic I call "the savior effect." After the first counselor

Right now I feel _____ .

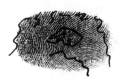

Guilty

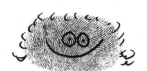

Satisfied with my decision

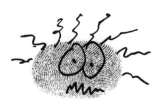

Scared

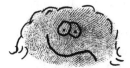

Mixed feelings
(some sadness, some guilt, and relieved
I won't be pregnant after today

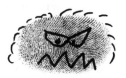

Angry

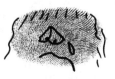

Sad

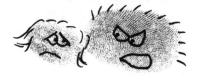

Pushed into the abortion
by someone else

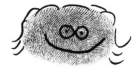

Sure that this is
my own decision

has left the office, the woman is probably thinking about what just occurred. When a fresh face walks into the room, she may feel relieved and choose to open up, glad to be saved from an imagined oppressor. Or she may have realized that if she really wants the abortion, she will need to communicate certain things to the next counselor. The second counselor may have no more expertise than the first one, but in the eyes of the client the second counselor may automatically take on the role of savior. The woman whose walls are impenetrable the first day she came can be requested to reschedule on another day. On the day of the rescheduled appointment, she usually seems a different person - relaxed and responsive. Sometimes she confides that she felt pushed by her parents or partner the first time, but this time it feels like her decision. Or she states she was petrified the first time but feels more comfortable the second time around.

Angry

Her anger is undoubtedly misdirected at you and/or the clinic. She may be angry with herself for being pregnant and needing your services, she may be mad at her boyfriend or parents, or she may handle fear like a wounded animal - with a display of ferocity. She may hurl complaints at you, such as waiting too long, too many forms to fill out, too hot, too cold, too crowded, and then appear disinterested and impatient in the session. If she snaps, "Look, I just want to get this the hell over with!" you can match the volume of her voice and snap, "I'm with you. I can't stand waiting around in a doctor's office! Let's try to get this over with as quickly as possible! I'll tell you briefly what I need and why, and then you give me a short reply, and we'll just zip this right along!" She may calm down because you aligned yourself with her, or she may rebel against being told to go fast. Either way, she is likely to slow you down. Her replies may become lengthier and her pace less brisk. If this happens, you can slow down accordingly.

Another approach to the angry client is to keep your voice steady, calm, and low. While the aim of pacing the client is to match her energy, volume, and tempo, this theory maintains that the angry client needs a calming influence and a steady anchor. Different clients respond to different approaches. Both theories, however, advocate setting firm limits on the client's angry behavior if it

becomes abusive. A client's behavior is abusive if she threatens, curses, ridicules, or insults you.

If the client becomes abusive, it's time to set limits. You might say something like, "Stop. If we are going to provide a service for you, we require the same respect from you that you will receive from us. You can expect not to be mistreated by any of our staff, and we expect the same from our patients." Usually after you set limits, she will settle down and explain why she feels angry. She may still seem defensive, and that's OK. You can work with a defensive manner but not one that is abusive.

Talkative

At first this client is a joy by being so expressive and communicative. Then you find the stream of talk gushes along interminably. The idea is to match her energy, give direction to her thoughts, and bring her back to relevant discussion when she digresses to Aunt Martha's arthritis. Constant chatter may reveal anxiety and a desire to put off the procedure by lingering with the counselor or to keep the focus off her real feelings. Other times people are just naturally talkative or relieved to find someone willing to listen.

Upset Due To Harassment From Anti-Abortion Protesters

Informing And Reassuring Clients

It is important to inform the patients when making their appointment that they may encounter protesters. Sometimes there's no more than a handful of them; other times there may be 50 or more. Letting clients know what to expect and what to do helps allay their fears. Some clients possess a fighting spirit and tell us, "Just let them come near me! I have a few choice things to say to them!" We caution all our clients to IGNORE the protesters because what the picketers want and thrive on is our attention.

During warm weather we instruct our patients to roll up their car windows as they approach the clinic parking lot to avoid literature being hurled into their open windows. I have seen protesters throwing not only their brochures into open windows as a car slowed to make the turn into our lot but also plastic fetuses as well. And while some of the protesters stand in front of the patients' cars to block their entrance, others rush up and plaster gory pictures on the windshields.

We reassure the patients that our security guard and trained volunteers will make sure they are safely escorted from their car into the clinic. The National Abortion and Reproductive Rights Action League (NARAL) trains escorts to help patients avoid being harassed by aggressive protesters, to de-escalate volatile situations, and to comfort frightened patients by talking and walking with them into the clinic. Our NARAL escorts' cool-headed teamwork is invaluable to both staff and patients.

What Are The Protesters Like?

When people ask me, "What are the protesters like?" I reply, "You've got to see it to believe it." Every abortion clinic has its own stories to tell about the protesters who harass their patients and parade around their building. On the Saturdays Hope Clinic has protesters, they often arrive in church buses from out-of-town and sometimes out-of-state. Some protesters are old; some are teenagers; but most are in-between. Some drag their children into the fray and in all kinds of inclement weather. We staff members have seen young children wearing no hats or gloves shivering by their mother's side in the middle of January holding little protest signs. We've shaken our heads at the sight of a mother juggling a picket sign in one hand and a bare-headed baby in the other, sweltering under a blazing July sun. We've heard them beg in loud, woeful voices, "Young lady! You in the striped T shirt - don't do it! The Bible says thou shalt not kill! Take that money and go and raise your child!" Some protesters keep up a continuous flow of preaching and quoting from the Bible. One of our sidewalk "preachers" works herself up into a frenzy. Whenever she sees a young woman and male companion getting out of their car and walking toward the clinic door, her voice reaches a shrill pitch, her face gets red as a beet, and she cries and wails as loudly as her vocal cords will vibrate: "Sir! You in the blue jacket! Be a man and marry her! Don't go into the place of darkness! Please! Please! Don't do it!" As soon as the door closes, she paces up and down, mumbling indistinctly, until the next couple comes into view. Then the whole scene repeats itself.

A few years ago a male protester carried a

fishing pole to extend his reach. Since he was not allowed on our parking lot, he'd stand on the sidewalk with his pole. At the end of the fishing line dangled a red paint-splattered baby doll he'd attempt to thrust in front of the faces of clinic patients walking on our parking lot.

One hot Saturday morning a large mob of protesters gathered across the street from the clinic in front of the Catholic hospital. They paraded up and down the sidewalk carrying aloft a baby coffin containing the remains of a human fetus. This display was accompanied by loud chanting and howling about the "sanctity of life" until the hospital had to silence their din for the sake of the hospital's own patients.

The protesters' intentions are to prevent or at least dissuade people from having an abortion and to harass providers. However, their lack of success is demonstrated by the percentage of people who keep their appointments despite the presence of the picketers. The percentage of patients who show up for their appointments is the same on Saturdays when protesters are present as on days when they are not there. Nationally the number of abortions performed each year does not fluctuate with the presence or absence of protests. The grim truth is that the picketers only succeed in scaring and angering people who are already nervous and anxious about undergoing a medical procedure. Imagine yourself making a difficult decision about whether to undergo chemotherapy or surgery for prostate or breast cancer, depending on your gender. Imagine your state of emotion as you head for the hospital that morning. Then imagine how you'd feel if a throng of religious fanatics swarmed around your car and shouted their beliefs at you, begging you not to carry out your decision, and brandishing color enlargements of advanced cancer tissue they claimed would be removed from your body. How would you feel? How would you feel if your daughter or son were the patient, and you were there for emotional support? Would the protesters change your mind about the treatment you painstakingly decided upon? Would you turn around and go home?

The Clients' Reactions To The Protesters

Some people are so frightened they take flight and turn back home. But they call back to make (and keep) another appointment. Years ago before we had guards and escorts, I saw a patient whose experience I'll never forget. She was a 40-year-old mother of four. Her medical history revealed she had diabetes, high blood pressure, and asthma. Her poor health and life of poverty left her looking years older than her age. She told me, "I tried getting in last Saturday, but my boyfriend dropped me off in front of the building. Some of those people with signs talked me into getting into a van and they took me to St. Mary's hospital (in another town). They showed me pictures of bloody arms and legs and told me they were babies all cut up from abortions. They told me I'd go to hell for having an abortion. I told them I wanted to go home and I had no way of getting there. They finally let me call my social worker. She was so mad with those people that she came and took me home herself! When I got home I called here and made another appointment. That was last week. This time my older brother came with me. When we got here and those people came at me, I stuck out my hand and hollered, 'Leave me alone, I'm comin' through!'" Upon our Director's suggestion, she chose to file a complaint with the Granite City Police Department. We hired a guard and built a new entrance to our building from our parking lot.

No matter what the protesters' intentions and tactics are, they cannot change the life situations that compel women to choose abortion over adoption or parenthood. Many clients express their anger about protesters who scream, "We'll help you! Don't kill your baby!" One of my clients stated, "The only way they can help me is to give me a substantial salary every year for the next 20 years while I raise this child into adulthood. A few maternity clothes and booties and diapers are NOTHING in comparison to what I'd need as the baby grows into a child, and the child grows into a teenager! And can they give me a man that will be a father to this child? I grew up in a one-parent home, and I do not intend on putting my own kid through that!" Another client put it this way: "All they're thinking about is a cute little baby. They're not thinking about me, and they're not thinking about the fact that cute little babies grow up. Children's needs get bigger and more expensive. Are those protesters going to be there for me 13 years from now when I'm still trying to raise this child? No! It will all fall on my shoulders!"

The people who come with the patient are sometimes as furious as she is about the picketers.

The escorts have averted fist fights between a patient's incensed boyfriend and an antagonistic male protester. Taunts hurled at the male partners are intended to shame and emasculate them. There have also been times when abusive partners have reluctantly brought their girlfriend or wife to the clinic, gone outside to chat with the protesters, and come back in using the protesters' rhetoric to upset her further.

Some of the patients who are already feeling guilty and ashamed feel tormented by the preaching and judgment of the protesters. These are the patients who break down in tears as they hurry into the clinic. Others - usually young teens - break into tears out of fear. One of the counselors who witnessed a flock of protesters swooping down on a young teen and her boyfriend, pecking at them relentlessly until she broke into tears and started running, stated it reminded her of Alfred Hitchcock's bone-chilling movie, *The Birds*.

Women vividly describe the sense of violation they feel: "These are absolute strangers to me, and here they are getting right up in my face, touching my arm, pushing pictures an inch in front of my face, trying to block my way, and shouting criticism at me!" No one enjoys having their personal space invaded. And any woman who is an incest or rape survivor, or who has ever been molested in her life, is especially affected by such intrusive behavior.

There are those patients and support people who view the protesters as minor irritants, and once they are safe inside the building focus on the present moment. These are the folks who use their sense of humor and pluck to get through life. They are enormously helpful to others in the waiting room and usually wind up putting the frightened teens at ease with their humor.

Total strangers often form a bond in the waiting room because they all went through the same ordeal and all have a common foe. It doesn't take long before our patients and their supporters refocus their attention on what's going on INSIDE the clinic.

Staff's Response To Clients' Reactions To The Protesters

Frightened, tearful patients and their support people are attended to immediately. I have walked into the clinic, and before my coat was off, took a patient and her Mom to my office, talking as we all unbuttoned our coats.

Most people who come through the protesters are angry. Some are irritated, some incensed, and others furious. When people are riled and their adrenaline is pumping, they are eager and ready to channel their angry energy into action. And that is exactly what we do. We let clients know what they can DO about it. Their bitter feeling of powerlessness is converted into political action. We let them know the same people who harassed them are also trying to revert federal and state laws to the days of illegal abortion by writing letters to their legislators. We ask if they'd like to voice their own opinions to the people who have the power to keep the antis from shutting down clinics. There is a flurry of letter-writing activity in that waiting room on Saturday as we pass out the stationery and pens. If there is a particular anti-abortion bill before the legislature, we let them know what it entails. What starts out as helpless outrage can become a potent force to keep abortion safe and legal.

Another helpful response to our patients and their supporters is letting them talk about what they saw and heard while walking into the clinic. Giving them the opportunity to vent in the group as well as in the individual session helps immensely. Once they've talked about what happened and how they felt and had their questions answered about their safety, they are ready to focus on the here and now.

Chapter Twelve

Exploring The Decision
On The Day Of The Abortion

IT'S HER CHOICE

As her counselor, you need to let her know you are there to support her in WHATEVER she has decided. Sometimes she has been given lectures by friends, family members, partner, doctor, or an anti-abortion activist posing as a counselor at a free pregnancy test center. She may fear you are going to try to talk her into or out of her decision. Once you have established your support for whatever decision she has made, you might ask, "Can you tell me a little about how you arrived at your decision?" If she feels unsure abortion is what she wants, or if she feels pushed into it, she'll usually tell you right away. Sometimes a woman may sigh, "Well, there is really no choice but to have an abortion," but what does she mean by this? Once she has explained her meaning, you may decide to point out there IS a choice, regardless of how grim the consequences may seem. If she insists, "This isn't what I want, but I don't see any other way," then an exploration of all the alternatives and their possible consequences may help her see the number of options from which she has to choose. She can also hear herself think out loud and hear her thoughts summarized and clarified. The more thorough she is in exploring the consequences of each choice, the more complete her decision-making process. Most people have already gone through this process before they see you, but some need it. The crux of the issue is choice - HER choice.

Sometimes this is the first weighty decision the woman has ever had to make by herself and for herself. Women in this culture are generally conditioned toward passivity and dependence on someone they perceive as stronger than they are - their male partner or parents. In some families the conditioning and reinforcement for dependence is strong, so she may be swimming in uncharted waters. By your very attitude you can convey to her she is capable of making this decision no matter how big or difficult it seems. Even though she may feel helpless, stupid, and vulnerable, you can point out her private pool of strength and the resources available to her for taking care of herself (e.g., affordable counseling, friends, prayer, pastoral counseling, support groups, books, and self-help materials). You can help to reframe a seemingly negative abortion experience into a personal victory: a growth experience. She can gain the knowledge that she is a person who can take control of her own life.

WHEN THE CLIENT FEELS COERCED INTO THE ABORTION

When you ask, "Can you tell me a little about your decision?" most women have no problem describing the set of circumstances that led to their decision and expressing confidence in their choice. On occasion the client declares, "I'm being forced into it!"

When a client makes this statement, let her know your doctors will not perform an abortion on someone who feels forced into it. It must be her own decision. Then go on to discuss what she prefers to do and if there is anyone who supports her plan of action. If it becomes clear she does not want an abortion, recommend she return home and follow her own plan. Then offer to talk to the person who has brought her to the clinic (usually the person accused of the coercing).

It is helpful to talk with the other person to allow them to vent their frustrations with you instead of blowing up at the client. They are usually angry because they're scared their lives will be negatively affected if she carries to term. When they can feel your empathy, their anger will probably diminish. Then you'll be able to explain your clinic policy to a more receptive audience. You might say something like, "In our years of experience, we have found that clients experience more physical and emotional complications if they feel pressured into the abortion. We do not believe in compromising our clients' mental and physical welfare. We have learned that clients who leave and choose to come back of their own accord fare much better during and after the abortion both physically and mentally. We care about the people who come to us, and we must use our best professional judgment for their welfare. I know you care for her, too, and are trying to do what's best." Sometimes reframing your clinic policy in a way that demonstrates your mutual caring for the woman helps build a bridge between you and them. You can also show you care about them by asking if they have anyone to talk to for support. When you adopt this approach, they are less likely to keep on insisting she have the abortion that day.

Sometimes they leave, but in an hour they're back asking to talk to you. The woman then tries to convince you she wants the abortion herself, all the while using the same words you heard her companion or parent spouting. The wisest course of action is staying firm with your initial decision. If they didn't receive a counseling referral the first time, now is a good time to offer one.

AMBIVALENCE AND THE BLAME GAME

The client who states she is being forced into the abortion sometimes makes the accusation because she feels guilty or ashamed and is using the other person as a shield. When you tell her no one can force her to have an abortion because the doctor will refuse to perform it, this client changes her tune. When you suggest she return home to reconsider her decision, she will protest and demand, "I want this done today!" It is the counselor's job to discover whether her insistence comes from her own genuine desire to have the abortion or her fear of repercussions from whomever she is blaming.

During the course of the session, you will need to assess whether she accepts the responsibility for the decision, denies future regret, seems to have manageable levels of guilt and adequate coping strategies, and a strong support system. You will also be assessing whether her words ring true or seem false and manipulative. The manipulator will often switch her story in midstream. You may become aware of double messages and your own mounting confusion.

One day a client stormed into my office, sat down on the edge of the chair and blurted out, "This is an abortuary and I don't want to be here!" She burst into tears and roundly blamed her boyfriend. When she heard she was free to leave at any time, she proceeded to tell me she "had to have it done!" She believed if only she had the abortion, then her partner would marry her. She talked at length, sobbing most of the time, decrying the immorality of abortion, and repeating she had no choice unless he stopped being so "cheap." She said he wanted to buy a house and have money in the bank before he became a parent. "Imagine putting material things before this child's life!" she said disdainfully. She had told no one else about the pregnancy but her boyfriend. It became clear she needed a support person and she and her boyfriend needed a lengthy couple counseling session. She said she refused to tell any of her friends or family because she felt ashamed.

When I recommended couple counseling before she went through with an abortion, and made it clear we were not going to perform an abortion on her that day, her stance turned 180 degrees. As I offered to bring him in and explain why I was sending her home, she said, "I think I'll go ahead and have it done. I'll be OK." I confronted her with the contradiction of this conclusion in light of everything she had just told me. She said, "Well, I didn't really mean all those things." I reiterated that having an abortion that day was not an option because I was concerned about her emotional and physical well-being. I told her she could either choose to stay or wait in the waiting room while I explained to her partner our clinic policy. She told me to go ahead and bring him in. After I had told them both about our policy regarding ambivalence, he looked frustrated and sighed. He looked at her and complained, "All the way here you kept agreeing with me this was best. Then you get here and give this lady the impression you don't want it done. Make up your mind!" She looked at me and said, "I'll have it done." She paused and then added, "As long as I won't die." He rolled his eyes and groaned audibly. We had gone over her fears already and she knew about the possible complications, so I announced she had the choice of coming back another day, but today I was relieving her of all pressure to decide. He rose to leave and she followed him out.

The next week she returned with a girlfriend and could articulate why she felt the abortion would be best for her own life. She said she did not want to struggle as a single parent and felt adoption would cause her more distress for a longer time than an abortion. She had told both her girlfriend and her mother, and they were supportive. She told me she had been upset that I sent her home, but was glad I had done it because today she felt much better about her decision. I asked if I could call her in a few weeks to see how she was doing and she said yes.

Three weeks later I called and she said, "Sometimes I feel good about the decision and sometimes I feel bad. It depends on how he's treating me. If he treats me good, then I feel good about the abortion. If he treats me bad, then I feel bad." She said she felt a little better when she talked to her girlfriend and mother. I asked if she had considered using the counseling referral I had given her. She replied, "No, but if I ever feel really bad, I will." She thanked me for calling and told me to thank everyone at the clinic.

AMBIVALENCE WITHOUT THE BLAME GAME

"I Just Don't Know What To Do!"

If the client appears distraught and undecided, go over all the options. If she waivers back and forth among options, then she needs more time and another counseling session on another day before she undergoes an abortion. If, however, she methodically rejects all other options and keeps returning to abortion as her best alternative, then explore her feelings and beliefs about abortion (See Chapter 6, Decision-Making and Ambivalence). Ask about any fears she has about the medical procedure and possible complications as well. Sometimes the client appears undecided when actually she is afraid. Here are some of the most common fears clients harbor about abortion.

THE APPEARANCE OF INDECISION AND UNDERLYING FEARS

Fear Of Doctors, Pain, and Medical Procedures

People who initially present themselves as undecided sometimes are blocked by fear of doctors, pain, and medical procedures. If that obstacle can be removed by relaxation and pain management strategies, the appearance of indecision sometimes vanishes altogether (See Chapter 17, Helping Clients Manage Pain And Fear Of Pain).

Fear Of Becoming Sterile

Other times people have been frightened by anti-abortion propaganda they've been subjected to in schools, churches, or at free "pro-life" pregnancy test centers. Two of the primary fears the propagandists play upon are 1). fear of sterility post-abortion and 2). fear of causing the fetus pain.

People need to know that sterility after an abortion is highly improbable if the abortion is done by a competent physician using sterile instruments, if the patient does not make sudden movements during the abortion, and if the patient follows the aftercare instructions faithfully. She needs to be told the ways in which sterility CAN occur and how the risks are increased or decreased by her following instructions (See Chapter 16, The Abortion Procedure – First Trimester).

Fear Of Causing Fetal Pain

Some women are scared the fetus will feel pain and cite anti-abortion literature, "counselors," and propaganda films as the main sources of their fear. Usually giving them the facts and the source of your facts is all that is needed to eliminate this fear.

Two legitimate references refuting the existence of fetal pain are Planned Parenthood of America's Rebuttal to the Silent Scream (1984) and Science and the Unborn (Grobstein, 1988). Planned Parenthood's panel of medical experts included a professor of neuroscience and the Director of Gynecological Cancer Research from Albert Einstein College of Medicine, the Acting Chair of the Department of Ob-Gyn from Columbia University, the Chief of Pediatric Neurology from Cornell University Medical Center, and the Director of Ob-Gyn Ultrasound, Columbia Presbyterian Medical Center. This panel of eminent physicians stated, "At this stage of the pregnancy (12 weeks) the brain and nervous system are still in a very early stage of development. The beginnings of the brain stem, which includes a rudimentary thalamus and spinal cord, is being formed. Most brain cells are not developed. Without a cerebral cortex (gray matter covering the surface of the mature brain), pain impulses cannot be received or perceived." Additionally, experts find that newborns at 26-27 weeks' gestation who survive have significantly less response to pain than do full-term newborns.

Clifford Grobstein, a professor emeritus of biological science at the University of California, San Diego, presents scientific facts about prenatal development in relation to ethical concerns. In Psychology Today (1989), he stated that saying a 12-week fetus feels pain and tries to avoid a stimulus it knows to be painful is "pure creative imagination." He went on to say the perception of pain is highly unlikely without both the cerebral cortex and neural connections to the cortex – neither of which are adequately developed until the third trimester.

Fear Of Death

Sometimes clients secretly fear dying on the table during the abortion as punishment for "killing a baby." The fear of death seems to be such a private terror that the client seldom brings it up directly. One 30-year-old client I saw appeared so ambivalent about her decision that she easily agreed to return home and reconsider her options. One week later she returned. The first words out of her mouth in the counseling session were "I was afraid I'd die. That's why I left." Not once had the issue of dying been brought up in all the time I had spent with her. Fear of death may be the underlying factor when clients express an extreme fear of the procedure, pain, or complications.

Occasionally a client will ask, "Has anyone ever died from this?" If a client has simply been frightened by anti-abortion propagandists claiming abortion is "dangerous" and "people die from it all the time," then a simple statement of fact is all that is needed. Yes, women have died from abortion, but The Center for Disease Control has recorded that natural childbirth has a 10-times-greater mortality risk than first trimester abortion and Caesarian childbirth has a 100 times greater mortality risk. However, if the client's fear stems from guilt, then exploring the source of guilt and ways of handling it will probably be more effective than citing statistics. Once my client had made up her mind God was going to forgive her, she no longer feared dying on the table.

Chapter Thirteen

How Women Cope After Their Abortion:

Implications for Pre-Abortion Counseling

POSITIVE REACTIONS

The vast majority of legitimate research on post-abortion emotions shows that abortion is NOT an event that causes severe repercussions for most women. The majority of women report feeling positive about their decision, relieved, and able to move forward with their lives (Adler, l979; Adler et al., 1990 and 1992; Berger, 1978; Dagg, 1991; David et al., 1978; Fingerer, 1973; Kalmar, 1977; Kummer, 1963; Major & Cozzarelli, 1992; Osofsky & Osofsky, 1973, Payne et al., 1978; Romans-Clarkson, 1989; Simon & Senturia, 1976; Smith, 1973; Zimmerman, 1977). These positive feelings may be mixed with some transient feelings of sadness, loss, or guilt. While some women feel nothing but relief and confidence in the decision, a few women predominantly feel depression and severe guilt.

NEGATIVE REACTIONS

The Myth Of The Post-Abortion Trauma Syndrome

What emerges in the research are identifiable factors that seem to predispose a woman to negative reactions after an abortion. The specific "negative reactions" that have been researched include depression, guilt, shame and regret. It has been alleged by anti-abortion proponents that a num-ber of women experience "post-abortion trauma syndrome." However, to date there has been no scientific evidence of such a syndrome (Adler et al., 1990; Adler et al., 1992; Blumenthal, 1991; Dagg, 1991; Romans-Clarkson, 1989; Stotland, 1992). The article, "The Myth of the Abortion Trauma Syndrome" published in JAMA refutes the existence of such a condition. The author, Nada Stotland, M.D. states:

> An extensive search of MEDLINE, Psychological Information Data Base, Sociological Abstracts, Health Information Data Base, and review articles and their bibliographies reveals that there is no specific abortion trauma syndrome described in survey populations or in individual cases in the psychiatric or psychological literature. A small number of papers and books based on anecdotal evidence and stressing negative effects have been presented and published under religious auspices and in the nonspecialty literature (DeVeber, Azenstat, and Chisholm, 1991).

Research is needed to determine the characteristics that differentiate the women who experience extreme negative reactions (of any kind) from those who do not experience such distur-

69

bance. Adler et al., (1992) suggests this kind of study would need a large sample due to the relatively few women who would show such a response.

The Myth Of "Going Crazy" Because Of An Abortion

Anti-abortion factions have promulgated the allegation that women go crazy in droves after an abortion. Study after study refutes this myth. Suffering from severe psychological repercussions (i.e. psychosis) is rare after an abortion, and in fact occurs much more frequently after childbirth. The incidence of **post-partum** psychosis (after birth) is five times greater than **post-abortion** psychosis. Two studies revealed 0.3 cases of post-abortion psychosis per 1,000 abortions and 1.7 cases of post-partum psychosis per 1,000 deliveries (Tietze U. Lewit, 1977; Handy, 1982). However, as with any major life event, some people's ability to cope may be taxed beyond their capacity, especially those who are already mentally ill. A literature review on psychological sequelae after an abortion reveals that women who have a mental illness or poor psychological functioning before an abortion experience a higher incidence of negative repercussions after an abortion (Payne, Kravitz, Notman, & Anderson, 1976; David, Rasmussen, & Holst, 1981; Dagg, 1991; and Major & Cozzarelli, 1992).

PREDISPOSING FACTORS FOR NEGATIVE REACTIONS

In the cases where women do react negatively after an abortion, there appear to be predisposing factors linked to those reactions. There is enough valid research from which we can attempt to assess a client's **potential** for negative reactions after an abortion. Counselors can use this information by 1). screening for these factors in pre-abortion counseling and 2). following a plan of action that may potentiate the client's successful coping.

Remember, despite our best efforts, no one has the infallible ability to foresee the client's future coping skills. The decision and subsequent coping is ultimately the client's responsibility. Research has identified the following in women who experienced depression, guilt, sadness, or regret after their abortion.

1. The women have no substantial emotional support from anyone, or those they told are opposed to the abortion, including those whose male partner has either rejected them, abused them, or offered little or no support. (Adler et al., 1990; Bracken et al., 1974; Freeman, 1978; Joy, 1985; Major & Cozzarelli, 1992; Mosley et al., 1981; Payne et al., 1976; Rizzardo et al., 1991; Robbins & DeLamater, 1985; Smith, 1983).

2. Mom and/or Dad are highly critical of Daughter's sexual activity and pregnancy, and/or they oppose the abortion (Bracken et al. 1974; Major & Cozarelli, 1992; Mosley et al., 1981).

3. They do not view the abortion as **their** decision, but feel coerced into it, and blame someone else for the abortion. (Adler, 1975; Bracken, Klerman, & Braken, 1978; Smith, 1973; Spreckhard, 1987).

4. They expect to cope poorly, including expecting to regret the abortion (Baluk & O'Neill, 1980; Fingerer, 1973; Major, Mueller, & Hildebrandt, 1985; Mueller & Major, 1989).

5. They are highly self-critical and blame their character rather than their behavior for the unwanted pregnancy (Major et al., 1985).

6. They have an existing mental illness prior to the abortion (Dagg, 1991; David et al., 1978; Weing & Rouse, 1973).

7. They are highly religious (Adler, 1975).

8. They feel very guilty and ashamed about having an abortion. (Dagg, 1991; Spreckhard, 1987).

9. They view themselves as worthless and suffer from low self-esteem. (Athanasiou et al., 1973; Freeman, 1978).

10. They express extreme ambivalence over the decision. (Adler, 1975; Dagg, 1991; Freeman, 1978; Osofsky & Osofsky, 1972; Payne et al., 1976).

11. They have chosen abortion due to genetic or medical indications. (Blumberg, Goldberg, & Hanson, 1975; Dagg, 1991; Donnai, Charles, & Harris, 1981; Niswander & Patterson, 1967; Peck & Marcus, 1966; Smith, 1973).

12. Their coping style is to block out and deny disturbing events and problems rather than think and talk about them (Cohen & Roth, 1984).

The following identifying factors are not based on systematic research but are observations I have made from years of experience at Hope Clinic and follow-up interviews with women post-abortion. I include them when listening for signs of potential negative reactions and poor coping in the pre-abortion counseling session.

13. The women have been prescribed anti-depressants or anti-psychotic drugs for depression, manic-depression, or schizophrenia, have recently quit taking their medications, have not discussed the pregnancy with their therapist, and refuse to do so in the future.

14. They are adolescents and are being isolated from all friends and from their boyfriend by over-controlling/overprotective parents after the abortion. These teens may feel imprisoned and helpless and can become suicidal.

15. They have a hard time nurturing or forgiving themselves, and/or they doubt God's forgiveness.

16. They believe having an abortion is the same thing as murdering a newborn.

17. They treat themselves poorly, rarely take care of themselves emotionally, and seek situations and people who mistreat them. They may presently be in an abusive relationship or have a history of abusive relationships.

18. They often experience symptoms of depression, have attempted suicide in the past but are not seeking help.

A STUDY OF POST-ABORTION REACTIONS AND WAYS OF COPING

From 1986 to 1989 I conducted telephone interviews with women who were willing to talk about how they felt after their abortion and how they coped. I interviewed a total of 100 women from the St. Louis metropolitan area who answered an ad in the newspaper. The phone interviews averaged 30 minutes, with some taking up to two hours. Most of the women had had their abortion one to five years ago, with some as long ago as 15 to 20 years.

Some of the 20 questions I asked during the interview included, 1). How long ago was your abortion? 2). What stands out in your memory? 3). What emotions did you experience the first few days after your abortion? 4). Did your feelings change over time? In what way? 5). If they said they felt sad, angry, guilty, or regretful, I asked: What were you telling yourself? What did you do to cope? 6). If they said they felt positive, confident, or relieved, I asked: To what do you attribute your well-being? The last two questions of the interview asked: What did you learn from your experience? What tips would you give other women to help them cope well after an abortion?

Defining Successful Coping

Those women who reported only positive feelings or mixed feelings with manageable levels of guilt or sadness I defined as "successful copers." Successful copers were in the majority. Even when they experienced some guilt or sadness, they described it as transient and unproblematic. A minority reported signs of depression, severe guilt, regret, and unresolved grief. I defined this group as "poor copers." One or more of the 19 high risk factors I listed above was evident in the poor copers.

Defining Poor Coping

To clarify my definition of "poor coping," I used the following descriptions of depression, severe guilt, regret, and unresolved grief. Parts of the descriptions were provided by the cited references.

Signs of **DEPRESSION** included thinking about death or feeling suicidal, sleeping or eating too much or too little, crying frequently, losing interest in enjoyable activities, losing ability to concentrate, performing poorly at work or school, not caring about personal appearance and hygiene, feeling constant fatigue, restlessness, irritability, excessive guilt or anger, and feeling worthless (DSM III-R).

Signs of **SEVERE GUILT** included fearing God would punish her, interpreting any misfortune, illness, or accident as signs of God's punishment, having nightmares about killing babies or saving them, engaging in self-punishing behaviors and continuous, self-deprecating thoughts (i.e. "I'm a murderer."), blocking out the experience, and avoiding anything that reminded her of the event.

Signs of **REGRET** included wishing she could go back in time and change the decision, believing carrying to term would have resulted in a more desirable outcome, and dwelling only on negative consequences she attributed to the abortion decision.

Signs of **UNRESOLVED GRIEF** included engaging in thoughts and behaviors that kept alive a strong emotional attachment and investment in the pregnancy, baby, or meaning she attached to the pregnancy; engaging in thoughts and behaviors that prevented her from redirecting her emotional energy into the here and now, moving adaptively forward, and getting on with her life (Rando, 1988).

Results Of The Study

The results from these interviews supported the findings in other research: The majority of women reported positive feelings or positive feelings mixed with some manageable, transient feelings of guilt or sadness as years went by, but no regret. Results showed that negative reactions were linked to lack of support, denying feelings rather than coping with them, and feeling coerced into the abortion.

All the women who had coped poorly and then received counseling for their distress reported a substantially improved ability to cope. In addition, despite negative reactions, most of the poor copers in this study did NOT regret their abortion **decision.**

The information was organized into coping methods that led to well-being and those that didn't. The responses fell into five categories:

- **Expressing vs. repressing feelings**

- **Taking responsibility vs. blaming others**

- **Accepting forgiveness vs. rejecting it**

- **Positive vs. negative self-talk**

- **Empowering vs. debilitating actions**

The following are responses from the interviews.

Descriptions Of Behaviors And Self-Talk That Foster Poor Coping After An Abortion

Repressing vs. Expressing Feelings

1. I isolated myself.

2. I stuffed my feelings down and pretended they weren't there.

3. I hid behind a facade of strength.

4. I listened to judgmental, anti-abortion people who condemned abortion and told me I was a murderer.

5. I talked to negative people who brushed me off with, "It's over. Why talk about it?"

6. I allowed people to make me feel guilty.

Blaming Others vs. Taking Responsibility

1. I let others think for me and make my decisions.

2. I let myself be shamed into making a decision I couldn't live with.

3. I kept blaming my boyfriend, thinking he'd feel guilty and sorry.

4. I blamed my parents.

Rejecting Forgiveness vs. Acceptance

I kept telling myself:

1. I'm bad for having an abortion.

2. I'm a murderer.

3. I'm a cold, selfish woman.

4. I shouldn't have done it.

5. I'm worthless.

6. I should suffer for this.

7. God will punish me.

8. God won't forgive me.

9. I was stupid and weak.

10. I had no right to take a life.

Debilitating vs. Empowering Actions

1. I turned to alcohol and drugs.

2. I put myself in hurtful situations, like having sex with men who treated me bad.

3. I punished every man that came into my life afterwards.

4. I stayed by myself and didn't talk to anyone.

5. I told certain people about my abortion who snubbed me and looked down on me.

6. I interpreted every bad thing that happened to me after the abortion as a sign of God's punishment.

7. I waited much too long before getting professional counseling.

One Unexpected Finding

One unexpected but not surprising finding emerged from the small group of poor copers who described the most severe reactions. All of them spontaneously revealed physical, sexual, and/or emotional abuse they had endured as children at the hands of their primary caretakers. It is not known if any of the successful copers also experienced abuse in their childhood as this specific question had not been asked. The connection between childhood abuse and poor coping after an abortion needs further investigation.

Descriptions Of Behaviors And Self-Talk That Promote Successful Coping After An Abortion

Expressing vs. Repressing Feelings

1. I talked to someone who was supportive

and understanding before and after the abortion. It felt good to think out loud and to receive their comfort and understanding.

2. I carefully selected who to tell and who not to tell, so I wouldn't have to listen to a lecture from someone who judged me.

3. If somebody said something mean, I considered the source.

Taking Responsibility vs. Blaming Others

1. I used my own mind – not what my church or anyone else thought about it.

2. I looked at all my alternatives and feelings before the abortion instead of waiting till afterwards.

Accepting Forgiveness vs. Rejecting It

1. I believe God forgives you even if you think you don't deserve it.

2. Everyone makes mistakes.

3. Why punish myself when I did the best I could under the circumstances?

4. You might be able to forgive yourself if you quit judging others.

5. I talked to my minister - I knew he wouldn't condemn me.

6. I prayed and asked God for forgiveness.

7. I looked at what I gained, not just what I lost.

8. I focused on all the reasons I chose the abortion.

9. I read that being "selfish" sometimes is good because it means you're caring for yourself.

10. Being responsible for the pregnancy doesn't mean having a baby you can't take care of.

11. God gave me my own life and he expects me to take care of it.

12. I decided to learn from my mistakes.

13. I don't have to make myself suffer just because I had an abortion. I did the best I could.

14. I talked to a counselor who helped me accept myself.

Empowering vs. Debilitating Actions

1. I wrote down all the reasons I had the abortion.

2. I took care of myself after the abortion and went on birth control pills.

3. I helped my girlfriend avoid a pregnancy by telling her where to go get birth control.

4. I grieved the loss, but didn't let it control my life.

5. I stopped pleasing my boyfriend and started doing what was right for me.

6. I hand-made gifts for my friends for Christmas to get back in touch with the giving part of me.

7. I put my best energy into school and made good grades for my future. The abortion was all about my future.

8. Years later I helped someone else in my situation.

9. I devoted my time and energy to the kids I already had.

10. I let myself cry at night, but kept it out of my mind while I was at work. I gave my feelings a time and a place.

11. I gave myself a rest from men for awhile - and decided to go more slowly getting to know a man before I had sex with him.

12. I avoided doing things that would make me feel like a hypocrite.

13. I read about grief and loss to help me cope.

14. I joined a volleyball team and made new friends. I wanted to feel happy again.

15. I prayed for peace of mind and forgive-ness.

16. I talked to my friends.

17. I got back into my normal routine.

18. I surrounded myself with people who love me.

19. I wrote a pro-choice letter to my senator to tell him how I felt about abortion.

20. I told myself I can take care of myself and I have control of my life.

IMPLICATIONS FOR PRE-ABORTION COUNSELING

Counselors can give the client the benefit of what is known about coping after an abortion by assessing her risk for negative reactions, sharing information about what helps and what hinders successful coping, and referring for counseling in high risk cases.

Screening For High Risk Factors For Negative Reactions And Poor Coping

Keeping in mind four main categories will help you ask questions that may reveal poor coping factors: decision, support, feelings, and coping.

Decision

Is she accepting responsibility for the decision or blaming someone or something else? Is she ambivalent about the decision, and if so, to what degree? The more ambivalence, the more risk of negative reactions afterwards.

Support

Whom has she told and what were their reactions? Always check out the support from her male partner. The more rejecting, abusive, or withdrawn he is, the more potential for her to become depressed, angry, and lonely. When a teenager reveals little or no support from parents who know about the abortion and who have forbidden her to talk to friends and boyfriend, this is a red light indicator! The weaker her support system, the more internal strength and coping ability she needs.

Feelings

When exploring feelings, listen for signs of extreme guilt, depression, unforgiveness from self or God, intense sadness and loss, or regret.

Coping

Ask how she **expects** to cope after the abortion. If she says she doesn't know, ask how she has coped with stressful events in the past. Does she believe she has been successful in coping with past stressful events? Two studies found that a reliable predictor of successful coping after an abortion is "self efficacy." Self efficacy is a person's belief in her ability to do what it takes to cope with difficulties. When women believe they have handled stress well in the past and will continue to do so after an abortion, they usually fulfill their own prophecy (Mueller & Major, 1989, Major et al., 1990).

Be alert to signs of self-defeating behaviors such as using denial, intending to forget the whole thing ever happened, or discounting the reality of the fetus by trying to perceive it as "just a blob." Take note if she tends to bottle up feelings and is shutting out support people by isolating herself or if she has no support. If she indicates she will probably hang onto guilt and negative thoughts about herself and has trouble forgiving herself or believing God will forgive her, poor coping is a possible outcome. Other self-defeating behaviors include bulimic, anorexic, or compulsive eating, drinking or drugging, avoiding counseling she seems to need for other problems, and quitting medications and other treatment for mental illness.

Counselor Limitations In Assessing The Client's Coping Ability

As an abortion counselor, you have to make an assessment based on what the client has told you in the limited time of one session. You do not have the luxury of getting to know the client gradually over a period of time and have no way of knowing what the client may be withholding. You certainly can't see into the future and know what, if anything, might cause her to regret her decision. You are simply required to make your best judgment given the considerable limitations of the situation.

There are times when a counselor spends well over an hour with a client who reveals signs of potential poor coping in the first part of the session. Then, as the session progresses, the client does a remarkable job of convincing the counselor she is sure of her decision, no amount of time or counseling intervention will change her mind, and she will be able to cope afterwards without regret. Any suggestion to leave and reconsider options is firmly declined by the client. The procedure and recovery may go smoothly. Then weeks, months, or years later she is sitting in a lawyer's office drawing up papers to sue the clinic for psychological damage because "they didn't tell me I would feel bad and regret it!" The allegation is that the clinic is responsible for the client's emotional distress and failed in its duty to warn the client of ensuing depression, regret, and suicidal thoughts and acts.

The Hope Clinic counselors co-sign a consent form with the client that states she understands research shows the majority of women experience feelings of relief and have no major regret after an abortion. It goes on to explain that some women MAY experience guilt, sadness, depression, and/or regret following an abortion, and that these feelings can range from mild to severe. If she needs further counseling following the abortion, she can call The Hope Clinic for Women for a referral. It also states she has received the booklet, How To Cope Successfully After An Abortion, and it describes the content and purpose of the booklet.

This 10-page booklet describes the full range of post-abortion feelings, defines each feeling, and gives useful strategies for coping. One section lists warning signs, such as symptoms of depression and post-trauma stress, and advises counseling. The last part explains what counseling is, how much it costs, and where to locate counseling services, including spiritual counseling. You can purchase this booklet by writing to The Hope Clinic for Women.

After The Assessment: Employing Strategies For Successful Coping

Going Home With A Counseling Referral Before The Abortion

Once you have made your best judgment and assessed the client to be at high risk of poor coping, ask yourself what quality of support does she have? And how accessible is her support person? A teenager whose parents were very unsupportive told me her married sister was her confidante, but her sister lived 800 miles away, and they didn't have the money to make lengthy long-distance phone calls. If the client has poor support, how willing is she to see a counselor afterwards? If she is at high risk of poor coping, has poor support, and seems unreceptive to seeking help for herself, then I recommend sending her home with a counseling referral BEFORE she has the abortion. When sending clients home, consider their length of pregnancy, any fee increases that may occur by the delay (something to try to avoid), and offer to explain to the person who brought her why you are sending her home. At Hope Clinic the number of clients we typically send home annually is between .5%–1% of our total number of patients.

Making An Agreement To Seek Counseling After The Abortion

If she refuses the recommended intervention and insists on having the abortion THAT DAY, you can proceed in several ways. You may decide to receive a verbal or written agreement that she will see a counselor after the abortion, and then document your initial recommendation and her refusal in her chart along with the agreement for post-abortion counseling. However, it has been my experience that clients who have been extremely upset from the beginning and refuse to leave upon our recommendation, are usually uncontrollable during the procedure, experience much more pain than normal, are likely to be distraught in recovery, more likely to disregard aftercare instructions, and are more likely to experience real or imagined complications.

Receiving A Second Evaluation From Another Counselor

The client may be given the choice to talk to a second counselor for another assessment if she does not accept the first counselor's recommendation. Sometimes it takes two counselors' recommendations before the client agrees to the prescribed course of action.

Those clients who have complied with our recommendation and have returned on another day appear immeasurably calmer, more at peace,

and confident in their decision. Physically they usually tolerate the procedure well and are not distraught in recovery. From start to finish the entire process goes smoothly. When I explain why I recommend sending her home, I include a description of the physical consequences others have experienced when they stayed and had the abortion. However, there are always exceptions, and some women proceed with the abortion after convincing the counselor they will be able to cope, and they do not want to leave. These women insist the abortion is their best option and can articulate why it is beneficial to their lives. At the end of the session, they appear relieved to be able to go through the abortion that day and no longer appear combative. They may tolerate the procedure well and recovery time may be spent without apparent distress.

Seeking Support From Significant Others Before The Abortion

Some clients may not need to see a counselor but may need to talk to someone they have not yet told. For example, a client stated she believed that if her mother knew she was pregnant, she'd probably want to help her care for the child rather than see her have an abortion. The client was morally opposed to an abortion and based her decision solely on the assumption that caring for both her and the baby would be an undue burden on her mother. At the end of the session, she concluded she was second-guessing her mother's thoughts and would be wise to check out the reality. She never returned.

Reconsidering Other Options By Doing "Homework"

Sometimes the client simply needs to take more time to reconsider options and resources for carrying to term. A client who was not averse to living on government assistance had not checked out her eligibility. She adamantly refused the idea of adoption and was very morally opposed to and extremely afraid of an abortion. She willingly left to check out her eligibility and returned one week later, more resolved and less afraid. In that week she had discovered the limited help she might receive from state aid. She also had reunited with her boyfriend, and he came with her to the clinic the second time around. She seemed more confident in her ability to view the abortion as a good choice and cope with a diminished level of guilt feelings.

Others need time to calm their fears. When fear of the procedure, pain, or complications is overwhelming, going home and returning on another day sometimes works wonders. When she returns, she states she is more familiar with the people and the place, knows what to expect, and feels more ready to go through it physically. She may have left with the "homework" of practicing relaxation and distraction techniques. As you can see, the "homework" recommendation needs to be tailored to the individual.

Learning Constructive Coping Skills And Using Handouts And Self-Help Booklets

Some clients who appear at risk for poor coping may not need to be sent home. If they have a good support person and seem receptive to learning new strategies for coping, you may decide to share this information in both verbal and written form, and give her a counseling referral. Besides talking about coping strategies that have worked and not worked for other women after an abortion, you can also give her a handout to read later. Because of time constraints, giving the client something for later may enhance her learning. The booklets, How To Cope Successfully After An Abortion and How To Cope With Guilt are two of several self-help publications we at Hope Clinic give to our clients.

Chapter Fourteen

Exploring The Client's Feelings About The Abortion

Before asking her about her feelings, ask yourself, "What do I need to know and why is it important?" Are your questions going to help her in the long run? Are they going to help you assess her risk of poor coping? She may become uncomfortable with some of your questions, withdrawing eye contact, sighing, fidgeting, changing the subject or becoming silent. Explaining why you need to know can be helpful if she regards your questions as unnecessary and intrusive. Keep your purpose in mind and stay focused.

Sometimes the counselor is the one who is uncomfortable asking certain questions, for fear of what she'll uncover. The direct question, "Do you believe abortion is killing a baby?" is one example. What do you do if she says yes? The next chapter on helping clients cope with guilt may boost your comfort level. Some counselors have voiced a fear that certain questions are "too personal." In the field of abortion counseling it is often appropriate and helpful to the client to ask questions about her relationship with her parents, the fight she had last night with her boyfriend, whether or not intercourse burns when she uses spermicides, whether she believes abortion is murder, and a host of other very intimate questions.

POSITIVE FEELINGS

Over the years at Hope Clinic I've counseled approximately 16,000 women before their abortion, and the majority state they feel positive and confident about their decision and expect mostly relief mixed with "a little guilt" or "a little sadness" afterwards but no regret. Some state they don't expect any sadness or any guilt whatsoever.

Many women have expressed feeling grateful that they were able to exercise their option safely and said they felt relieved they would soon have their life back to normal again. Some have been so sick and debilitated from extreme nausea that they are looking forward to feeling well and regaining their health. Some state they have felt so depressed because of the dreaded consequences of carrying to term that they look forward to feeling hopeful and normal again. Other women have exclaimed, "I'll feel like a ton has been lifted off my shoulders!" and "I feel like I'm being delivered from hell!" They have expressed thankfulness that all the suffering that would have befallen themselves, their parents, partner, or children they already have is NOT going to happen. While no one expresses happiness at undergoing surgery, many express relief at the end result: not being pregnant anymore under their set of circumstances.

"I DON'T KNOW HOW I FEEL"

Sometimes when you ask such a broad question as, "What are your feelings about having an abortion?" the reply is "I don't know." They may honestly not know what they believe or how they may feel. It is sometimes hard to know how you're going to feel after any major life event. On the other hand, they may not want to express their worst fears and would rather push it out of their minds.

Help Her Get In Touch With Her Feelings

Describing the range of emotions women have reported after an abortion may help her identify her own. "Relief, confidence in a good decision, and feeling back to normal are common. Some women feel guilty, sad, angry at themselves or someone else, depressed, or regretful. Some women say they feel both positive about the decision and a mixture of other feelings as well. Did you hear anything that sounded close to what you think you'll feel?" Usually she is able to identify one or more feelings that fit her.

Another way that helps to clarify her feelings is posing one or more of the following questions to her.

1. What did you believe about abortion before this became a personal issue? What do you believe now? Do you view abortion as "killing a baby?"

2. What emotions do you expect to feel afterwards: immediately afterwards and as time goes by?

3. If she says she expects to feel regret ask, "Do you mean when you look back on the decision you'll wish you had never had the abortion, but instead had the baby?

4. If she says she expects to feel sadness, loss, guilt, shame and/or depression ask, "How intense do you imagine the feeling will be afterwards? Do you expect it to be manageable? What do you normally do when you feel sad, guilty, etc.? What else can you do to comfort yourself? What can you tell yourself?"

I have found that mentioning the results of the following research serves to bolster the client's belief in her own judgment. Fingerer (1973) studied women's expectations of how they would probably feel after their abortion. Results showed that the woman herself was more accurate in her judgment than what anyone else thought - including her friends and family members who accompanied her to the clinic or a Ph.D. in psychology.

What's The Point Of Exploring Feelings?

If she says she feels guilty, sadness and loss, and expects regret or depression, you need to find out 1). if she expects to feel overwhelmed by intense feelings or be able to cope, 2). if her usual ways of coping are constructive or unconstructive, and 3). if she needs additional counseling before and/or after the abortion.

SADNESS AND LOSS

If your client states, "I feel sad," what exactly does she feel sad about? One woman might answer,"Because my boyfriend left me. He doesn't care." Another might reply, "I keep wondering if it would have been a girl or boy and what it would have looked like." Both are common replies, yet there are many other reasons why a woman would feel sad during or after an abortion. Just knowing other women have experienced the same thing can feel consoling.

Possible Causes

The cause of her sadness will guide you to appropriate ways of helping her. If she feels a loss (loss of a dream, her innocence, a relationship, the baby) she needs to grieve, and naming the loss is important to her grieving process. Because she is choosing to end the pregnancy, she and her significant others may not believe she deserves to grieve. "It's what you wanted, isn't it?" they or someone else might ask her. Talking about the process of grieving can be helpful because l). you are acknowledging her loss, 2). you are offering her knowledge, and 3). knowledge is power.

Strategies For Coping With Sadness And Loss

Ask what other losses she has experienced and what she did to comfort herself. If she describes repression or self-defeating behaviors, you can offer to describe what has comforted other women after an abortion. Having a good cry, being with or talking to their partner or a close friend, being alone for a while, or engaging in a pleasant activity are some ways women have taken care of themselves.

During my study on how women cope after an abortion (1988), when they stated they felt sad I asked specifically, "What did you tell yourself that helped you cope?" Here are some of the replies:

1. I told myself what's past is past. Look to the future!

2. How could I have raised that child with enough of anything? I can barely take care of myself. I did the right thing.

3. I can always have a child in the future, and that one can be planned.

4. Look at what I would have missed if I had had the baby.

5. Having that abortion gave me another chance, and I'm going to make the most of it.

6. Caring for myself is as important as caring for others. My life counts too.

7. Just because I feel sad doesn't mean I made a bad decision.

8. Quit dwelling on the what-ifs and get on with your life.

9. I don't have to keep dwelling on thoughts that hurt me.

10. I am a survivor.

Some women are afraid they might regret their decision if they are feeling sad about it. It's true that if her sense of loss outweighs the expected benefits from the abortion, she may indeed regret her decision. On the other hand, just because a person feels sad about a decision doesn't mean it was not a good decision. Some people feel relieved to hear that good decisions are sometimes sad - a divorce, placing an aged parent in a nursing home, moving, ending a relationship, or ending a pregnancy. The more they desired mother-

hood and the more they became attached to the pregnancy, the more likely they will feel a loss. However, keep in mind that not all women feel sad about an abortion. Some women describe no attachment whatsoever to the pregnancy or to the idea of parenthood at that time, and feel no loss.

Trigger Events, Dates, Places, People, And Things

Talking about "trigger" events, dates, places, and things that provoke sad feelings is also helpful because she won't be caught unaware. Things like walking through the baby department in a store, seeing a diaper commercial on TV, or standing in line behind a woman holding a darling baby are common triggers. Her due date, the anniversary date of the abortion, or the birth of a friend's baby are times that may trigger sadness. Any sadness her partner shows can also trigger her own sadness. As time goes by, seeing a child the approximate age as hers would have been can provoke a twinge or wave of sadness. Can she think of any other trigger? Let her know that she need not dread those events. Once she already knows she might feel sadness under those circumstances, she can prepare her strategies for coping if and when it happens.

You can also challenge her to look for situations and events that trigger good feelings about her decision. For example, she might see a haggard looking woman in a store with screaming toddlers and a crying infant and think "Thank goodness that's not me!" Or as she is talking to a girlfriend who is living the life she didn't want to suffer through, she can think "I made the right decision!" On the day she graduates from high school or college she can feel grateful she gave herself the gift of her education by postponing parenthood. Any important event she might have missed had she carried to term is an opportunity for affirming the wisdom of her decision.

Reading Materials

Because of time constraints in a pre-abortion counseling session, you can also give her reading materials she can look at later. My booklet, How To Cope Successfully After an Abortion has a section on strategies for coping with sadness and loss. Giving her the title and author of the paperback book, How To Survive The Loss of a Love by Colgrove, Bloomfield, and McWilliams provides her with an excellent resource. I particularly like the way it describes the ups and downs along the bumpy path of the grieving process.

GUILT

When a client states, "I feel guilty," it is not necessarily because she believes abortion is killing. While this is the issue for many women who state they feel guilty, it is not the source of guilt for others. Let the client know you do not want to assume what she is feeling guilty about. Ask her to tell you more to help you understand.

Reasons For Guilt

1. **"I feel guilty about getting pregnant in the first place."** Some women state they are NOT feeling guilty about the abortion per se because they don't believe aborting a fetus is the same as killing a baby. However, what they MAY be feeling guilty about is failing to prevent the pregnancy. Some feel guilty for not using any birth control while others feel badly for not using a **better** contraceptive than condoms, spermicides, withdrawal, or rhythm. If she is over 21, she often uses her age as an indicator she "should have known better!" But is there an age we can look forward to when we reach perfection, make no more mistakes, and take no more risks? If so, I certainly haven't reached it yet.

She may attribute the pregnancy to her "stupidity." First, if there was any "stupidity" involved, then it must have been both his and hers, not just hers. A man has just as much responsibility to contribute to the contraceptive effort as a woman. Granted, she has more to lose if the effort fails, but they are both equally responsible.

Second, saying "I did it because I was stupid," probably isn't accurate and certainly isn't helpful. She might mean, "I feel foolish for taking a risk." Explore what she means by "stupid." People do things for reasons, usually to satisfy a desire or a need. Everyone takes risks and for a lot of different reasons. When she discovers what prompted her to take a contraceptive risk, then she can decide how to satisfy her needs in the future without having to repeat history. For example, one woman thought about the circumstances under which she took a risk with birth control. She discovered she was feeling lonely and needy, and when a former boyfriend called, she invited

him over. Her need to be wanted overwhelmed her better judgment. They had sex using withdrawal. For the future she decided to be more protective of herself when she felt lonely. Instead of walking into a situation in which she feels vulnerable and is tempted to engage in unprotected sex, she said she'd get together with a female friend. "That way I'm with someone who appreciates me and I won't get hurt by some thoughtless impulse." This was one of several options she considered.

Finally, she can choose to continue criticizing herself or she can make a conscious decision to take better care of herself the next time. We all make mistakes, and the best we can do is learn from them. For instance, if she was using methods that were not very effective, what prevented her from using a more effective method? There may be any number of fears and other obstacles that need to be surmounted before she feels free to obtain and use better contraceptives. You can help her identify these obstacles and help her solve the problem.

2. **Some women say they feel guilty because they usually tell their mothers "everything," but this time they have chosen not to tell.** "I feel like I'm hiding something," she may say. What made her decide not to tell her mother? Do her reasons reflect an attempt to protect their relationship or protect her mother from unnecessary worry? Is it shame? What does she stand to gain if she tells her mother, and what does she stand to lose? Would she feel better telling her mother before she goes through with the abortion? Some women resolve their guilt by telling themselves, "I'll tell her later on when the time seems right."

From another standpoint, does she think she should know everything her mother has ever done, or are there times when it is appropriate for a mother to keep something private from her daughter? Is the reverse also true? If she feels sad because she perceives a loss of closeness, are there ways she can continue to feel close to her mother?

3. **A substantial number of women who feel guilty say they feel "SELFISH" for putting their own emotional or physical welfare before that of the fetus or significant people in their lives.** Culturally, women are taught to value others before themselves. Putting themselves first can create an uncomfortable feeling of guilt.

So when women put their health, education, or life goals before motherhood, they may feel selfish. Some also feel selfish if they put their own welfare above the desires of their partner or parents.

Acknowledge that women often feel selfish if they put themselves first on a long list of people to care for. Ask if she believes it's bad to make something out of her own life before she tries to give anything to another human being. If she already has a family and doesn't want any more children, is it bad to want time of her own? If she feels it IS bad, then does she feel she should choose another option besides abortion? If she feels it IS bad and still chooses abortion, what are her coping strategies after the abortion?

Inform her that most mentally healthy people care for themselves first some of the time, and they put others before themselves some of the time. It all depends on the situation. Does this hold true for her? If so, it appears that this is one of those times she feels it's important to care for herself. Removing the label of "selfishness" and relabeling the abortion as an act of self-care can help her let go of self-criticism.

Some women are ingrained with the belief that putting themselves first in any circumstance is BAD, and are unable to view it any other way. To strengthen her self-esteem and belief in her worthiness, she could consider therapy. If she seems unwilling to pursue therapy, her guilt may diminish once she has reestablished herself as a giver of care. This strategy does not solve her self-esteem problem, but it may restore her self-image. It may be helpful to explore with her what she can do to show special caring for others after the abortion. Some clients decide to engage in a day of special activities with their kids. One woman intended to volunteer a few hours that week at her mother's nursing home. Another woman said she wanted to make a special dinner for the friend who took off work to bring her to the clinic.

4. **"I feel guilty because I'm taking the easy way out."** The women who make this statement usually don't seem to be having an easy time of it, and you can point this out. However, she might mean that she feels more able to cope with an abortion than with adoption or parenting. Assessing our ability to cope with choices we make and acting in our best emotional interest is taking

care of ourselves. In addition, is taking the hard road necessarily **better**?

One young woman told me she always took the hard path because her father repeatedly told her it built character. I agreed that tackling challenges could certainly build character. I also observed that making choices based on easiness or difficulty may not always be the best criteria to use for making good decisions. I asked if she could think of a situation in which the BEST decision might be easier than another choice. She thought for a moment and said, "Well, this past semester in college I had the choice of taking a class with a professor who was known to be hard and flunked half the class or with a professor everybody liked. Of course I took the hard professor. I got a C in that class and hated every minute of it. I know if I had been in the other professor's class, I would have made an A and enjoyed it. The C grade has really brought down my grade point average." We evaluated the ease or difficulty of coping with abortion, adoption, and parenthood. Then I asked her to evaluate each option using the criteria of consequences to her, the potential child, and significant others in her life. She came to the conclusion that 1). abortion was not easy, but it was the least difficult and 2). abortion led to the least negative consequences for the most people, including herself.

5. **"I feel guilty because I don't feel guilty."** Some women think they SHOULD feel guilty, and if they don't, it means they're cold-hearted. There are many good-hearted women who do not feel guilty about having an abortion because they don't believe they've done something wrong. What does she think she should feel guilty about? What does she suspect are the reasons she does not feel guilty?

6. **"I always feel guilty about everything."** The woman who habitually feels guilty for everything is in need of therapy. This is a deep wound that won't heal with just a bandaid. Ask if she has ever had or considered counseling. Assess her knowledge of what counseling is all about and her receptivity to it. In addition, explore what she plans to do after the abortion when she experiences guilt.

7. **"I feel guilty because I'm killing a baby."** Some women believe strongly that a fetus at any gestational age is the same entity as "a baby."

Others are simply parroting what they've heard from an anti-abortion free pregnancy test center, from their parents, or their church, and admit they have never given it much thought themselves.

Clarifying Their Beliefs

One way to establish whether or not the client really believes having an abortion is the same thing as killing a baby is to ask the question, "Do you believe going through an abortion at your stage in the pregnancy is the same thing as carrying to term, giving birth, and then shooting or smothering the baby?" If the woman says no, ask what is different about those two acts. Most women respond, "In an abortion the baby isn't formed yet and it can't live on its own, but after birth, it's living on its own." If the woman says yes, she believes having an abortion and shooting a newborn baby are one and the same, the guilt is generally much more severe. She may need to go home and rethink her decision, or receive additional counseling before having an abortion.

Another question that stimulates the client's own thinking is, "Why do you think when a woman has a stillborn baby, there's a death certificate and a funeral, but when a woman has a miscarriage at your stage in the pregnancy, there is no funeral and no death certificate?" No matter what she responds, she has had to put her own thought into the answer. Her beliefs become more her **own**.

Sometimes when a client states she feels guilty about "killing a baby," and is invited to think about it from a different perspective, she may express confusion. What she has believed on a superficial level may become questionable when examined on a deeper level. You may want to bring up various criteria people use to form their beliefs about abortion.

Criteria People Use To Determine If A Fetus Is "A Baby"

1. **PHYSICAL APPEARANCE**: Many people focus on the physical aspects of the fetus. They compare the **size, shape, and appearance of the body** to that of a newborn. They may ask you,"How big is it? What does it look like?" Ask her what she imagines it to look like. How big does she think it is? Then clear up any misconcep-

tions. Tell her the size and weight of the fetus and what body parts are present and those that are not. How does that information make her feel? Does she want to see a picture of it? Of course, most pictures distort the actual size of the fetus. Looking at an 8 x 10 glossy of an eight-week fetus is very different than seeing the real thing. People may look at the 8 x 10 photo and say, "Oh, it's a baby!" and then see the real thing and ask, "What is it?"

Does the information change her mind about having the abortion? How does it help or hurt? Let her know you have nothing to hide from her. If fetal development is an important issue to the client, then she needs to know the truth BEFORE she goes through with the abortion.

Sometimes it is simple human curiosity, but it may be self-punishment that prompts questions about fetal development now that the reality of the abortion is at hand. Making herself feel worse by visualizing the fetus dying or in pain can all be part of her self-inflicted punishment for her "sin." When a patient works herself up into a frenzy of guilt by visualizing the worst just before and during the abortion procedure, she is more likely to lose control physically, screaming, crying, jerking suddenly on the table, and possibly injuring herself. If so, she will have successfully orchestrated a nightmarish abortion experience for herself to recall again and again. She will also have punished and exhausted the medical staff with her uncooperative, hysterical behavior. If you suspect a client may be prone to this type of response, bring it out into the open. This self-punishing behavior is predictable from someone who exhibited the following in counseling: a very dramatic demeanor, crying, expressing fear with no capacity for being comforted, expecting you to make it all better for her ("tell them to knock me out!"), not listening to or participating in any of your instructions for relaxing, tending to blame others for her misfortunes, and viewing abortion as "killing a baby."

Depending on the client, you may inform her that some people ask questions about the appearance of the fetus right before the abortion because they feel guilty. If she seems to agree this is the case, then assess her ability to cope in ways that will not endanger herself during the procedure. She may need to find some form of constructive "atonement" to perform AFTER the abortion, or to leave the clinic and choose another alternative.

2. **DEVELOPMENT**: Some people select a vital function or an ability they know babies possess and ask if the fetus also possesses the same, such as "Does it have a heartbeat?" or "Is it moving?" Some women ask these questions to find out if it's alive. To them as long as it's alive, it must be a baby.

3. **VIABILITY**: An important question to many people is "Can it live outside my body?" They feel if it can't live outside their body and breathe on its own, then it's not the same as a baby that's already born and living. To these women, lung development is a critical factor in determining when a fetus becomes a baby.

4. **BIRTH**: Some say until it's born, they don't believe it is the same as a baby. They may say "as long as it's inside me, it's not a baby yet."

5. **THEIR INTUITION**: Some women rely on an inner feeling rather than a physical aspect of the fetus to formulate their own belief. They explain with unshakable conviction, "From the moment I knew I was pregnant, it was a baby!" For them, no other criteria matters. Sometimes these women also assign a gender to the baby and have been thinking of it in terms of " a little boy" or "a little girl." To them there is no doubt that abortion is "killing their baby." Others say their intuition tells them the fetus is NOT a baby.

6. **RELIGIOUS TEACHINGS**: Some people focus on religious teachings and may use Biblical quotes to "prove" abortion is or is not killing a baby. A Catholic client told me, "It doesn't matter what stage of the pregnancy I'm in, it's a baby from the moment of conception because that's when it has a soul." One client expressed her certainty that abortion was NOT taking a life because, "My Daddy is a Baptist preacher and he always says you do not become a living soul until the Lord God breathes into your nostrils the breath of life. That happens once you're born!" Other clients who believe abortion IS killing a baby have recited a passage from Jeremiah, "Before I formed you in the womb I knew you and before you came forth from the womb, I sanctified you." Although some Bible scholars refute that this passage has anything to do with abortion, she might view it as proof of her belief. Others who believe in reincarnation have told me the soul that is presently inhabiting their fetus's body will go back to the Source and choose another body at another time because "souls never die."

Not Knowing What To Believe And Still Feeling Guilty

If the client has not explored her beliefs until the day of her abortion in the pre-abortion session, she may or may not be able to come to a conclusion. Some women have solidified their initial belief while exploring other perspectives; others have modified or changed their beliefs with new information, and still others have concluded they don't know what to believe.

If she expresses confusion about whether she believes abortion is killing or not, then explore:

1. The level of confidence she has in the decision.

2. Her susceptibility to regretting her decisions.

3. The degree of guilt, if any, she expects post-abortion.

4. Her support system.

5. The degree to which she is affected by what others think.

6. Her degree of exposure to anti-abortion sentiments and religious condemnation. The woman's view of the reality of her situation and her reasons for the abortion often override the **possibility** that she may be taking a life.

What's The Point Of Exploring Her Beliefs?

Your purpose in exploring the client's belief is not to convince her that abortion is or is not killing. SHE is the one who will need to live with whatever decision she makes. Your purpose is to sort out what she really believes about what she is doing, and how she feels about it. Are her actions congruent with her beliefs? Are they in conflict? If they are in conflict, does she need more time or counseling before going through with the abortion? How does she expect to cope after she has the abortion? When you know what she believes and how she feels about her decision and herself, you can better assess what she needs from you and whether she needs additional counseling prior to the abortion, a counseling referral post-abortion, both, or none.

Religious Guilt

Some people fear God is not going to forgive them. They have a habit of interpreting any misfortune that comes their way as a sign of God's punishment. Does the client believe God is All-Merciful and All-Forgiving? If yes, then why would God single her out as the exception? She can decide to have faith that she is forgiven and discontinue doubting God's ability to forgive. If no, what are the limitations she believes God places upon forgiveness? What is necessary for her to be forgiven?

Some women feel religious guilt because to them "a baby is a gift from God and here I am getting rid of it." First, she can choose to accept the gift and not have an abortion. However, if she strongly believes the abortion is best for her life, does she believe God is All Wise and All Understanding? If yes, then does she believe God understands why she is returning the gift back into His hands? God also gave her the gift of a brain and expects her to use it to make the wisest decisions she knows how to make.

Some people think God waits to forgive only after they have suffered for their sin. People have a tendency to view God as they view their parents (Borysenko, 1990). Parents tend to punish their children first for their wrongdoings and only then forgive. This is done in hopes of teaching them not to do it again. Some parents do not forgive, but cut their children off from their acceptance and love. People who believe God balances the scales of justice without mercy or love may need the following resources to help assuage their guilt and fear.

Pastoral Counseling

When you refer a client for pastoral counseling, know the attitude of the minister, priest or rabbi to whom you are referring. Hope Clinic counselors refer to Missouri Religious Coalition for Reproductive Choice (RCRC) in St. Louis because they have a list of pro-choice religious counselors, ministers, priests, and rabbis who are trained and willing to do post-abortion counseling.

Women who are struggling with religious guilt are often fearful God will punish them and won't forgive them. Any difficulty in conceiving a wanted pregnancy or any subsequent pregnancy that results in a miscarriage, stillborn, or fetal abnormality may be attributed to God's punishing them for the abortion. Pastoral counseling serves to reassure them that God is an infinitely loving, forgiving God. Does a loving God kill or maim someone's children to punish them for what they believe they did wrong? Whether or not she ever has an abortion, there will be good and bad things that will happen in her life. How she interprets any misfortune is up to her. She can choose NOT to label misfortune as "punishment for the abortion," or she can choose to increase her guilt and attribute unfortunate events to the abortion.

Some people use quotes from the Old Testament and from Revelation to substantiate their fear in a punishing, wrathful God. Almost anything can be supported or refuted by Biblical quotes taken out of historical context. When someone is convinced she will be (or needs to be) punished, she and the minister may formulate a constructive penance for her repentance. Some faiths teach that the way to forgiveness is realizing a sin was committed, feeling sorrow for the sin, and repenting. "Repenting" might include prayer, going to church, and/or doing good deeds. If she keeps thinking her repentance is never enough, she may need more than what pastoral counseling can offer. She may need therapy.

Many faiths teach there is immediate forgiveness as soon as the person asks. Nothing else is required. The parable of the Prodigal Son may help restore her faith in a loving, forgiving God. In this parable Jesus likens God to a father who has two sons. One son leaves home with his inheritance and squanders it on riotous living. When he becomes destitute, he realizes his wrongdoing, feels guilty and ashamed, and decides to go back home and beg his father's forgiveness. As the son is walking down the road to his father's house, his father looks out the window and sees him coming. The father immediately runs to meet him with arms outstretched. Without ever having to beg, suffer punishment, or prove his remorse, the son is immediately forgiven and welcomed back.

I interviewed ministers and priests from various Christian faiths and asked them, "What is necessary for God's forgiveness when a woman has an abortion?"

A Catholic priest said, "God is infinitely merciful. He forgives the instant she has the abortion." However, the same priest told me, "Abortion is forgivable but never justifiable. Even if the child or the woman must suffer, suffering is preferable to killing. Suffering can be a growthful experience." Then he said she must feel truly sorry and remorseful for her sin. I asked, "What if she feels the abortion was the best decision?" He replied that abortion is NEVER the best decision and that she is operating from distorted thinking. He added that God's forgiveness is not dependent upon her emotions, however, so even if she does not feel regret, God has still forgiven her.

A Baptist minister from RCRC told me, "God's forgiveness is immediate, unconditional, and final. It is a gift that we don't have to earn or beg for." He also stated there was NOTHING in the Bible that stated abortion is killing. He felt his role would be to support any decision a woman felt was best and help her find peace with any decision she made.

A Unity minister recited part of a favorite prayer to me about the nature of God's forgiveness: "God does not strike a bargain; God gives. God does not forgive me because I am good; God forgives because HE is good. God is love."

In the interviews of the clergy from the Mormon Church, Pentecostal, Christian Scientist, Jewish, Methodist, Lutheran, Presbyterian, Church of Christ, Episcopalian, Science of Mind, Catholic, Baptist, and Unity, they all stated God forgives for an abortion. Some stated there was no Biblical basis for equating abortion with murder. However, the Mormon, Pentecostal, Christian Scientist, Missouri Synod Lutheran, and Catholic all stated abortion was killing a person. There was only one faith that stated God's forgiveness depended upon the judgment of the "elders" within their religion: the Jehovah's Witnesses. I was told by two elders from different fellowships that if a woman wanted forgiveness, she would have to confess to the body of elders in her fellowship. Then they would pray and know whether God

forgave her or whether they should cast her out of the fellowship.

Helping Clients Cope With Guilt

1. What exactly is she feeling guilty about? One way to find out is by writing," I am feeling guilty because..." and finishing the sentence with as many answers as she feels are true for her, or by talking about it to an understanding listener.

2. Is there anything to gain by holding on to the guilt? If so, how can she get what she wants in another way? When will she decide to do what it takes to let go of guilt? What might she gain by letting go?

3. What are some of her good characteristics? She may be focusing on her faults to the exclusion of her goodness. If she can't think of anything, she may need to ask a good friend. If she continues to "yes-but" any evidence that she is a good person, she is probably suffering from low self-esteem and could benefit from therapy.

4. What can she learn from the experience? Learning from the past can help fortify her for the future and propel her forward.

5. If she believes in God or a higher power, is she willing to ask for help in letting go of the guilt? How can she get in touch with God's forgiveness? Reading the New Testament or holy books from her faith, engaging in prayer, meditating, and talking to a compassionate minister, priest or rabbi are all ways to reconnect with a forgiving, loving God.

6. What is she saying to herself when she is feeling guilty? Self-forgiveness depends on the self-talk she engages in and what she does for herself. If she tells herself, "I don't deserve forgiveness," then she'll stay stuck in guilt. She'll be more likely to move past the guilt if she tells herself, "I'm human and I sometimes make mistakes, just like everyone else. I forgive myself and I move on." Self-talk and affirmations must be believed to be effective. People who have a history of abuse in their background and/or addiction will probably need therapy to build self-love and feelings of worthiness.

Resources For Coping With Guilt

1. Referrals to pastoral counseling.

2. Referrals to secular counseling.

3. References from the Bible on the nature of God's forgiveness and love: (Luke 23:32-43, Luke l5:11-32, John 3:15, I John 2:1-2, I John 1:8-9, Hebrews, 4:14-16, Matthew 18-22-23, and Isiah 43:25). These references are also listed in my booklet, How To Cope Successfully After An Abortion.

4. Hope Clinic has a variety of self-help booklets. One of the booklets is entitled, How To Cope With Guilt. The booklet on guilt lists 14 different ways people try to cope with guilt in their lives. It explains why some of the ways are hurtful and keep the client stuck in guilt, and why other ways are more constructive. It can be purchased by writing to The Hope Clinic for Women.

5. Two other booklets I recommend are: Personhood, the Bible, and the Abortion Debate by Dr. Paul Simmons. (To obtain it, contact The Religious Coalition for Reproductive Rights, l00 Maryland Avenue, N.E., Washington, D.C. 20002) and The History of Abortion in the Catholic Church: The Untold Story by Jane Hurst. (To obtain it, contact Catholics for Free Choice, 1436 U Street, NW, Washington, DC 20009, 202/986-6093.)

6. Guilt Is The Teacher, Love Is The Lesson by Joan Borysenko (1990) is an insightful and beautifully written book on the subject of guilt, forgiveness, and spiritual healing.

Memorable Religious Clients

Not all religious clients feel guilty about their decision to have an abortion. Some have prayed long and hard about what to do and feel God has helped guide them in the decision.

One woman I counseled told me her family prayed together every night and went to church every Sunday. She also did volunteer work with handicapped children "for the Good Lord." She stated, "I never thought I'd be having an abortion, but my husband and I have been praying a lot together over this decision. We feel that God has sent me this cross to bear because some time in the future I may be able to help someone else in my situation."

One strict Southern Baptist woman told me, "I always thought abortion was killing, but I have three small children and the only money we have to live on is welfare. I can tell you what killing is - it's trying to raise three children on food stamps!"

A Southern Baptist minister came to the clinic with a member of his congregation in support of her choice. I spoke with him and he said, "Regardless of what ministers believe or preach, we're not here to place judgment. I figure if there's anything to forgive, that's up to the Almighty. My place is to be there when one of my congregation members needs me. I know this girl's situation and how hard it was for her to make this decision, and I'm right behind her!"

One Catholic woman in her forties went to Mass before coming to the clinic for her abortion. She explained that when she was a child, her father was a laborer and worked hard to support his five children. They were raised strict Catholic, but her father ate meat on Friday because he said he needed more than fish to keep him going. Her mother told the children to pray hard for their father's soul because if he had an accident on the job and died before receiving the Last Sacrament, he'd go to hell for breaking the church law. Then sometime in the sixties, lo and behold, the church decided it wasn't a sin after all to eat meat on Friday!" She concluded, "Now who's to say some time in the future the church won't decide it's not a mortal sin to have an abortion. So I'm doing what my father did - I'm doing what I feel is necessary to keep me going." Then she related all her reasons for the abortion.

The following letter came to us from one of our clients. "Making a decision of this magnitude can put us closer to God than we may have ever been before, embracing, maybe for the first time in our lives, the fact that all of God's creation does not fit into geometric blocks of absoluteness: Good or Evil, Right or Wrong, Acceptable or Unacceptable. With each new situation that arises, we are each responsible for using every ounce of our God-given talents - mind, heart, and soul - to make the best possible choice for everyone involved, including partner, family, friends and the potential human being you carry. This is truly a no-win situation - a mistake, an accident, and NO, God does not want us to suffer a lifetime for committing a "sin" like seeking warmth, gratification and comfort and making love to another human being ...not MY God, anyway! I know this is much more of an evaluation than you might have been after, but it has taken four years and two abortions to sort through these feelings. I appreciate you allowing me to express them. There is enough suffering in this world. And I truly believe that every woman going through this procedure does suffer. But why should we suffer even more by feeling estranged from our God? Women who seek abortions are NOT Godless - just unfairly burdened. Thank God, and all Her Angels, there are people like you to share and ease that burden!"

REJECTION FROM THE PARTNER

"I've been feeling bad because my boyfriend left me." Grieving over the loss of a boyfriend can be all too common after an abortion. The relationship may already have been floundering and this was "the last straw." If her boyfriend ducked out after she told him she was pregnant, she's probably suffering from feelings of rejection or betrayal. She may also feel guilty and ashamed if she thinks it was her fault he left.

What does she feel toward him? Anger? Sadness? Does she still love him? Wish he'd come back? Never want to see another man as long as she lives? Does she fear getting close again, physically or emotionally? She may feel a need to tell you all about it, and the best help you can offer is to listen. I also recommend to my clients two of my favorite books on the subject of healing from a broken relationship: Letting Go by Dr. Zev Wanderer and Tracy Cabot and How To Survive the Loss of a Love. I've mentioned the latter in the section on Sadness and Loss. The former uses a behaviorist's approach to picking up the pieces after a broken love relationship and gives concrete suggestions for restoring self-esteem and detaching oneself from the ex-lover.

Some women may need additional counseling after the abortion to help them grieve the loss of the relationship and restore self-esteem. Counseling is also indicated when a client describes a pattern of choosing men who "love 'em and leave 'em."

ANGER

When women describe feelings of anger, they are usually feeling angry at: 1). themselves "...because I didn't use birth control," "I gave in to my boyfriend's pressure"; 2). male partner "...for getting me pregnant, not using a condom, pressuring me to have an abortion, thinking the abortion is no big deal"; 3). parents "...because they won't let me see my boyfriend again," "they don't let me talk to anybody about the abortion," "they're pressuring me to have an abortion"; 4). God "....because I prayed I wouldn't wind up pregnant"; 5). fate "...these things are always happening to me"; 6). circumstances "...if only I had more money and my boyfriend was responsible, I'd have the baby"; or 7). contraceptive failure "...I was trying to prevent the pregnancy by using contraception, and it failed me".

You can help by letting her get it all out, and in some instances help her think what she could do differently next time. For example, one woman stated, "I was mad that I got sexually involved too soon before I knew him for what he was - irresponsible!" She vowed to go slower in her next relationship and wait to become intimately involved until she knew the man better. Her anger served her well because of what she learned and decided to do.

When women are angry with their boyfriends, sometimes they are simply blaming them for what they both did. Other times her anger is right on target. As one woman related, "I thought he was acting responsibly by using condoms, but then after I get pregnant, he has the gall to tell me he deliberately put holes in the condoms to get me pregnant! I could kill him!" Some women in situations like this understandably want revenge. But revenge has a way of backfiring, so help her release her rage in harmless ways. One way might be for her to write the coldest, angriest letter imaginable, telling him what she thinks of him and what she'd like to see happen to him. She can imagine him having to listen to every word. She might want to read the letter aloud to a friend and have a good laugh over it. Then, the next step would be to examine her own behavior and the risks she took with him and with her well-being. She can decide how to take better care of herself the next time. Finally, she needs to refocus her attention away from him and onto caring for herself. One woman said the way she finally let go of hating him for his callous, uncaring attitude was to simply believe, "Someday he'll be on the other side of the coin."

Some people may be able to forgive the offender eventually, but it takes time and doesn't necessarily come easy. However, there is no need for her to criticize herself if she cannot forgive him. It is "good enough" to let go of anger by expressing it safely and taking care of herself. If she continues to feel angry and can't seem to let go, she needs to see a counselor.

When teens feel angry at their parents, they need an outlet to avoid turning the anger inward and becoming self-destructive or depressed. Teens usually do find release from feeling frustrated and angry at parents by talking to their friends. If an adolescent states she doesn't have any friends, she may keep a journal and prefer to write down her feelings. She may need encouragement to seek counseling or call you back if you have developed a good rapport.

FEAR OF SEX

Naturally, if you get burned once, you're not likely to want to touch whatever burned you again. Thus, we hear clients state, "I'll never have sex again!" Some laugh as they make their declaration, but others are dead serious.

Results of our post-abortion evaluation forms show that many women welcome physical **affection** directly after an abortion. However, not nearly as many say they desired sexual intercourse; and a small minority express an aversion to being touched at all. These feelings normally do not last forever but can easily last several weeks post-abortion. Letting the client know many women echo her sentiments, and that she doesn't have to have sex until she feels ready usually brings a smile. This may be a time she needs to rebuild trust - in herself, men, or the reliability of contraception.

REGRET

Some people use the word "regret" when they really mean "sad." Define it and see if "regret" is what she really means. "Regret" means she'll wish she never had the abortion even if placed in the same situation at the same point in time. If the answer is yes, she really means she'll regret her

decision, then strongly suggest she go home and reconsider her choices.

If Only...

People who regret their decision often indulge in dreaming up "if only's" and then using these as a form of punishment and suffering. For example, some of the women in my study who experienced regrets after their abortion explained that if only they had kept the baby, their lives would somehow be better! Knowing herself, is it likely she'll think about the if only's? "If only's" come from hindsight, and rather than being used as a valuable growth experience, they keep people feeling disappointed in themselves. It is quite possible that the thought, "If only I kept the baby, my life would be better" may not be true at all. However, such a thought will keep her feeling bad about her decision and provide an excuse for not making her present life happier.

From time to time as we grow older, we will pause to reflect on events of our past. If our lives are not going as well as we'd like, it may be tempting to think, "If only I had made different decisions, I'd be better off." But is it fair to judge our past decisions based on what we know now? Who can see into the future? We all must base our decisions on the limited knowledge we have at the time. There is an endless number of regrets we could torture ourselves with, but we can use our time and energy instead for creating joy in the present and planning for the future. Gaining wisdom from hindsight is constructive, but using "if only's" to foster misery is a self-destructive practice to avoid.

Reasons For Feeling Regret

Some people who experience regret feel remorseful that they did not live up to their values. For example, some women criticize themselves for lacking the strength to have given birth to the child and then to have placed it for adoption. Thus they regret what they consider "weakness." There are also women who feel ashamed of themselves because they believe abortion is an unforgivable act, and they can't bear to own up to their part in the abortion. These women talk themselves into believing they "didn't know what they were doing," and often blame the doctor, "legalized abortion," the clinic staff, or their partner or parents for the abortion. This is a way of fooling themselves and is a defense to ward off intense feelings of self-hatred and self-destruction. However, there is a better way of coping.

If She Fears Regret – A Counseling Scenario

In pre-abortion counseling, if she says she fears she may regret the decision, she can STOP, think, and alter the course of her actions before it's too late. If she says she is certain today that her decision is the best of all her options, what could change her mind in the future? One of the most common responses to this question is addressed in the following scenario.

Client: "I'm afraid when I have my first baby I'll look back and regret I never had this one."

Counselor: "What are the reasons you're choosing NOT to have this one?"

Client: "Because of all the suffering I'd put myself and the child through, not to mention the burden on my family."

Counselor: (After the client has elaborated on the "suffering" she was referring to) "What do you want it to be like when you have your first child?"

Client: "I want it to be at the right time when I've got enough money to provide for a child and a home and when it would have a father. Then everybody would feel happy - even my parents. I want it to be a happy time...Not something everybody is dreading."

Counselor: "So if you had this child as your first, it wouldn't be anything like what you want and hope for. And so by having this abortion, you'll have the chance to have that dream come true...when the time is right."

(The expression on her face indicates she hasn't thought about it in that light.)

Counselor: "That's not to say you won't think about this one and feel sad that the timing wasn't right back then."

Client: She looks sad, nods in agreement, and says, "I'll probably wonder if it would have been a girl or a boy and what it would have looked like."

Counselor: "Many women experience normal human curiosity like that. And it sometimes makes them feel sad. What can you tell yourself to comfort yourself when you're having your first baby and feeling a little sad about not having this one?"

Client: "I can tell myself that it wouldn't have been right to have had this baby because I couldn't have provided for it, and it wouldn't have had a father."

Counselor: "So you can feel sad and reassure yourself you made the best decision for you and the child instead of regretting the abortion and doubting yourself."

(She nods and appears relieved.)

Remembering Her Reasons For The Abortion

Another way of helping her avoid needless regrets is to suggest she find some quiet time to write down exactly why she chose to have an abortion. She needs to include every reason she can think of and describe in detail what her set of circumstances were. The closer to the time of the abortion she performs this task, the more accurate and vivid it will be. Then she needs to put the paper in a safe place where she will always be able to find it. Memory has a tendency to fade with time. If she ever wonders why on earth she didn't have the baby, she can reach for that paper and jog her memory.

Chapter Fifteen

Exploring The Client's Support System

Nobody exists in a vacuum. Asking about the people the client lives with and those she has told about the pregnancy can help you understand her situation. Their reactions may have an impact on her decision and/or her feelings about her decision and herself.

Research has repeatedly shown the beneficial effects of receiving emotional support both before and after an abortion. In my study on post-abortion emotions, almost all the women who coped well had talked to at least one supportive person. Those who coped poorly had either little or no support from others in their lives. Those who coped the worst, suffering from depression, shame, or post-trauma stress after their abortions said they continued to suffer until they finally spoke to a professional counselor, therapist, pastor, or psychiatrist. These were the women whose partners left or abused them, who received abuse or no support from anyone else they told, or who isolated themselves. However, the majority of women chose to involve someone in their lives who they knew would be supportive. Most stated all they really needed was an understanding friend, family member, or partner to talk to and were able to find such a person. In cases where women suffer depression after an abortion, studies have shown a significant link to a lack of emotional support (Mosley, Follingstad, Harly & Hickel, 1981). Post-abortion depression and griev-

ing have been specifically linked to the male partner's lack of support (Mosley, 1981, and Joy, 1985) and, for adolescents, lack of support from parents (Bracken et al, 1974).

DISCUSSING SIGNIFICANT OTHERS IN HER LIFE

In the pre-abortion counseling session, we need to ask:

1. Who knows about the pregnancy? (Specifically inquire about the partner in the pregnancy and parents, for anyone living with parents).

2. What were their reactions?
   • What did they say? How has she reacted to them?
   • Have those relationships (male partner, parents) changed in any way? How?
   • Are they supportive to her in her decision? How have they shown their support?
   • Are they objecting to her decision? What do they want her to do? What has she told them? How does she feel about their objections?
   • Are they trying to make her feel bad about having an abortion? What are they doing and saying? How does she feel and how does she react? Specifically, are they successful at "making her feel guilty?" What does she tell herself? What

CAN she tell herself instead, and who else can she talk to for support?

3. Regarding the significant people in her life she has chosen not to tell, what made her decide not to tell them?

• How does she feel about not telling? (Some adolescents who report a "close" relationship with Mom start crying when reporting this is the first thing they haven't shared with her. Discussing pros and cons of telling, validating privacy and separation needs, and talking about "growing up" may be helpful).

• Would she feel better about her decision if certain significant people knew PRIOR to the abortion procedure? (There have been some clients who chose to leave the clinic after the counseling session and went home to tell their partner or parent because they discovered they would feel more comfortable if this person knew what was going on. When they returned on another day, they appeared much more at ease.)

• Has she been thinking she will tell them afterwards? How does she think they'll react after the fact? Has she considered the possibility that they'll react angrily? What does she and the other person/persons stand to gain or lose by her telling them afterwards?

4. Does anybody she lives with know about the pregnancy? Are they supportive? If they are not supportive, is there somewhere else she can stay today and tonight after the abortion where she will receive support?

MALE PARTNERS

Impact On The Woman's Well-Being

Many studies report a significant correlation between post-abortion emotional well-being and high levels of male partner support (Bracken et al, 1974; Freeman, 1978; Joy, 1985; Mosley et al, 1981; Payne et al, 1976; Robbins & DeLamater, 1985; Smith, 1973). Conversely, when women's relationships with their partners are unstable and lacking in mutual support, they report higher levels of depression and anxiety (Mosley et al, 1981, and Payne et al. 1976). Another unfavorable outcome, post-abortion regret, has been associated with the partner's opposition to the decision or outright abandonment (Freeman, 1978). From the results of these and other studies, it seems clear that male partner support or lack of it can strongly influence women's feelings after their abortion.

Results Of Hope Clinic Study: Why Women Tell Or Don't Tell Their Male Partners

In 1985 The Hope Clinic and two sociologists from Washington University in St. Louis completed a study on abortion patients who told their male partners about their pregnancy and abortion decision (Plutzer & Ryan, 1985). We asked why they chose to tell and what their partner's responses were. We asked those who chose not to tell why they didn't. The results gave us useful information.

Of the 2,300 abortion patients who were surveyed, most described their relationship as "steady and ongoing," 12% were married, 10% were in unstable relationships, 23% had broken up, and 1% were raped. Ninety percent (90%) of the women in the study chose to tell their partner about the **pregnancy**. Of that number, 85% of the men were told about the **abortion**. The 5% drop was due to some men abandoning the woman after learning about the pregnancy, and some women deciding not to further inform the man because of his negative reaction to the idea of abortion.

One client sat down and removed her sunglasses that had concealed two black eyes. She needed no question from me to explain her condition. She pointed to her face and stated flatly, "This is what I get for telling my boyfriend I was pregnant and wanted an abortion. He told me I wasn't gonna kill any baby of his! He beat me up pretty bad. Blacked my eyes and kicked me in the stomach. Said it was all my fault."

The women who told their partners gave the following reasons: "It's his responsibility too;" "I wanted to know how he felt;" and "I thought he should know." Of the 90% who told, almost one-fourth reported having mixed feelings about telling. These women described the nerve-wracking task of facing a variety of anxiety and fears: fear of the unknown, fear of the man's insistence she have the baby, fear of his anger, fear she'd burden him with one too many problems, fear he wouldn't care, and fear that he'd deny paternity. For some women, these fears came true.

Nearly one-fourth of the men who were told behaved in unsupportive ways. Reactions from unsupportive partners included denying paternity, blaming her, withdrawing, abandoning her, showing indifference, attempting to persuade her to place for adoption or give the baby to him, and verbal or physical abuse.

Some clients broke down and cried as they described outrageously cruel responses they had received from their partners. One of the women tearfully told her story: "I had been deeply in love with this man for three years," she began. "We were planning to marry, or so I thought. When I told him I was pregnant, he didn't say a word. I didn't know what to think. He grabbed his car keys and said he was going drinking. He never came back that night, but two days later I received a phone call from a strange woman. She sounded angry and told me she was two months pregnant by MY boyfriend, and that he had been seeing her for the past year and a half! She was having his baby, she informed me, and he would be living with her from here on out. I almost passed out. I finally got ahold of the S.O.B. and we had it out. The worst of it all was - he wasn't a bit sorry. He simply didn't give a damn!"

More than one woman sadly explained that her partner demanded, "You're not going to kill my baby! You're going to have it!" But then he offered no financial or emotional support, much less marriage. The same man was seen going out with a new girlfriend the very week he had issued his ultimatum against the abortion.

Some teenagers fought back tears or exploded with anger as they told about an ex-boyfriend who denied paternity and then spread the news of her pregnancy throughout high school. One girl confided, "I can hardly get myself to go to school anymore. I'm tired of the way everyone's whispering behind my back. One girl had the nerve to call me a whore right to my face! I know it's terrible to say, but I've been wishing I were dead."

Several other women reported that their partner had made it very clear he wanted nothing to do with her or the pregnancy. However, once she had "fixed her problem" he'd gladly resume a sexual relationship with her. One woman looked me dead in the eye and asked, "Isn't that the ultimate insult?!"

On the positive side, a slight majority (51%) of the women who chose to tell received supportive reactions from the partner. "Supportive behaviors" included, "He shared his feelings with me;" "he asked about my feelings;" "he listened to me;" "he agreed with my decision;" "he drove me to the clinic;" "he paid for the abortion;" "he wanted the baby but told me he'd support any decision I made;" "he told me what I wanted was more important than what he wanted;" "he told me he'd back me 100% in whatever I chose to do." Indeed, it is not uncommon for our waiting rooms to be filled with men who have accompanied their partners, especially on Saturdays when they are off work. Occasionally he will ask to join her in the counseling session prior to the abortion. Sometimes he asks if he can be with her every step of the way. It is heartwarming to see the boyfriend or husband holding his partner's hand and expressing concern about her safety and their future birth control efforts.

More than one woman described how her partner called her every day to see how she was feeling and expressed how sorry he felt for "getting her pregnant." Some men chose not to leave the clinic until they knew she was fine and completely finished with the process. One young man greeted his girlfriend after her stay in the recovery room with a red rose and warm embrace.

The married women had a higher percentage of receiving support than the unmarried women. However, 8% of married women decided not to tell for one or more of these reasons: "It's not his and the marriage would collapse if he knew; he'd make me have the baby; he's against abortion; he's abusive."

In general, the women who chose not to tell their partners gave the following reasons: "He would oppose my decision; he wouldn't care; he didn't need to know; he'd get mad; we don't see each other any more; I was raped; he has too many problems already."

Most women who describe their relationship as "steady and on-going" tell their partners and get some measure of support. However, some tell and wish they never had. Those who don't tell are operating from fear, independence, or a protective stance toward the partner.

Knowing what, if anything, has transpired between her and her partner will help you assess what support she may need from you and from others. It may also give you clues to her emotional state before and after the abortion.

Sometimes the client knows what she wants from her partner: "to understand what I'm feeling and going through." If he is available and she is willing to bring him into the session, you can facilitate communication between the two by asking her to tell him what is important for him to know. Then ask him to repeat back to her what he heard her say. Once she feels heard, you can ask him to tell her anything that is important for her to know, and ask her to repeat back to him what she heard. Unless they are at odds with each other, this technique is usually quick and simple as well as effective.

If she does not want him to join the session for fear it would "embarrass" him, you can give her the pamphlets, After Her Abortion (Baker) and For Men About Abortion (Wade) to give to him. Clients are usually pleased to receive anything that helps bridge the gap between their experience and their partner's.

After Her Abortion addresses the man's feelings about the situation, and focuses on some of the most prevalent:
• feeling guilty about the pregnancy and/or abortion,
• frustrated or angry if his partner is blaming him,
• scared the relationship will end,
• withholding feelings to appear strong or to avoid influencing her decision,
• angry if he wanted the baby and she wanted an abortion, and
• confused about what to say and do to show his support.

The booklet lists ways he can show he cares about his partner during and after the abortion experience, and educates him about the physical and emotional changes a woman undergoes when she is pregnant. It helps him understand that an abortion can be physically painful, and that he can help her prevent an infection by abstaining from sexual intercourse for two weeks afterwards. The booklet concludes by suggesting ways they can **both** participate in the birth control effort to help protect against another unplanned pregnancy.

After Her Abortion can be purchased by writing to The Hope Clinic for Women.

The booklet, For Men About Abortion was written by a psychologist who provided counseling in an abortion clinic for both men and women. From his years of counseling men who accompanied their partners to the clinic, Roger Wade has written a thorough, down-to-earth discussion of feelings many men experience before, during, and after an abortion, and informs them how to show support for their partner. The booklet also provides a summary of the abortion procedure and aftercare instructions, and ends with suggestions for how a man can actively participate in preventing another unplanned pregnancy. You can purchase the booklet by writing to Roger Wade, P.O. Box 4748, Boulder, CO 80306.

Involving The Male Partner On The Day Of The Abortion

Counseling Session With The Supportive Partner

When I called Janet's name, she asked if her boyfriend, Brian, could come with her into counseling. I told her I needed to see her by herself first, and then we could certainly include him. Once in my office, I explained that I needed to see her alone to make sure she wasn't being pushed into the abortion by her partner. She smiled and assured me the decision was hers, explained why she felt abortion was her best option, and then informed me Brian had told her he'd stand by any decision she made. She described him as "caring and supportive." She stated he insisted on paying the whole fee and taking off work to be with her on the day of the procedure, and had expressed his sadness that she was the one who "had to go through everything."

When she brought Brian into my office, he appeared nervous and alert, and reached over to hold her hand. He scooted his chair closer to hers. I explained what the purpose of the counseling session was, and I asked how he was feeling about the decision. He stated he left it up to Janet, but that he agreed they were unprepared to provide for a child at this time in their lives. His explanation was identical to what Janet had told me. Then he asserted he would have done whatever it took to raise the child if Janet had wanted to carry to term. Brian was halfway through pre-med school and had a long way to go to achieve his goal of being a physician. Janet was studying to be an elementary teacher and had three years to go.

He had taken books out of the medical library for them to read about the abortion procedure. He seemed knowledgeable but wanted to know if Janet would be in any pain. I went over the possible sensations Janet might experience during and after the abortion. While I was talking, he was rubbing the back of Janet's neck with one hand. He asked what he could do for her afterwards, and I suggested he ask her. He cupped her hand in his and asked the question. She smiled and said, "Just what you've been doing, and a steak dinner when we leave here!" He laughed and said, "Oh, don't mention food – I'm starved." She told me, "He said if I couldn't eat anything before we came, then he wouldn't either!"

Brian then asked if he could be present during every step of the abortion process, and I explained what parts he could be present for and why he could not be present for others, due to our state regulations. He seemed disappointed, but she reassured him she'd be all right. I suggested I act as their messenger and keep him informed of her progress. They both seemed pleased. Then he asked, "When can she start her birth control pills?" We launched into a discussion about the Pill. Before they left, I commented that theirs seemed to be a strong, loving relationship. They smiled broadly, held hands, and she said, "Some day we're going to be married and have children, but just not right now." He echoed her sentiments, saying, "Once I'm out of med school and into my residency, we'll be able to provide for a child and take care of it the right way."

Of course, not all partners are as supportive and sensitive as Brian. Most unsupportive partners don't choose to come with the woman to the clinic, so we usually don't see them. However, sometimes an unsupportive partner does come, and either the woman asks to bring him into the counseling session, or the situation seems to warrant it.

Counseling Session With The Unsupportive Partner – First Scenario

Here are two versions of the same session: the first version is one in which the partner is brought in with the client after the counselor has talked to the client at length by herself. The second version shows what might have happened if both the client and her partner were spoken to alone first and then together.

Pam dragged herself into my office, sat down and said, "I'm depressed." She explained that she wanted to be a mother and felt this was her last chance. She stated, "I'm 34 and I've lived with my boyfriend, George, for 11 years. I've had two other abortions and in both cases he was the father. The first time we both wanted the abortion, but the second time **he** wanted the abortion more than I did. This time he wants the abortion and I don't. But I'm scared of what would happen to our relationship if I don't have the abortion." By this time she was dabbing tears from her eyes. She looked tired. I asked, "What do you fear would happen to your relationship if you don't have the abortion?" She surprised me with her reply. "I know he would marry me. We've already talked about marriage, but he does not want the financial responsibility of supporting a child." Wanting to know if I was hearing correctly, I responded, "So you're saying he would marry you even if you had the baby, but he would resent having to pay for the support of the child?" She answered, "Yes, and I'm afraid he'd get fed up real quick and ask for a divorce. Then I'd be on my own with a child. I am petrified of being a single parent." I asked what petrified her about single parenthood. She replied, "I've seen my best friend and my own sister's struggles, and I say 'no thank you.' I don't want that kind of life. They're barely making it. They never have any money; they work all the time, and hardly have time to see their own kids. It looks like hell to me." I asked if he left her, would she have any financial and emotional support from her family. She said, "Yes, I'd never be alone or homeless. My Mom helps my sister as much as she can, but it's not the same as having a husband." She stated she has talked to her mother whom she described as "pro-choice" and who has said she'd support any decision her daughter made. I asked about her father, and she snorted, "Hmm! My father left us when I was eight. He tried to come back into my sister's and my life since we've been adults, but what do you say to him now? I'm not even sure where he lives." I reflected, "So you knew as a child what it meant to be left." "Yes. I saw what my mother and me and my sister went through. I don't want to live through it again," she asserted.

97

I then turned to discussing her relationship with George. "What has he told you exactly about his feelings if you carried to term?" She stated he has given her mixed messages, occasionally saying he wants the baby, too, but doesn't feel they can afford it. Other times he asserts he doesn't want to support the child. "Money," she said, "is a major thing with him." "In what way?" I wanted to know. "He was really poor as a child and has had to work hard for every nickel. His parents never gave him a dime. He works 60 hours a week sometimes. We split all the expenses, except he pays for the house. It's in his name. He talks about money as his only security," she replied. "Some people think of having a child as security," I commented. "How do you view having a child?" She smiled broadly and answered without a moment's hesitation. "I would feel fulfilled. I've always felt I'd make a good mother and would enjoy mothering a child." I then asked how she would probably feel if she had an abortion. The smile vanished and she replied, "Like I felt after the other ones – sad and like I lost some part of me. Only this time would be worse. I never felt guilty about the other abortions, just sad." Then I added, "And how would you feel about placing the child for adoption?" to which she replied, "I could never part with it once it was born. Then I'd be a mother. Adoption is out of the question. I either have this baby and keep it, or I don't have it at all."

I reflected to her what I had heard and seen so far. "The only time I've seen you stop crying and in fact saw you smile was when I asked how you'd feel to have this baby. She smiled a little and waited for me to go on. I continued, "The dilemma seems to be your fear of his leaving and your fear of single parenthood." She nodded. "What is the probability of his leaving if you carried to term?" I asked. She responded, "I'd say a 50-50 chance."

I asked if he was with her, and she said yes. I suggested we bring him in and find out where he stood, especially since she said he had sent her conflicting messages. She agreed. George entered the room, sat down on the edge of the chair and folded his arms. I explained that we both felt it was important to hear how he'd feel if she carried to term. He was loud and clear: "I do NOT want this child or ANY child EVER!" Pam looked embarrassed and shaken. He went on stating his goal in life was to be financially secure and independent and did not want any of his "hard earned

money going to the on-going support of a child." I asked Pam if she would ask George what he'd be willing to offer her if she carried to term. She asked in a small voice, "What would you do if I had the baby?" He answered, "You'd have a house to live in, but I couldn't promise I'd be around much. I can tell you right now I would be very unhappy." Pam became teary. He turned to her and angrily told her to go ahead with the abortion as "they" had planned. She turned away from him, burying her face in a tissue. He said, "Well, you wanted to know where I stand, and I've told you."

I commented that since he gave an honest answer, Pam had some solid information which might help her make a decision. I commented further that it was obvious their needs were directly opposite to each other, with Pam ready to be a mother and George not ever wanting to be a father. I asked George to return to the waiting room and told him Pam would join him shortly. After he was gone, Pam looked relieved. She said she wanted to go home and talk to her mother again. I supported this plan of action and offered a counseling referral. She seemed grateful for the referral. Because George seemed so controlling, I asked if George had ever hit or shoved her, and she denied any physical abuse. I also asked if her mother might be home now, and she said yes. She left planning to see her mother once she arrived home. Pam never returned.

Counseling Session With The Unsupportive Partner – Second Scenario

When I asked Pam, "What is the probability of his leaving if you carried to term?" and she replied, "A 50-50 chance," I might have requested to see George by himself first, and then to bring them together. This may have eliminated his aggressive and defensive behavior when brought in the middle of HER session. After bringing him into the office by himself, the following dialogue may have occurred.

Counselor: George, thank you for being willing to meet with me. The reason why I asked to speak with you is because when the woman expresses a desire to know what her partner wants and doesn't seem to know the answer, then it usually helps for the counselor to talk to both of them separately and then bring them together. That way each person has had an opportunity to state what they want and then to communicate it clearly to the other person. Once she has all the facts, she can make a clearer decision. Would you be willing to do this?

George: I thought we already went over this. Isn't she going to have the abortion?

Counselor: You may have already gone over it with her, but what you want is still unclear to her. Would you be willing to tell me what you think should be done about the pregnancy?

George: I don't want it. I told her I never wanted to be a father.

Counselor: (Waits in silence).

George: I've worked hard for every penny and every last thing I have - my house, my car, the clothes on my back – and I don't intend to see my hard-earned money going for the support of a kid I don't even want!

Counselor: (Aligning with him) Making your way in life has not been easy, and everything you have you've earned by yourself.

George: (Interrupting) And I don't see why I have to give it all up for a kid I don't want.

Counselor: I don't either.

George: (Looks surprised at this response).

Counselor: You're very clear. You do not want Pam to have this baby because you don't want the obligation of paying child support, and you don't feel it would be fair to you to be pressured into parenting. When men are this clear about not ever wanting to become a father, my question to them is, "What did you do to prevent the pregnancy from happening?"

George: Well, I thought she was on the Pill. How was I to know that she missed a pill?

Counselor: At first glance it seems impossible to know if she had taken her pill, but some men help their girlfriend by asking if she took it, or they help her choose a time of day that might help trigger her memory. Some use condoms along with her taking the Pill. I'm bringing this up because it is important for men and women to own their part of the responsibility in creating the pregnancy.

George: (In a muffled voice) I know it takes two. I'm just mad she messed up.

Counselor: Even if she hadn't missed any pills, no contraception is 100% effective, so any time people consent to have sex, a pregnancy is always a possibility. Both people are taking the chance.

George: (Looking down and not saying anything).

Counselor: (Stays quiet).

George: Well, I'm mad at myself too. I'd give anything to go back in time and do something different to prevent the whole thing from happening. I don't know why she thinks I might want her to have the baby.

Counselor: What did you tell her?

George: Well, just what I've been telling you. But I have to admit when she gets all sentimental about it and asks me, "Don't you want it, too?" I've told her yes because it seems to calm her down. She's not as upset about the abortion when I tell her that.

Counselor: So that is probably how her confusion resulted. You were trying to calm her down by telling her what she wanted to hear. She seems to have interpreted it as you expressing a desire for the baby.

George: It was a damn lie, but when she gets mad at me for not wanting the baby, she starts to change her mind about the abortion.

Counselor: The last thing you want is for her to change her mind about the abortion.

George: (Looking very nervous again). Is she going through with the abortion?

Counselor: I can't answer for her. What I can tell you is that our doctor will not perform an abortion on anyone who feels pressured into it. It has to come from the woman's own free will. I'll be honest with you. She may leave here without the abortion.

George: (Runs his hand through his hair and shakes his head).

Counselor: You said you didn't want to have to give up everything you've worked for to parent a kid you didn't want. I can certainly understand that, but parents don't have to give up EVERYTHING for their kids. What is the most you'd be willing to give your son or daughter if Pam decided to carry the pregnancy through?

At this point, George talks about allowing Pam to live in his house if she continues to pay half of all other expenses. I ask specifically about doctor bills, food, diapers, and baby clothes. He commits only to paying for groceries but nothing related to the baby. I ask about non-monetary care for the baby, such as feeding, holding, and bathing him or her. He says, "I can't see it." I then tell George that when I bring Pam in to join us, I will ask her to ask him what he wants and what he is willing to give by way of support if she has the baby. I commend him on his crystal clear communication with me.

When I see them together, **both** Pam and George have had the opportunity to be heard and to hear themselves state what they want and don't want. George has been prepared for the possibility that Pam may leave without the abortion, and Pam knows caring for the child may be left up to her.

PARENTS

Impact On Their Daughters' Well-Being

Studies have shown young women are more likely to experience a favorable outcome after an abortion if their parents are supportive (Bracken, Phil, Hackamovitch, & Grossman, 1974, and Mosley, Follingstad, Harley, & Heckel, 1981). Bracken et al. (1974) discovered a correlation between a favorable outcome and a high level of anticipated parental support. In the same study women under the age of 22 were more heavily influenced emotionally by parents' support than by male partners' support.

Some adolescent clients have stated, "I don't know what I would do without my Mom. She told me she'd support me 100% no matter what I chose to do about the pregnancy. She's with me today." A client is likely to perceive her parent/ parents as completely supportive if the parents

have told her they would support and help her with any decision she makes, and then reinforce their words with action.

Emotional Impact Of Unsupportive Parents

Mosley et al. (1981) found higher levels of hostility, anger, anxiety, shame, and depression in young women whose parents were unsupportive than in those women whose parents were supportive. Depression, anger, and shame were more acute in women who described their relationship with their mothers as "negative."

Another study's results found that women who told their families and then found their family members to be less than completely supportive were significantly more depressed than those who did NOT tell their families. The women who did NOT tell their families scored almost as low on depression post-abortion as those women whose families were told and were completely supportive (Major, Cozzarelli, Sciacchitano, Cooper, Testa, & Mueller, 1990). The same study found that women who told a significant other and then discovered he or she was not supportive experienced poorer short-term post-abortion adjustment than those who chose NOT to tell certain significant others. Long-term post-abortion adjustment was not studied.

The majority of the women who coped poorly after their abortion in my study had told one or both parents and received emotional abuse or total lack of support in return. Poor copers who told their parents about the pregnancy were frequently shamed, punished, and degraded , and they reported being labeled "whore," "trash," or "baby-killer."

At Hope Clinic there have been a few patients who have called back asking to talk to a counselor. When they have called, their reasons have usually been relationship difficulties with the male partner, guilt, or problems with unsupportive parents. One of the most serious post-abortion situations arose when a teenager threatened suicide - not because of the abortion - but because of her parents' behavior. Her older sister made the initial call asking what to do because her sister, Alicia, was being treated like a prisoner. Their father had nailed the door to Alicia's room open to deprive her of privacy. Their mother took her to school and picked her up immediately afterwards. Alicia was forced to drop all extra-curricular activities at school and was forbidden to have contact with her friends and boyfriend. She stated Alicia had written her a note threatening suicide, and she didn't know what to do. The older sister went on to explain she had moved out herself when she was 16 due to her parents' oppression. She said she had to sneak her sister out of the house in order to make this phone call to me. When she put Alicia on the phone, the girl sounded teary and depressed. She confirmed what her sister had said. She stated the abortion decision was what she wanted and was not the problem. She used the word, "prisoner" and stated she had been thinking about taking a bottle of pain pills, but had written to her sister instead. After talking to both of them, they agreed on a strategy to seek help from both her school counselor and the county mental health department.

FRIENDS

Friends can have an important impact on a woman's emotional state before, during, and after her abortion. Many women state they need someone to talk to who will support them no matter what. If their partners withdrew, opposed their decision, abused or abandoned them or simply didn't understand their feelings, many women turned to their best friend for support. Most Hope Clinic patients confide in their boyfriends and one close girlfriend. Support from friends can be enough to counterbalance the negative effect of an unsupportive partner (Mosley et al., 1981). A common refrain is "I don't know what I'd do without my best friend!" On the other hand, clients have said, "I've found out who my true friends really are. One of my good friends did nothing but criticize me and tell me I was killing my baby. I didn't appreciate her passing judgment on me." Some friendships have been broken and others deepened.

On the first page of the booklet, <u>After Her Abortion</u>, I validate the importance of a friend's willingness to listen and show she/he cares. I offer information about how they can continue to demonstrate their support after the abortion and inform them about circumstances that may complicate a woman's post-abortion reactions. There is a section addressing the special issues of those who may be morally against an abortion but loyal

to their friend. A best friend of one of the women I counseled declared, "I don't believe in abortion, but showing compassion for my friend is more important to me than any beliefs I have about abortion. So here I am."

WOMEN WHO DON'T TELL ANYONE

The Super-Independent Woman

Some women are not accustomed to conferring with others about their problems and usually work things out on their own. They may describe themselves as "loners" and prefer to keep to themselves, or they may have one good friend. Some have a strong sense of independence and inner strength. Although most women who cope well after an abortion utilize their support system, people who choose not to tell anyone **may** also cope well. In fact, telling people who turn out to be unsupportive of the abortion can lead to greater distress than choosing **not** to tell someone (Major et al., 1990).

Keeping Secrets Due To Shame

Some women avoid talking to friends about their problems due to shame. Those who feel ashamed often project their feelings onto others and assume everyone else will feel ashamed **of them**. They tend to repress painful feelings and events in their lives. Keeping a pregnancy secret from everyone because of shame may be an emotional time bomb waiting to go off.

Strategies For Combatting Shame

These clients may need your guidance in selecting someone who will be supportive. When they **do** choose to reveal their "shameful" act to someone, they tend to choose the very people who harshly criticize and judge them. It's a good idea to refer them to a counselor before and/or after the abortion. Healing from lifelong shame is not easily accomplished without professional help. In addition to the counseling referral, explore which of her friends might be supportive. If she has no idea how any of her friends feel about abortion, help her learn how to find out about their attitudes in ways that won't hurt her. For example, bringing up a TV program on abortion and talking about the issue in general terms is safer than revealing her own personal experience.

This client is likely to be easily affected by what others think, particularly anti-abortion propagandists whose specialty is provoking guilt. Explore the degree of exposure she'll have to such propaganda. For instance, ask a Catholic teenager if she attends a Catholic school. If so, it is highly probable that her religion teacher will bring in speakers and films on the topic of abortion. One Catholic student told me her English teacher as well as her religion teacher discussed the "sinfulness" of abortion in class. Childhood development classes are another source of abortion discussions in high schools and colleges. If the client is a church-goer, January and May are times of the year that some ministers and priests traditionally preach against abortion. January 22 marks the anniversary of legal abortion in the United States and May brings Mother's Day. Finally, sometimes a family member is extremely anti-abortion and lets his or her opinions fly at every family gathering. One woman stated her aunt was always picketing clinics and at the Thanksgiving meal tried to talk her into going by bus to march in Washington, D.C. Eliciting strategies to cope with impending, sensitive situations may be helpful to her.

Of course the best antidote to the attempts by others to inflict shame is strong self-esteem. In one counseling session there is no way to change a person's lack of self-esteem. However, you **can** teach her about self-talk and thought substitutions. You might ask, "What has your teacher said that resulted in your feeling bad?" She replies, "When she said abortion is a grave sin." You then ask, "When she said abortion is a grave sin, what did you think about yourself?" She replies, "I'm a terrible sinner." You again inquire, "When you think, `I'm a terrible sinner,' what could you tell yourself that would be comforting?" She answers, "I could tell myself everyone is a sinner, including the teacher," or "Jesus always forgives sinners," or "The Church thinks abortion is a sin, but God understands why I felt it was necessary." You can help her see there are numerous substitutes for the negative thoughts that provoke guilt and induce shame.

Let her know if she discovers her negative thoughts are overshadowing her comforting thoughts, she can use the counseling referral you gave her. Using thought substitutions are only one way of fortifying herself against things people say to inflict guilt. Counseling will give her more options. She may also want to read more about the effects of negative and positive self-talk in the book, Feeling Good by David Burns.

Chapter Sixteen

The Abortion Procedure –
First Trimester

DESCRIPTION OF A FIRST TRIMESTER ABORTION

Clients need to know about the procedure, aftercare, and possible complications. Keep in mind there are variations from clinic to clinic, including who performs the abortion (nurse practitioner, physician's assistant, or physician). The following describes the abortion procedure at Hope Clinic and has been worded to avoid inaccurate, scary impressions.

"When the nurse calls you into the procedure room, you will find yourself in a room that looks like a doctor's exam room. The nurse will stand by your side throughout the entire procedure and will help you feel as comfortable as possible through the procedure. Let her know how she can best help you relax. What works for one person may not be helpful to another. Some women find comfort in holding her hand; some want her to tell them what the doctor is doing step by step; others prefer for her to chat with them about anything other than the abortion - their school, job, or children. Most women find the slow, deep breathing exercises relaxing and helpful, and the nurse will breathe along with you. Keep in mind the whole procedure only takes between five to 10 minutes.

You will be lying down on the table with your feet propped up in the foot rests (stirrups). You will have your blouse on and will be draped with a sheet from the waist down. You won't be able to see what the doctor is doing unless you make an effort to stretch your neck, so just lie in a relaxed position and focus on the nurse by your side.

The doctor will first do a pelvic exam to determine the length of pregnancy and position of the uterus. Although this exam takes but a few seconds, relax your abdominal muscles by taking a deep breath in and slowly exhale, and you will feel more comfortable.

The doctor will then apply an antiseptic solution to the outside of the vagina. This will kill germs and will feel cold but will not burn or sting. Then the same instrument that is used during a Pap smear (a speculum) will be gently inserted to hold open the vagina so the doctor can view the cervix. The cervix is the opening to the uterus (it's helpful to show a diagram of the cervix and uterus). If you breathe in slowly and exhale very slowly when the doctor inserts the speculum, it will not feel as uncomfortable as when you tense up. This is a good tip to remember the next time you have a Pap smear, too.

Once the speculum is in place, the doctor will apply the antiseptic to the cervix and then numb the cervical area with a local anesthetic. At this point you may feel a pinch or some pressure, and some women say they do not feel much of anything. This is especially true for those who are distracted by talking to the nurse. It only takes a minute or two for the anesthetic to take effect.

From there the doctor will open or "dilate" the cervix, making it wide enough to insert a small plastic tube called a vacurette (if the woman's pregnancy is between eight to 10 weeks, the width of the vacurette is approximately the size of the tip of a woman's little finger). While the doctor is dilating the cervix, you will probably feel some cramps. Most women describe the cramps as "uncomfortable;" some women say they are "mild" and others say the cramping is "painful." What helps is breathing slowly and steadily to relax the body and help stay focused. Dilating the cervix takes about a minute. Then you're ready for the last step.

This is the time the doctor slips the vacurette into the uterus through the opened cervix, attaches the vacurette to the tubing that is connected to the machine, and turns on the vacuum aspirator. When it is turned on, you will hear the motor – it's a good sound to listen for, because you know the procedure is more than halfway finished. You may feel a tugging sensation in addition to some cramping that will last about 60 seconds. Once again, the cramping varies - from mild to very strong, so continue your slow deep breathing with the nurse. After the doctor turns the aspirator off and removes the vacurette from the uterus, he/she checks to see if there is any tissue left. If so, then the doctor may slip the vacurette back into the uterus for a few seconds. The doctor will take a few more seconds to clean the inside of the vagina with a piece of gauze, then remove the speculum, and it's finished.

(At the Hope Clinic the doctor inserts a sterile tampon before removing the speculum, but this varies from clinic to clinic.)

You are then ready to sit up, wrap your sheet around you, and head for the recovery room. In the recovery room, you will be relaxing in a comfortable recliner. You may be experiencing cramps at this time because your uterus is contracting back to a normal, non-pregnant size. You may receive a pain pill for the cramps, and the nurse will take your blood pressure and pulse, and offer you some refreshments. Your stay in the recovery room is about one hour. During that time, the nurse will check your bleeding and ask about any cramping you have. During recovery, your cramps will probably go away, and by the time you are ready to leave, you should feel fine. You might still have some cramping, but it should be manageable and not painful. You will probably be bleeding, but the flow should be moderate, not heavy.

Most people are amazed how well they feel afterwards. And while some women do report the procedure was painful, it is more common to hear women saying the procedure was not as bad as they expected.

POSSIBLE COMPLICATIONS AND AFTERCARE INSTRUCTIONS

The following is Hope Clinic's combined written and verbal description of possible complications and symptoms we want our patients to be aware of after the abortion. We stress the importance of calling back and talking to our doctor if they notice these symptoms. Aftercare instructions vary to some degree from clinic to clinic. The patient should follow the instructions of the doctor who performed her abortion.

We tell our patients that with every medical procedure, from a tooth extraction to open heart surgery, there are always possible complications. A first trimester abortion is a very safe procedure. Complications following an abortion are POSSIBLE, but NOT PROBABLE, especially if the doctor is experienced and if she follows her aftercare instructions to the letter. Here are some signs she needs to watch for. ANYTIME she has a question or suspects a problem we ask that she PLEASE CALL US.

Hemorrhaging

Some women bleed after the abortion; others do not. Some bleed a few days; others spot off and on for two weeks. Some pass small blood clots. Cramping is not uncommon. All of this is normal. What is not normal is if she is bleeding "too much." This means soaking three or more pads in an hour's time, non-stop, and/or passing bright red blood clots. Bleeding this heavily is defined as "hemorrhaging." She needs to CALL US to check it out. She is given a 24-hour emergency line to use when the clinic is closed (after hours or Sundays), so she ALWAYS has access to our doctor.

We want her to talk with OUR doctor before she calls any other doctor, hospital, or clinic. Other doctors who are not experienced in performing abortions will not be able to give her the same kind of knowledgeable answers to her questions. They lack the experience and expertise of our doctors who specialize in abortion care. Possible causes of hemorrhage can include perforation or "tear" in the uterus, or incomplete abortion where fragments of tissue remain in the uterus. The solution lies in having an OB-GYN (preferably the abortion clinic doctor) do a pelvic exam and ask the patient questions to help determine the cause. The solution will depend upon the cause.

Infection

Another possible complication is infection. Signs to watch for include running a temperature of 100.4 or higher, having a foul-smelling vaginal discharge, and/or severe abdominal pains that may or may not be accompanied by fever. An infection, if left undiagnosed and untreated, can result in septicemia (blood poisoning) or sterility. If she experiences any of these symptoms, she needs to CALL US IMMEDIATELY. She can help prevent an infection by following these instructions:

1. Don't have sexual intercourse or douche for two weeks.

2. Take the antibiotics we have prescribed as directed until the capsules are gone.

3. Our doctors prefer that our patients use sanitary pads. For first trimester abortion, they may use tampons, but they must not use tampons that don't come with an applicator. We do NOT permit the use of tampons after a second trimester abortion, however, because the cervix has been dilated wider and the risk of infection is increased.

4. She may take tub baths or showers.

Missed Abortion

Another possible complication is a "missed abortion." A "missed abortion" occurs when the embryo is missed and the woman is still pregnant after the abortion. Although rare, this can happen and is one of the reasons why it is so important she has a post-abortion check-up. Signs of a missed abortion are symptoms of pregnancy and an en-

larged uterus, which a doctor can detect by a pelvic exam. There are several reasons why an abortion might fail: 1). If the pregnancy was earlier than seven weeks, the embryo may be too small to be detected, so the doctor may not know for sure if the abortion was complete. At Hope Clinic the tissue is sent to a pathology lab at the end of the day, and the lab contacts us immediately if there were no products of conception present. We would then contact the patient. 2). Another reason is if the pregnancy is in the fallopian tube. This is called an "ectopic" pregnancy. The patient would be told immediately if this was suspected. 3). If there is a twin pregnancy that is not known at the time of the abortion, it is possible for one embryo to remain in the uterus. At the two-week checkup, the doctor could tell she was still pregnant, and she would need to call us right away. 4). Sometimes a woman has an abnormal uterine or cervical structure that makes it difficult to remove the embryo. These and other unusual cases may cause the abortion procedure to be unsuccessful. The solution would be repeating the procedure (at no additional expense to the patient).

Incomplete Abortion

An incomplete abortion is one in which there are some fragments of tissue left in the uterus. Signs of incomplete abortion are usually prolonged spot-bleeding past two weeks, hemorrhage, infection, or severe cramping. The solution is to return to the clinic and have the vacuum aspiration procedure repeated at no expense to the patient.

This is perhaps the most common of all the possible complications, although it still occurs in only 1% of the cases. Even an experienced doctor can miss a tiny fragment of tissue. Our doctor uses an instrument that looks like a long-handled spoon called "a curet" to feel the walls of the uterus immediately after the vacuum aspiration. The doctor can usually tell if all the products of conception have been removed. Even when the doctor checks the tissue afterwards, nobody can be 100% certain there are no small fragments left. Again, she needs to call the clinic if she is experiencing the symptoms.

Laceration Or "Tear" Of The Cervix

The doctor would be aware immediately dur-

105

ing the procedure if the cervix was torn. This can happen if the patient moves suddenly on the table. A tear can occur from the instrument (called "tenaculum") that holds the cervix and uterus while the doctor dilates the cervix. The solution would be a stitch or two to close the tear immediately following the procedure.

Reaction To The Local Anesthetic

Although exceedingly rare, some individuals may have a severe reaction to the local anesthetic, such as convulsion, shock, or cardiac arrest. Our doctors and nurses know what to do in these situations. While possible, it is highly unlikely to occur, especially if she has had a local anesthetic before (in a dentist's office, most likely) and had no adverse reaction.

Perforation Or "Tear" Of The Uterus

Another rare complication is a perforation, which is a puncture or tear in the uterus. If she lies still during the abortion without making sudden movements with her hips, the doctor can work as safely as possible. In this way she can help keep the risk of a perforation very small.

The signs of a perforation are excessive bleeding, drop in blood pressure, and sometimes abdominal pain. The doctor may be able to tell immediately during the procedure if a perforation occurred, but if it is a small tear, it may not be symptomatic until the patient is in the recovery room. Symptoms in the recovery room can include low (and dropping) blood pressure, pale complexion, continuous heavy bleeding, and sometimes heavy cramping. The solution may include an overnight stay in a hospital for observation. If the perforation is small, it will heal by itself like a scratch on the skin heals. However, if large enough, it may need stitches. And if the perforation is so large that hemorrhaging occurs, the uterus may need to be removed to save the patient's life.

To keep this in perspective, remember serious perforations are extremely rare (less than 1%), especially since abortion is legal and performed by competent physicians. Perforations were common during the days of illegal abortion, as were the other complications. Also, there is a 30 times greater chance that a woman would need major surgery during childbirth (C-section) than she would during an abortion (Hern, 1990).

Resuming Physical Activities

She does not need bedrest after an abortion. Of course, she shouldn't start a gymnastics class or join a weight lifting course immediately after an abortion, but any physical activity she is used to, she can resume immediately. She may go back to work or school the next day following the abortion.

Cramping

Cramping is normal after an abortion because the uterus needs to contract back to a non-pregnant, normal size. Some women have mild cramps or none at all. Others experience cramping that is easily relieved by pain pills from one to seven days after the abortion. What is NOT normal is severe cramping that is unrelieved by the pain medication we have prescribed. In that case, she needs to call us RIGHT AWAY. Possible causes include incomplete abortion, perforation, a retroverted (tilted backwards) uterus, or P.A.S.

P.A.S. (Post-Abortion Syndrome)

Sometimes blood pools in the uterus, forms large clots, and then the uterus contracts hard to push out the clots. This is called P.A.S. (Post-Abortion Syndrome) and can be very uncomfortable. Solutions include taking pain pills, firmly massaging the lower abdomen, and allowing the uterus to continue to push out the clots, or coming back to the clinic to let the doctor remove the clots with the vacuum aspirator.

For a more extensive list and explanation of all possible complications, read Dr. Hern's book, Abortion Practice (1990).

Death

First trimester abortion is 18 times safer than childbirth. The average mortality rate for a first trimester abortion (6–12 weeks) is .36 per 100,000 and for childbirth 6.6 per 100,000. (Henshaw, 1990).

Chapter Seventeen

Helping Clients Manage Pain
And Fear Of Pain

"WILL IT HURT?" RESULTS OF TWO STUDIES ON WOMEN'S REPORTS OF PAIN DURING AN ABORTION

One of the first questions women ask about the procedure is, "Will it hurt?" The most accurate answer to the question may be "Some women say it does hurt and others say it does not. Many women describe it as `uncomfortable' rather than `painful.'"

Preterm Clinic Study

In a study of 2,000 first trimester abortion patients at the Preterm Clinic in Massachusetts, 46% reported "moderate" pain, 32% reported "severe pain," 20% reported feeling less than "moderate" pain, and only 2% reported "very severe" pain. These patients had received no other medication than a local anesthetic of 20 ml. 1% Lidocaine (Stubblefield, M.D., 1989).

Hope Clinic Study

In 1993 Hope Clinic conducted a pain survey of 900 patients. Our purpose was to determine which drug or combination of drugs had the most effect on reducing pain during a first trimester procedure:
- Valium taken by mouth pre-operatively
- Valium pre-operatively plus intravenously-

administered Nubain (non-narcotic muscle-relaxer and pain reliever)
- Orudis (pain pill) and Valium pre-operatively
- Orudis and Valium pre-operatively and Nubain I.V. push.
- Darvocet (narcotic pain pill) and Valium pre-operatively and Nubain I.V. push. (A local anesthetic of 10 ml. 1% Lidocaine was used in all cases.)

We offered the medications in each of the above categories for a two-week period and then switched to the next category for the next two weeks, and so on. However, we always allowed our patients to decide if they wanted: 1). no drugs; 2). only pre-operative medications; or 3). Nubain as well as pre-op drugs. Because we did not want to deprive our patients of their choice of pain management, we had no control group, and no randomly assigned categories. In addition, for a variety of reasons there was not an equal number of subjects in each category.

The patients were not told before their procedure that we were conducting a pain survey. At the end of their recovery time (one hour), the nurse asked them to fill out a questionnaire. A few patients declined, and it was not forced upon them. In the questionnaire, patients were asked to indicate whether they felt relaxed, pretty calm, nervous, or very nervous right before the procedure; and they marked the statement that most closely described the level of discomfort they felt during the procedure.

We discovered that 64% of the people who perceived themselves as "pretty calm" or "relaxed" chose both the pre-operative medications and the Nubain. Of the people who reported they were "nervous" or "very nervous," 77% chose both the pre-op medications and the Nubain. Of the total population, 72% chose the Nubain along with the pre-op medications. So, when given the choice, the majority chose to take extra medications to manage pain.

The majority of the total population (62%) described the procedure as "uncomfortable but not painful" regardless of the drugs they received. Of all the categories of medications used, one resulted in the most significant reduction of pain: the combination of Valium and Nubain. However, more Valium was NOT more effective in pain reduction.

Another significant (but not surprising) finding emerged from our study. When people perceived themselves as "pretty calm" or "relaxed," they reported less pain **regardless of the category of drug combinations** than those who said they were "nervous" or "very nervous." The majority of the calm group described the procedure as "uncomfortable but not painful." There was no significant difference in perceived comfort between the calm patients who took all the drugs we offered and those who only took a Valium. Sixty-three to 67% described the abortion as "uncomfortable but not painful."

For the nervous group (including the "very nervous") the combination of Valium and Nubain reduced pain more effectively than the other combinations of drugs in this study. The majority (60%) of the nervous group who chose the Nubain combination described the procedure as "uncomfortable but not painful." When nervous women did not choose the Nubain, only 50% described the procedure as "uncomfortable but not painful." The other 50% reported the abortion to be "painful" or "extremely painful."

Keeping the flaws of the study in mind, it appears that the key to pain reduction is relaxation. And for those who cannot relax, Nubain

and Valium affords some pain relief.

Another effective combination we have tried since this study is Versed (derivative of Valium) and Nubain. Other providers have reported effective relaxation and pain relief with this combination, too.

THE EXPERIENCE OF PAIN

People's perception of what they feel varies and is closely linked to the way they manage their fear of pain. When fear increases, muscles tense up and everything they feel may be intensified.

Observations of women's reactions during an abortion support the research on pain that concludes there are three components to the experience of pain: physical, emotional, and cognitive. During an abortion, the woman may feel the physical pressure from the speculum, the pinch of local anesthetic, or the cramping during dilation and aspiration. Those women who are thinking and saying, "I can't stand pain and I can't relax" generally appear to feel more pain than those women who think and say, "I know I can put up with this for five minutes" and make conscious efforts to use various relaxation and distraction techniques.

THE CONNECTION BETWEEN GUILT AND PAIN

I have witnessed the powerful connection between severe guilt and a painful abortion procedure. The woman who is visibly upset in pre-abortion counseling, expresses extreme guilt and remains upset throughout the session is likely to experience pain and be uncooperative in helping herself relax during the abortion. This can occur even when she vehemently says she wants the abortion. Our experience with these patients led Hope Clinic to establish a policy of having extremely distraught patients reschedule their procedure on another day after the counseling session. On the day they return, they are remarkably more resolved in their feelings about their decision and calmer about the actual procedure itself. We do not reschedule **every** patient who expresses guilt...only those who seem extremely distraught, inconsolable, terrified, and self-punishing. One woman I talked to years after her abortion said she "made the abortion worse than it needed to be." She said she felt so guilty she thought she should "suffer and pay the price, so I tensed up and made it worse for myself." Another woman told me she had talked herself into a state of terror thinking she was going to die on the table for committing "the sin of abortion." She described herself as a devout Catholic. She had also been subjected to tales of horror by one of the anti-abortion pregnancy testing centers.

INTERVENTIONS FOR MANAGING PAIN

Emotion, thoughts, and sensation can keep snowballing and increasing pain unless there is some form of intervention (Barber et al, 1982, Worthington et al, 1981). Interventions that help manage pain include anesthesia, pain relievers and muscle relaxers, breathing exercises, mental imagery, distraction, focusing on something else, knowing what to anticipate, hypnotic suggestions of comfort, positive reinforcement, and the human touch. At Hope Clinic we use a variety of these techniques.

Pain Relievers And Muscle Relaxers

We continue to search for medications that are safe, effective, fast-acting, inexpensive, have few side effects, and wear off quickly for easy recovery. To date we have not found the ideal drug that fulfills all six criteria, but we are still actively searching.

Keeping abreast of research in the field of abortion and in the area of analgesia (pain relief) is important. One study administered 275 mg. of Naproxin (Anaprox) by mouth one hour before a first trimester procedure showed a significant reduction in pain (Suprato and Reed, 1984). However, the study advises caution because uterine contractions may be reduced and thus it may possibly cause uterine atony (the uterus won't contract properly and hemorrhaging can result). Hemorrhaging did not emerge as a problem in this study.

Another study compared the effects of using local anesthetic only, local plus i.v. sedation, local plus pre-operative instructions on what sensations to expect during the abortion, and local plus i.v. sedation and the pre-operative instructions (Wells, 1992). Those women who had the i.v. sedation (Valium and Fentanyl) reported less pain, regardless of receiving pre-operative information on what sensations to expect. However, those

women who received the sensory information appeared more cooperative during the procedure, and the physician was able to complete the procedure more quickly.

For more information on using medications for pain and relaxation, see the articles, "Sedation and Analgesia Options for 1990" by David Robinson, M.D. and "Control of Pain for Women Undergoing Abortion" by Phillip Stubblefield, M.D., printed in the 1990 National Abortion Federation publication, Pain is a Four Letter Word: Minimizing Patient Discomfort. To purchase this publication, write to National Abortion Federation, 1436 U Street, NW, Suite 103, Washington, D.C. 20009.

Anesthesia

Local Anesthesia

A paracervical block (injecting a local anesthetic such as Lidocaine into the cervix), is normally used to reduce the pain of dilating the cervix. However, the block is not able to deaden all the nerves affected during an abortion. To try and block all the nerves would risk puncturing and tearing the uterine artery and vein and the ovarian artery and vein (Stubblefield, 1989). The local anesthetic helps reduce pain but cannot eliminate all pain during an abortion. The patient is awake when given a local anesthetic, thus reducing the risk of heart and respiratory failure associated with general anesthesia. Some patients say the local "hurts" like a pinch or a stick, some say it feels like pressure, and others hardly feel anything.

The way in which the local is administered and the time the physician allows it to work can greatly affect the level of pain felt during the abortion (Stubblefield, 1989). E. Glick, M.D. described his technique for administering a paracervical and lower uterine field block anesthesia at the 11th conference of the National Abortion Federation in Salt Lake City, Utah, in 1987. He modified the way in which the block is given to further reduce the pain from stimulation of the vacurette during the abortion. Phillip Stubblefield, M.D. describes Glick's technique in detail in his article, "Control of Pain for Women Undergoing Abortion," cited above.

The amount of Lidocaine used also has an

effect on pain. One study showed patients receiving 150 mg. of Lidocaine experienced less pain than those who received 100 mg. of Lidocaine. In the same study when the physician waited five minutes after administering the Lidocaine, the patient experienced less pain than if the physician waited less than five minutes (Stubblefield, 1989).

General Anesthesia

Many women ask, "Can I be knocked out?" Some abortion providers offer general anesthesia. They report the majority of women want this option. However, many clinics do not provide general anesthesia because of the two to four times greater risk of death (Peterson, Grimes, Cates, Jr., and Rubin, 1981). Using local anesthesia rather than general greatly reduces the risk of uterine perforation, cervical injury and the need for blood transfusion, cervical suture, and major surgery (Grimes, Schulz, and Cates, Jr. 1979, Hern, W. M., 1990). The relative safety of a general anesthetic depends on the expertise of the anesthetist, the health of the patient, the type and dosage of the medications used, and knowledge of the patient's medical history.

There are times when the only way a patient can undergo an abortion is with a general anesthetic. The patient who moves uncontrollably on the table during the speculum insertion even when heavily sedated and given adequate time to compose herself is not a safe candidate for a local anesthetic. This is a patient who needs a general anesthetic.

Referring for a General Anesthetic

Occasionally, a client must be referred for a general anesthetic and reassured that some women simply require a general. She certainly does not need to feel "bad" about not getting through it awake. Most of the patients who need a general are very young - under 15 years of age - and they often feel ashamed they couldn't get through it. Their parents are often disappointed and upset and need the same reassurance that their daughter is not odd or bad for not getting through it. You need to know where the closest clinics are that provide abortions under general anesthesia.

MANAGING FEAR OF PAIN

People who are terrified of pain usually make statements like, "I'm a big baby. I can't stand pain. I won't be able to hold still. I'm scared stiff." The underlying fear is that they will lose control because the pain will be too intense. To help them, you can assert that they CAN stay in control during the procedure, they just need to be equipped with a good strategy. Just as a person needs to be equipped with a boat to sail on a lake, people need to be equipped with strategies for staying in control.

Pleasant Imagery, Relaxation, And "Analgesic Imagery"

A number of studies have been conducted to determine which cognitive strategies offer the most help in increasing one's pain tolerance and pain threshold. In several of these studies, the use of pleasant imagery has been shown to increase a sense of control and reduce feelings of helplessness (Meichenbaum and Turk, 1976) and increase tolerance to a painful stimulus (Avia & Kanfer, 1980, Grimm & Kanfer, 1976, and Worthington & Shumante, 1981). In the study by Worthington & Shumante, subjects who were trained in pleasant imagery had longer tolerance times for pain than those who were not trained in imagery. And when subjects created their own imagery, they experienced even greater pain tolerance and less self-reported pain than those who were told what to imagine. Furthermore, subjects who planned specific images ahead of time actually used the images in 82% of all instances. This contrasted with the subjects who had planned helpful self-talk but only used their strategy in 26% of the instances.

One study by Wells (1989) specifically researched management of pain during an abortion using three intervention strategies and one control group: 1). pleasant imagery; 2). relaxation techniques; and 3). analgesic imagery. One group of women were given 10 minutes of instruction and practice in pleasant imagery and were given the choice between a beach or mountain scene; the second group practiced rhythmic breathing and systematic muscle relaxation techniques, and the third practiced imagining numbness in their hand and in their uterus. A fourth group was asked to think about previous experiences of pain and apply former ways of coping with pain during the abortion procedure. The group using pleasant imagery had the lowest reported pain sensation and lowest distress scores. The group using analgesic imagery reported the highest rating of pain sensation and distress, even over and above the fourth control group.

Intervention For The Patient Who Cannot Tolerate The Procedure

At Hope Clinic if a patient cannot tolerate a pelvic exam or speculum upon first attempt, the doctor leaves the room and allows the nurse to help the patient relax. When the doctor returns and tries again, and the patient still cannot lie still, the patient is given the choice to get dressed and speak to a counselor or have a seat near the recovery room. If she chooses to sit by the recovery room, after 20 mintues or so has elapsed, she will be asked if she feels ready for her procedure. We will change doctors for a "fresh start." If she still is unable to relax enough for a safe procedure, she will be asked to get dressed and see a counselor. The counselor will give her the following options: she can return home, practice various relaxation techniques over the next few days and return to Hope Clinic; or she can receive a referral to a clinic that offers a general anesthetic. Those who choose to return are instructed to practice techniques for managing fear. They are taught slow deep breathing in conjunction with visualization, and/or a distraction technique. The counselor also talks to the support person who came with them, eliciting their understanding and support.

Visualizing A Successful Procedure

The counselor instructs the client to take some quiet time, find a comfortable place at home and take some slow deep breaths. The counselor demonstrates the breathing and asks her to practice with her. Then she is asked to imagine herself walking into the Hope Clinic and feeling relaxed, going up to the front desk and talking to the friendly receptionist, sitting in the waiting room knowing in a few minutes it will all be over with. At any time if she starts to feel tense, she is to take another deep breath and feel relaxed. She imagines the nurse or counselor helping her onto the cushioned table, she hears her talking to her in a soothing tone, and the warmth of her hand holding hers. They are both breathing easily and slowly together. When the doctor comes in, she knows he will expertly and safely perform her abortion. Breathing slowly and easily, she will relax all her muscles. In a few seconds the pelvic exam is over. She feels herself relaxing while the speculum is being inserted. When she feels anything uncomfortable, she breathes in and out slowly and easily and is able to take control back into her hands. She feels the cramping come and go. When she hears the aspirator's low humming, she knows she is almost finished. She feels the cramping but relaxes her muscles and knows it is almost over. The aspirator is turned off, and once she feels the speculum slip out, she feels relieved and confident that it is over, ready to relax in a comfortable recliner in the recovery room. She hears the doctor tell her it's over and everything went smoothly.

Pleasant Distraction Technique

Another way to prepare the patient for the procedure is to ask her to think of some place she'd love to be. Once she has described a very pleasant place or an activity she'd love to be engaged in, you can ask her to think about it in as much detail as possible. Ask her some questions about what she sees, hears, smells, and feels while in her special place. Suggest that she daydream about this place during the time she leaves the clinic and the time she returns. Let her know that she will be more in control, more comfortable, and successful in getting through the procedure while she is imagining herself in this place and talking to the nurse or counselor. The more senses involved and the more vivid the imagery, and the more powerful a distraction this image will be during the procedure.

ASSISTING THE WOMAN DURING THE PROCEDURE

Most people are nervous before undergoing any medical procedure. The goal of the assistant is to help the woman relax and stay in control. There are a number of ways to do this.

First, the assistant's general friendliness and warmth adds greatly to the patient's comfort level. Smiling, looking confident and at ease, and talking to her in a relaxed manner all set the tone.

There are a number of helping styles and techniques that may help the patient through the procedure. Everyone is different, so the more flexible you are, the better. **SOME** women:

1. Want the assistant to tell them what the doctor is doing every step of the way.

2. Don't want to know what the doctor is doing because it makes them more uneasy.

3. Want to know when they are likely to feel something uncomfortable, but not every step of the procedure.

4. Don't want to hear anything about the procedure and prefer to listen or talk to the assistant about anything else.

5. Want quiet to concentrate by themselves.

6. Want to hold hands and appreciate the assistant's touch.

7. Dislike holding hands or other touch.

8. Are adept at visualizing something pleasant and talking about it.

9. Are easy talkers and keep themselves distracted by talking about a vacation they took, a hobby they enjoy, their kids, etc.

10. Prefer to listen to relaxing music on headphones.

11. Focus on a picture on the ceiling above them.

12. Are intent on helping themselves by following whatever the assistant suggests to them.

You can elicit their preference for what will probably help them while they are in the counseling session and make sure the information is passed along to whoever assists them in the procedure room. Or the assistant can ask her for her preferences.

Many people regress to a childlike state when they are feeling vulnerable or are in pain. However, it is a disservice to them to infantilize them by calling them sweetie or honey or talking in a tone of sympathy. Treating them respectfully, empathically, and speaking in a positive, confident manner helps to offset their feeling of vulnerability.

GIVING THE PATIENTS CHOICES

Some people will already know what will help them cope with pain and fear of pain and simply

need the assistant in the procedure room to follow their lead. Others haven't the foggiest idea of how to help themselves relax. Suggesting a few of the ideas presented above and letting them choose what they would like to try will probably have more success than imposing the best theoretical strategy.

Chapter Eighteen

Clients Who Pose A Challenge

THE CLIENT WHO SPEAKS NO ENGLISH

Occasionally the counselors at The Hope Clinic see clients who do not speak English. Due to our location in the Midwest, these clients are few in number. Those we do see are usually Asian. At the time of the appointment we require that they bring someone who can interpret for them. They usually bring their husband or a friend who has a **little** better grasp of the English language than they do. Sometimes the client's husband and she both state she can't speak English, but once in the counseling session, it is revealed that she can understand more than she can speak. In one of my sessions I learned the woman could not speak English but could read and spell enough to enhance our communication together with the interpreter. Communicating with non-English-speaking clients can include using pictures, visual aids, simple English, drawing, and increased use of nonverbals that may at times resemble mime or charades. Communicating does **not** include the natural tendency to speak louder and louder when she or the interpreter doesn't comprehend. Louder isn't clearer.

When clinics are located where a significant number of clients are from a specific ethnic culture, they usually hire at least some bilingual staff. They may also enhance their staff's knowledge about cultural differences in beliefs about abortion and gynecological practice by inviting a guest speaker. For instance, one client from a small town in India appeared mortified to learn a male doctor would be performing the abortion. I offered to find her a clinic that had a female doctor on staff, but she wanted to get the abortion over with that day. I did not minimize her anguish, but empathized with her embarrassment. Then we made a pact that she would just look at me and the female nurse during the procedure. When we were in the procedure room and the doctor walked in, she instinctively threw the sheet over her face. Periodically, she lifted the sheet just enough to see our faces as we talked in soothing tones. We knew it didn't matter what we said, but the sound of our voices, facial expressions and holding her hand meant everything.

In pre-abortion counseling, it is helpful if you have a film of the procedure, but even if you don't, you can still convey the process to her in ways she can understand. When describing the actual procedure, it is important to speak in simple terms and pause after every other sentence, asking the interpreter to explain to the client what you've just said. Deliberately refrain from using idioms, local expressions, and medical terminology. This requires you to think about every word you utter. For instance, when explaining the local anesthetic or relaxing medications, don't say "You won't be knocked out." The term, "knocked out" is not readily understood. Instead, say, "You will be awake during the abortion." If you do use a term or expression that draws a look of confusion from the client or interpreter, you can use that visual cue to further clarify. Using a number of facial expressions and gestures helps include the client, even if she speaks no English at all.

Use your sense of drama when describing anything she doesn't seem to understand. For one second-trimester Korean client and her husband, I described "I.V. medication" in mime or "charades." I outlined the pole, bag of fluids, and tube in the air and acted out the pleasant transformation that occurs once the relaxing medications enter the bloodstream of a nervous person. They watched intently, then exclaimed, "Oh yes, yes!," laughing in recognition. On another occasion I was asked what was the difference between "cramps" and "pain." So I held my abdomen and frowned for "cramps" and then grimaced and doubled over, clasping my middle for "pain." Again, the reaction was laughter and nodding up and down.

I have discovered that most non-English speaking people do not recognize the word, "cramps." To convey this term, I usually ask if she ever has pain during her period (they usually know what "period" means). I then let her know "pain on period" is called "cramps." If she has never felt menstrual cramps before but has had a baby, I will refer to pain during childbirth as "big pain" and pain during an abortion as "smaller pain." I definitely want these clients to be prepared for some pain, so they won't panic if they feel pain they were not anticipating.

Another term most non-English speaking people do not recognize is "tampon" simply because they have never used or seen one. I keep one in my office to show them. Many understand the term, "sanitary napkin" but not "pad."

Regarding birth control, most of our foreign clients know what "condoms" are, but some know it by the word "prophylactics." Many know about the Pill but have never used it. I have yet to see recognition of the diaphragm, IUD, or spermicides. One couple I saw had no comprehension of any of the methods I showed them. They did not even understand the term, "birth control" or "contraception." Finally, I asked them, "In your country, when a man and woman want to have sex but do not want to make a baby, what do they do?" He looked at her, said something to

her, and they started to laugh. She covered her face with her hand in embarrassment, laughing, and he said "sex only on period." I asked if they had tried to use that method this time, and he said, "Sometimes," grinning. I knew that explaining the details of rhythm was beyond me under the circumstances, so I settled for a little reflection: "So it doesn't always work." I asked, "Would you like something that DOES work so she won't get pregnant?" The response was a strong affirmative. I was lucky enough to find a doctor in our referral file who spoke their language, so I gave them strict instructions not to have sex at all until after the two-week checkup and after they talked with this doctor. I gave them a note to give the doctor at the checkup.

Had this couple spoken Chinese, Laotian, Vietnamese, Thai, Arabic, Persian, or Spanish, I would have been able to give them a birth control booklet entitled **How To Have Intercourse Without Becoming Pregnant. These** booklets are available from Alliance for Perinatal Research and Services, Inc., 321 South Pitt Street, Alexandria, VA 22314, 703/765-6300.

The general idea when communicating with a client and her interpreter is to take it slowly, think before speaking, and express yourself non-verbally as much as possible. At the end of your counseling session, both the interpreter and the client need to sign the consent forms for the abortion. Their signatures indicate that the woman understands the procedure and possible complications.

THE ABUSED WOMAN

Potential For Post-Abortion Depression And Guilt

When a woman is engaged in an abusive relationship, her chances for experiencing depression and guilt after the abortion may be increased. Many of the conditions inherent in abusive relationships have been linked with reports of depression and guilt following an abortion: isolation and lack of support, low self-esteem, lack of reciprocal love, and pervasive feelings of shame and guilt (Mosley, Fillingstad, Harley, and Heckel, 1981, Payne, Kravitz, Notman, and Anderson, 1976, Joy, 1985). It is important that this client has strong support from a friend or reliable family member and that you give her a counseling referral.

The Abuser's Behaviors And Responses To The Pregnancy And Abortion

An abusive man attempts to isolate his partner from her friends and family in his effort to control her feelings, thoughts, opinions, and behaviors. Among his arsenal of manipulations to control his partner are implied or real threats, physical and/or emotional abuse, and double messages of love and hate. If his partner has an abortion, it may become a favorite piece of ammunition in his relentless attacks on her self-worth and womanhood. An abusive man often deliberately instigates sex without contraception, wanting her to become pregnant. He may cajole her into having unprotected sex or rape her.

The abuser's response to the resulting pregnancy may be any of the following: 1). insisting she carry to term to form greater ties between them; 2). rejecting both her and the potential child; 3). demanding she have an abortion; or 4). alternating between rejecting the pregnancy and wanting her to carry to term. The latter can increase the woman's ambivalence, which is another factor linked to post-abortion depression and guilt (Payne et al, 1976).

When the woman chooses to have an abortion under threat of abuse, she may feel coerced and view herself as "having no choice." When feelings of coercion exist, a high potential for post-abortion regret exists (Bracken, Klerman, & Braken, 1978). During the interviews I conducted with women years after their abortions, those who described the most traumatic reactions, including deep regret, were invariably abused or neglected as children and some became pregnant by an abusive partner.

Even when a woman states her abusive partner agrees with the abortion decision, he cannot be relied upon for support afterwards, no matter what the appearances are at the time of the abortion. All too frequently an abuser bides his time and then uses the abortion as a club to beat down whatever shred of self-esteem she still possesses. In his arsenal of weapons to tyrannize and shame her as a woman, an abortion can be one of the most powerful. His accusing her of "murdering **his** child" or "killing her baby" and labeling her an "unfit mother" can rip through her sense of womanhood. Many abused women feel worthless to begin with, and he simply reinforces her belief.

Instead of or in addition to his accusations of murder, he may tearfully tell her he really wanted the baby, even after he provided the impetus for the abortion. In this case, she may feel doubly bad for hurting the man she loves and "killing their baby."

Because of an abused woman's increased risk for depression, guilt, and shame after her abortion, it is important to discover whether or not the client seeking an abortion is in an abusive relationship. The client will seldom tell you directly, but some clues will be sprinkled throughout her dialogue. The following are red-flag statements revealing the probability of an abusive relationship. After each quote is a brief explanation why the statement indicates an abusive relationship. Keep in mind not everyone who makes such statements is an abused woman; rather, these statements warrant further exploration.

Client Statements Indicating An Abusive Relationship

1. **"He told me it wasn't his."** Abusers refuse to accept responsibility for their own actions and habitually blame others for their behavior.

2. **"He'd kill me if he knew I was having an abortion."** Abusers are prone to violent outbursts of anger, especially when their partners step out of the bounds of their control. If she does something he doesn't want to happen, he feels a loss of control over her and explodes.

3. **"He has a temper."** Abusers have a short fuse. What might **annoy** one man will **enrage** an abuser. His temper flares up quickly and appears uncontrollable in its intensity.

4. **"He didn't want to come today because he was too tired. Last night he went drinking with his buddies."** OR **"He dropped me off and went to a tavern."** Abusers are often addicted to alcohol or other drugs and will "party" and drink when under stress. It also provides a chronic excuse for inexcusable behavior ("I couldn't help it - I was drunk.")

5. **"I didn't tell him about the pregnancy because he'd make me keep it."** An abuser often impregnates his partner deliberately, thinking a child will bind her to him. Abusers also threaten "I'd never let you kill a kid of mine! You'll never

115

have an abortion. I'll see to it you have the kid!" The issue is control.

6. **"He doesn't mean to do those things. I'm the one who starts the fights."** An abused woman often vacillates between complaining about his ill treatment and defending him. She accepts blame for his behavior and believes his accusations that he wouldn't behave badly if only she didn't provoke him.

7. **"He won't take NO for an answer."** A reply like this in response to your instructing her not to have sex for two weeks after the abortion spells trouble. Abusers often use sex as a way of controlling and humiliating their partners. Rape is common. On the other side of the coin, sex with him can also be the only time she feels close to him and loved. After a fight, making up often involves passionate lovemaking. Saying no to him for two weeks may seem an interminably long time.

8. **"I want to keep the baby, but I don't want to make him mad."** Here she is pacifying him to avoid his anger at the expense of her own desires. Asking what he does when he gets angry will help clarify if he is abusive. Throwing things at her, hitting, punching, shoving, grabbing, kicking, or breaking things (especially her treasures) are all signs of abuse. However, so are behaviors such as belittling, name-calling, verbally threatening harm, threatening to leave (especially if she depends on his income for her survival), or threatening to harm her loved ones, including her pets.

9. **"When we first met he treated me great! Now he seems to be changing. Sometimes he acts nice to me and other times he's really mean."** This is a description of the Dr. Jekyll-Mr. Hyde phenomenon so characteristic of abusers. They behave romantically and attentively, lavishing gifts and attention. This part of the abuse cycle is called "the honeymoon phase" and is followed by a deterioration of their mood and behavior. Criticisms, accusations, and eruption of abuse occur in the next phase followed by some form of repentance and empty promises "never to do it again." The cycle begins again when the woman forgives and they make up.

10. **"He is so jealous. He always thinks men are looking at me and I'm flirting with them. He even calls me at work to see if I'm there. He doesn't even want me to spend time with my** **family or friends."** Extreme jealousy, paranoia, and possessiveness are all characteristics of abusers. The issue of control is at the root of this behavior.

11. **"He told me it's all my fault I got pregnant."** This is a common statement and indicates his lack of responsibility and tendency to place all blame on her.

12. **"He threw my pills away," "He said he was using a condom, but he wasn't," "He said he'd pull out, but he didn't,"** or **"Afterwards he told me he poked holes in the condom."** These are statements that indicate his deliberate attempt to impregnate her against her will.

13. **"He had a rough life as a child, and his Dad used to beat up on him,"** or **"He's rich and spoiled by his parents. He always gets his way and knows he can have any woman he wants."** or **"He only does these things because..."** Abusers **are** often spoiled or abused as a child, and both the woman and the abuser use his past history as a way to excuse and rationalize his behavior.

14. **"Yes, we've broken up a lot of times before, but this time I really mean it!"** The relationship usually has numerous break-ups and make-ups. They are addicted to each other, and a final severing of ties is next to impossible without significant internal and external changes, as needed to end any addiction.

15. **"Even though he has done all these things to me, I still love him."** Again, the addiction she has to the relationship blocks her ability to leave him, except for short periods of time when they break up.

These are some of the most commonly made statements by abused women in the pre-abortion counseling session.

For an in-depth description of the characteristics of abusive men, abused women, and the dynamics of the relationship, read Susan Forward's book, <u>Men Who Hate Women and the Women Who Love Them.</u>

Counseling The Abused Woman In A Pre-Abortion Counseling Session

One of the priorities in any abortion clinic is the

patient's physical safety and well-being. An abortion is a surgery with possible complications, and women who are at high risk of physical abuse from a partner are also at high risk of incurring complications. For example, a woman whose partner will probably rape her right after the abortion procedure is at high risk of serious infection, especially if left untreated. A woman trapped inside the house with no access to treatment may wind up sterile from infected and scarred fallopian tubes or dead from septicemia (blood poisoning). The abortion counselor must assess the risk of sexual assault by asking if he has ever forced sex on her. What is his response if she says no to his sexual advances? If it appears she is at high risk, then they need to explore temporary shelter away from the abuser for at least one week after a first trimester abortion, and two weeks after a second trimester abortion to avoid risking uterine infection.

The woman is at risk of uterine hemorrhage if she is beaten shortly after the surgery. Special precautions should be taken if the woman is undergoing a second trimester abortion, since the risk of hemorrhage is greater than in first trimester. The first part of a second trimester procedure is the insertion of a sterile dilator (Laminaria, Dilapan, or Lamicel) that gradually opens the cervix overnight. The night of the laminaria insertion is particularly risky for a woman who is staying with her abuser. If he assaults her sexually or otherwise, the dilator could puncture her uterus, causing internal hemorrhage, shock, and possibly death. It is critical that the woman stay overnight with someone other than her abusive partner.

As a counselor in a one-time counseling session, you will probably have little or no impact on the woman's ability and motivation to leave an abusive partner permanently. Of course, your hope for her is to take care of herself. But if she is not emotionally ready to get help, you cannot impose help on her. What you can do is teach her ways to take care of herself after the abortion and thus minimize risks of serious complications. You need to let go of any goal to convince her to leave the abusive relationship. In letting go of this goal, you will be refraining from engaging in potentially controlling behavior. This does not mean you cannot make any impact on her life. While your goal needs to be the same as for any other client in the pre-abortion session, you can offer

three services that may be useful to her in the future.

1. You can give her information about abusive relationships. Once you hear a red-flag statement, ask more questions about his behavior. Extreme jealousy, attempts to isolate her from family and friends, the Jekyll-Hyde phenomenon, verbal abuse, and repeated break-ups and make-ups are as indicative of an abusive relationship as reports of physical violence. As you ask the questions, she will often look surprised and ask, "How do you know so much about him?" She may have thought her relationship with her partner was unique and is often surprised to discover there is a whole body of knowledge about abusive relationships. Knowledge CAN be powerful. It all depends on what she chooses to do with the knowledge.

2. You can offer referrals to shelters and counseling services specializing in abusive or addictive relationships. Your referrals MAY make a difference. It all depends on what she chooses to do with the referrals.

3. You can offer her empathy and humane treatment when her world has usually been filled with the opposite. Empathic and humane treatment nourishes the human spirit.

Anything else is icing on the cake. If by chance, the pre-abortion counseling session is her first encounter with a counselor, she MAY feel less fearful to seek the help she needs and see a counselor. If by chance, she has had one bad experience in counseling and finds the time she has spent with you satisfying, she MAY try counseling again with someone else.

She may feel empowered by the whole experience of taking back the control of her body. Even though abused women may be more likely to experience depression and guilt after an abortion than unabused women, it is not the case for every abused woman. One of the abused women in my interviews stated the relief she felt in knowing she would not have to be pregnant and not have to have another child outweighed her guilt. Twenty years after her abortion she told me, "I regret staying 15 years with that man, but I can't say I ever regretted the abortion!" More research is needed in this area to determine what factors enable some abused women to cope well after an abortion and cause others to cope poorly.

THE CLIENT WHO HAS MORE THAN ONE ABORTION

Repeated Abortion: Is It Safe?

Most health professionals wonder what may be the possible effects of repeated abortion on subsequent pregnancies. Many family planning workers and clients fear irreparable damage to the reproductive organs that might render the woman sterile. Of course, the anti-abortion forces reinforce this fear by citing references to only those studies which support the contention. Many studies refute it, and the fact is a great deal of the research results are inconsistent.

In Abortion Practice (Hern, 1990), a thorough review of the literature on repeat abortion and subsequent pregnancy outcome reveals conflicting results. Twenty-three articles researching repeated abortion cited in Abortion Practice studied secondary infertility, ectopic pregnancy, miscarriage, premature delivery, and low-birth weight infants and congenital defects in subsequent pregnancies. Many, but not all, concluded there were no adverse affects from repeated abortion. Reasons for conflicting results from one study to the next included failure to control for confounding variables such as: 1). smoking and alcohol use during the subsequent pregnancy being carried to term; 2). maternal health factors; 3). method of abortion used; 4). method of cervical dilatation used; 5). time intervals between multiple abortions; 6). pregnancy order; 7). number of prior abortions; 8). first or second trimester prior abortions; 9). existence of post-abortion infection or other complication after one or more previous abortions; 10). prenatal care; and 11). maternal age, marital status, and socioeconomic status at time of delivery.

For instance, one study that showed no relation between a history of induced abortion and ectopic pregnancy revealed a five-fold increased risk of ectopic pregnancy for those women who had a post-abortion infection or retained tissue over those who had no such complications. Another study that controlled for method of abortion showed repeated D&C abortions DID produce an increased risk of subsequent miscarriage and low-birth-weight infants, whereas repeated vacuum aspiration abortions did not.

A large study of 6,541 women in the state of Washington from 1984-87 investigated the effect of one or more abortions on the risk of low birth weight (Mandelson, Maden, and Daling, 1992). This study controlled for the number of previous abortions and confounding variables such as smoking, maternal age, marital and socioeconomic status, and prenatal care. Results showed that women with four or more induced abortions tended to be older than women with one or no abortions, and were more likely to be unmarried and smokers. Older age, single marital status, and smoking increase a woman's risk of delivering an infant of low birth weight without her having a history of one or more abortions. Once these confounding effects were adjusted, results showed little, if any, increased risk of low birth weight with one or more abortions. There was also no evidence of increasing risk of low birth weight with increasing numbers of abortion.

What does this information mean to us and to women seeking another abortion? The most accurate and fair answer we can give to a woman who expresses concern about possible risks to future childbearing would be: "A lot of the research to date has shown conflicting results. Some research has associated repeated abortions with an increased risk of future miscarriage, premature birth and low-birth-weight. However, other recent studies have shown no increased risks for women with one or more abortions. What this means is that you MAY have an increased risk, but remember that a healthy pregnancy outcome also depends upon your age, general health, alcohol use, smoking, number of previous miscarriages, prenatal care and nutrition, pelvic structure, hormones, and number and interval of previous births. There are many more factors involved in a successful pregnancy outcome than previous abortion." She needs to ask herself if ANY possible risk is enough to change her mind about having another abortion.

Finally, the late Christopher Tietze, M.D., world renowned researcher and statistician in the field of abortion, summed up his perspective of repeated abortion sequelae research:

"While these data seem to indicate that having an induced abortion may increase women's risk of an adverse outcome in later pregnancies, we do not yet know to what extent, or how particular groups of

118

women (such as very young women, who have a higher risk of these problems, even without having an abortion) may be affected. In addition, the risks to subsequent pregnancy should be compared with the many documented health, social, and economic consequences, especially to a teenager, attendant upon carrying an unwanted birth to term. Further research is essential to clarify the degree of risk to subsequent pregnancies from D&C and from vacuum aspiration , and to pinpoint the mechanism of action, so that techniques which eliminate or at least minimize risks can be identified and developed. Meanwhile, we should remember that the replacement of illegal abortion by legal abortion has vastly decreased the risk of complications that include infertility, serious morbidity, and death..."

Are Repeat Clients Using Abortion As Birth Control?

There seems to be nothing that riles people more or raises their self-righteousness to loftier heights than the belief that women use abortion as birth control. How often do we hear the allegation that "all those women who have all those abortions are using it as birth control!"

I don't know who "all those women" are because after counseling thousands of women for 17 years, I have yet to see them. Let me lay the myth to rest and set the record straight: women who have more than one abortion are usually using a method of birth control MOST or SOME of the time, but just not ALL of the time or 100% perfectly. They sometimes THINK they're protected, but because of inadequate knowledge or something their doctor told them, they are not.

Most are exasperated with their fertility, birth control methods, and/or their risk-taking behavior (and their partner's), and are highly motivated to prevent another pregnancy. The only universal truth that can be said about women who have multiple abortions is that they are FERTILE.

Do Repeat Clients Differ From First-Time Clients?

The articles, "Repeat Abortion: Is It A Problem?" (1984) and "Abortion, Childbearing, and Women's Well-Being" (1992) were published in Family Planning Perspectives and provide some answers to the question, "Do repeat clients differ from first-time clients?"

In "Repeat Abortion: Is It A Problem?" the research took place in Canada at the Montreal General Hospital. Five hundred eighty women seeking abortions were interviewed to obtain the following information: age, marital status, number of abortions, education, socioeconomic status, religion, number of children, quality of relationship with partner, contraceptive use, and frequency of intercourse. A 240-item true/false inventory was administered to assess the patients' degree of emotional disturbance on 15 scales that measured incidence of insomnia, headaches, health concerns, hypochondriasis, somatic complaints, depression, self-deprecation, disorganized thinking, feelings of unreality, impulsivity, mood fluctuation, neurotic disorganization, panic reaction, and perceptual distortion. The results of the psychological tests and the demographic data were divided by one variable into two groups: those clients who had more than one abortion and those who were seeking their first abortion. The results from both groups were then compared. Women having more than one abortion were older, had more children, were slightly more educated, were less likely to be married than first-timers, and reported slightly less satisfactory relationships with their partners. In addition, the repeat clients were MORE likely to have used contraceptives at the time the pregnancy occurred than the first-time clients, and they engaged in intercourse more frequently than the first-timers. No other factors were statistically different between the two groups. The two most significant factors that differentiated the repeaters from the first-timers were age and frequency of sex. These two factors alone can create the probability that a fertile woman will have more than one unplanned pregnancy in her lifetime. The article concluded by stating:

"Thus, our study indicates that repeat abortions are not the consequence of women's psychological maladjustment or negative attitudes toward using contraceptives. The important problem is that health care personnel involved in providing abortions may find it difficult to accept that a large number of women who are sexually active and who use imperfect birth control techniques can be expected to have repeat abortions. The challenge rests in communicating these findings to those who work with abortion patients, so they may counsel these women with more confidence, knowing that repeat abortion is due more to probability of pregnancy than to psychological problems."

In "Abortion, Childbearing, and Women's Well-Being," a seven-year longitudinal study was conducted on 5295 American women and measured self-esteem scores on women who had one abortion, repeated abortions, no abortions, and one or more unwanted births.

Results showed self-esteem scores for women having multiple abortions (two or more) did not differ significantly from women who had one or no abortions. Women who had one or more unwanted births had significantly lower self-esteem scores than women who had one or more abortions. And women who had a greater overall number of births had significantly lower self-esteem than those who had fewer births.

Counseling The Client Who Has Had More Than One Abortion: Issues And Concerns

The following is a list of questions and concerns to explore with the client in the counseling session.

1. Discuss this pregnancy and abortion decision first, unless she immediately brings up her other abortion(s).

2. Acknowledge previous abortions and ask where they took place. There are differences among clinics in terms of medications, procedure, counseling, aftercare instructions, and staff professionalism and friendliness. Ask her to describe each abortion physically. If any of her experiences were painful, does she fear the same now? Let her know that she may experience each abortion very differently. If she fears pain, focus on relaxation tips for overcoming fear of pain (See Chapter 17, Managing Pain and Fear of Pain). Her emotional state, support system, and reasons for the abortion all affect how she experiences the abortion physically. Many women have described

very different pain levels with each abortion they experienced.

3. How did she feel emotionally after each abortion?

4. What did she do after her abortion that seemed to help her cope?

5. How are her circumstances different this time? How does she anticipate she'll feel emotionally after this abortion?

6. People often fear that the risk of complications increases with each abortion. The Center for Disease Control in Atlanta, Georgia has not found any increase in abortion-related complications for repeat patients. As long as she lies still on the procedure table for the doctor and follows the aftercare instructions, it is as unlikely for her to experience a complication as it would be for a first time patient.

7. Some people also fear that repeated abortions inevitably lead to sterility and complications in future childbirth. First, reassure her that having an abortion (with no complications) does not result in infertility. Do let her know this even if she doesn't ask. I have discovered that women sometimes neglect birth control after an abortion simply because they think they have become infertile. The "right-to-life" factions perpetuate this myth through their literature, sermons, and TV spots. Then give her the most recent research findings on the effects of repeat abortions on subsequent full-term pregnancies. Subscribing to Family Planning Perspectives is one way of keeping up on the latest world-wide abortion research. This journal can also be found in the serials departments of some university libraries.

8. Trace birth control history with each of her pregnancies (including those that resulted in miscarriages and full-term births). Were any of those pregnancies **planned**? Discuss any problems she or her partner has with birth control. Are there any patterns of risk-taking? Risk-taking includes omitting birth control periodically, using rhythm or withdrawal, or knowingly using the method incorrectly. If there is a history of repeated risk-taking, you may decide to point this out to her in a caring way: "Correct me if I'm off target, but it seems each pregnancy was a result of both you and your partner taking risks with your well-

being." Usually that kind of statement brings a moment of silence. The client has probably not thought about it in terms of both parties neglecting her well-being. She usually views it as something "stupid" she has done. Let her know that people do things that SEEM stupid for reasons they are not readily aware of. There are many reasons why people take risks with birth control even when they know they are fertile. For instance, some people take more risks with contraception when they are:

- Feeling depressed, lonely, or angry at themselves or others.

- Planning a career change or returning to school.

- Experiencing a loss in their lives, perhaps a death in the family.

- Going through a divorce or separation.

- Using alcohol or drugs.

- Seeing their friends or relatives having babies.

- Feeling tired of waiting for the right time in their lives to have a baby.

These are just a few possibilities. For a more thorough exploration of contraceptive risk-taking, see "Attitudes Toward People Taking Contraceptive Risks" in Chapter 2. Sometimes the client feels ready and willing to examine this area of her life. Depending on your time limitations, you can choose to explore this with her thoroughly or simply stimulate thought and refer her for further counseling.

- At some point, if she hasn't brought it up herself, ask her how she feels about having x number of abortions. For example, "Some women say this feels OK to them, others say they feel guilty or embarrassed. I'm wondering how YOU feel about it?" This lets her know she's not alone in her predicament and validates a variety of feelings.

There are a number of women who express feelings of guilt and loss of self-esteem. They are often thinking they can make ONE mistake, but more than once is unacceptable! Let them know

that most, if not all, human beings make mistakes more than once (unless they have reached sainthood). However, people will keep repeating history until they discover WHY they keep taking the same risks and find new ways of meeting their needs. Once they know the motives behind their actions, they can choose to change their behavior, unless they have an addiction. Changing an addictive behavior requires therapy.

Can she think back to each time she got pregnant and discover any patterns? Were the situations similar? I posed this question to one client who thought for a moment and then replied, "All of my abortions fall in the same month – August." Three years in a row from ages 16 through 28, she wound up pregnant in August. I questioned further, "Is there anything that happens repeatedly each summer?" She replied, "I run out of my prescription for the Pill, and I don't get it refilled." I asked, "Is there anything else that happens that might keep you from getting your pills refilled?" She replied, "Well ... my boyfriend returns to college out of state each August, and he always wants me to get married and go with him. I think I want to do that, but then I keep winding up thinking of my mother. I know she would never approve of that. Each time I get pregnant it's all the more reason for me to go with him. He always wants to keep the baby. But then after it's too late and I'm already pregnant, I just can't get myself to leave home and follow him." We then talked about her ambivalence toward leaving Mom and gaining independence, her ambivalence toward marrying this young man, and her conflicting desire to go to college and leave both of them. She was playing out the conflict of doing what her boyfriend wanted, doing what Mom wanted, and doing what she wanted in the ritual of forcing the issue with a pregnancy each summer. So far, three times running, Mom always won (and she didn't even know about any of the pregnancies).

We talked about ways she could handle the conflict:
- Continue to get pregnant again next summer and the summer after next.
- Talk to a good friend or preferably a counselor about her three-pronged conflict. Make a conscious decision about what to do without having to go through another pregnancy and abortion.
- Buy next year's calendar and write in red, "Watch out for pill prescription and getting pregnant" on the month in which it usually happens.

That way it will be no accident – she can make a conscious choice. I then referred her to a counselor to talk to after the abortion.

I have found that if the partner is the same in all the pregnancies, then "forcing commitment" is sometimes the issue. Each time one client got pregnant, she said she was hoping THIS time they could get married and have the baby. But each time he wasn't ready. The first time he wasn't yet out of school. The second time he felt he wasn't financially able to afford a new family. Each time she agreed with him, but the third time he had just bought a new truck and said they should wait until he could buy a house. Now he said he had too many bills. She said she was feeling foolish and angry. I asked how else she could check out his readiness to settle down without getting pregnant. She said, "I guess I could ask him WHEN will it ever be a good time?" I stated, "I can understand that confronting him head on is taking a risk of being rejected, and that's scary. I'm wondering what would feel less hurtful to you – hearing him say he may never be ready or finding out by going through another pregnancy and abortion?" There was silence and then she replied, "As much as I hate going through these abortions and as bad as I feel about it ... it would be worse to think he was rejecting ME than to think he was rejecting the pregnancy. Isn't that awful?" She broke down and cried. After awhile she told me she has been hanging on to false hopes and that deep down she has known that the only way she'll ever have a family is to find someone else. "He's the type that will never be ready for marriage. He'll always come up with another excuse. It's just so hard to let go because I still love him!" she cried. After empathizing with the difficulty of letting go, I referred her to the book, Letting Go by Wanderer and Cabot and to a counselor for after the abortion.

These are just two examples of the issues that may underlie a client's repeated risk-taking with birth control and repeated pregnancies. The fact is, most repeat clients use birth control some of the time or even most of the time, just not all the time perfectly. There are always reasons why even good contraceptors take occasional risks.

9. When you are counseling, if you are under severe time constraints, plant some seeds for thought, encourage further counseling, and give her a referral. Sometimes it is helpful to project her thoughts into the future. You can subtract her age from 50 (common age of onset of menopause) and inform her she could easily have x number of years of fertility ahead in which to prevent or plan a pregnancy. Most people are thinking of the here and now, and it is a sobering thought for a 16-year-old to realize she has 34 years left in which to control her fertility. You can inform her that within 34 years, if she used no birth control at all, she could have 20 abortions, several children, and miscarriages besides. Then you need to increase her feelings of control by asking, "What age would you like to be before you start a family?" She might reply, "About 23, after college, and I've got a job and I'm married." Then subtract her present age from this ideal age and reflect to her, "So you've got about seven years in which to use birth control before you have a baby. Is that right?" Seven years may be a more manageable length of time in which to exert concentrated effort on birth control than an "indefinite eternity."

Then ask, "What birth control method would you like to use after the abortion?" If she replies, "the Pill", let her know there are many different kinds of pills on the market and each may affect her differently. So if she ever experiences any nuisance side effects, she can tell her doctor and be switched to a different brand instead of simply quitting the Pill. In addition, if she does ever want to go off the Pill, she will be unprotected immediately and will need another effective method of contraception if she does not want to get pregnant. Since many women quit the Pill for a variety of reasons, she needs to know not to rely on rhythm or withdrawal, as so many do. There are many men and women who switch from a reliable method to an unreliable one simply because they don't know how risky it is, and because rhythm or withdrawal is readily available and easy. Help her avoid the pitfalls.

10. When reviewing contraceptive history with the repeat client, you may find an enormous amount of frustration with birth control methods. Some of these clients have used everything but nonetheless wound up pregnant. The feelings of loss of control can leave the client feeling helpless and depressed. A study of Boston women showed that depression post-abortion was higher for those who had been using contraceptives. The researcher, Dr. Ronnie Janoff-Bulman, explained that getting pregnant while making the effort to prevent conception represents an upheaval of the

client's world, which had previously made sense to her.

You can empathize how unfair it seems to put forth effort to no avail, while others may leave their fate to chance and "not get caught." Point out that being a very fertile woman is part of her identity. Very fertile women are fortunate when they WANT to be pregnant, because it isn't hard to conceive. She needs to consider using the most effective methods (The Shot, Implants or the Pill), and she may need to double up on contraceptive methods. She and her partner can use two at the same time to cut down on the probabilities of a pregnancy. It is less likely that two methods will fail at the same time.

11. Sometimes the woman will allude to a growing sexual dysfunction due to fear of pregnancy. "It's to the point I'm afraid to have sex with my partner!" When a woman is fraught with anxiety before, during and after sexual intercourse, sex can become physically uncomfortable or painful. In addition, the relationship with her male partner can suffer miserably. She has a lot to lose, and so anxiety and fear mount.

12. Although it seems hopeless, she has several options to increase her sense of control over her fertility. She can re-examine the timetable she has fixed in her mind for having a baby, and choose to modify her life to accommodate having a baby sooner. This way, the sooner she completes her family, the sooner she can be done with the hassles of contraceptive methods by having a tubal sterilization. This is not a viable option for everyone, but for some it is very helpful and enlightening. One client, age 27, getting remarried in May, had stated, "I really wanted to be married for a year before I have my last baby." But after four abortions - one for every method she had used – and after reconsidering when to have that last child, she said, "Maybe it wouldn't be so bad after all to have a baby in the first year of my new marriage. At least I'll be married. It would be better than having another abortion as far as I'm concerned. Not ideal, but better. Then I can go ahead and get my tubes tied and be done with this mess!"

She can reconstruct her view of birth control to include new ways of using the available methods. A discussion of this can be found in my booklet, I'll Never Have Sex Again. It explains ways to combine and switch methods to increase effectiveness and avoid "birth control burnout." This is for the fertile person who needs on-going, super-effective, non-permanent contraception. Some of these ideas may be met with a negative response (" It's so much effort!"). How many more abortions is she willing to have? How many unwanted births? Make the statement that she needs ONLY to put the amount of effort into birth control it would take to get what she wants. No more abortions will require the most effort. One more abortion will require some effort, and so forth. You may decide to ask, "Have you ever worked hard for something and actually achieved what you were working for?" If so, how did she feel when she got what she worked for? Was it worth the effort? What would it be worth to have sex without the fear of pregnancy? What is it worth to avoid another abortion? She may decide the cost of all the effort is too much to pay and take the chance on another unplanned pregnancy, and that is HER choice. On the other hand, she may decide the effort is well worth the rewards.

Example Of Counseling The Woman Who Has More Than One Abortion

The following is a session with a super-fertile woman who tried numerous contraceptives and still wound up pregnant. Her story is characteristic of the repeat patient in that she has had times in her life when she diligently used birth control and times when she and her partner took risks. Super-fertility, risk-taking, and the passage of time added up to two births and three abortions for Sondra. This example shows the exasperation some women reach when they are extremely fertile, sexually active, and trying to use the imperfect contraceptive methods available today.

Sondra, age 26, divorced, with two children, sat down and immediately said, "I am so disgusted with birth control, I don't know what to do anymore. I guess I have to join a convent and forget about men!" She said this is her third abortion since the age of 17.

The first time she conceived as a teenager, she thought she couldn't get pregnant if she had sex right after her period. From then on she or her partner used various forms of contraception, but not consistently. She said she was sick and tired of birth control and had tried "everything." We discussed her contraceptive and pregnancy history, and she concluded by stating she wanted to remarry some day and have one more child. Until then, she said she didn't know what to do and was feeling exasperated.

Sondra: I'm nothing but a baby machine!

Counselor: It certainly sounds like you're a very fertile woman!

Sondra: Why, I LOOK at a man and get pregnant!

Counselor: That's an important piece of information to know about yourself. Less fertile people can take risks with birth control now and then, and they may get pregnant. For a very fertile woman, taking even a small risk with birth control will probably lead to a pregnancy.

Sondra: Yeah. It's not fair! I have a friend who doesn't use birth control and she never gets pregnant.

Counselor: It's just like some people who can eat a lot of food and they don't gain weight. Their body burns up all the calories. But others gain weight so easily, they say, 'I can LOOK at a cookie and gain five pounds!'

Sondra: My sister is like that.

Counselor: Once a person knows they gain weight easily, or know they are very fertile, they can use the information in ways that will take care of themselves.

Sondra: I tried, but it's no use.

Counselor: Yes, you did try. And I KNOW you were successful some of the time. Do you know how I know you were successful part of the time?

Sondra: (After a pause). Because I don't have 10 kids by now?

Counselor: Exactly. Or to be more precise – 10 kids and 10 abortions. In countries where there is no access to birth control, very fertile women easily have 14 abortions in their lifetime. They'd look at you with only two children and three abortions and marvel at how you prevented so many other pregnancies.

Sondra: (Looks surprised and reflective).

Counselor: Here's how all birth control methods work: they cut down the chances of a pregnancy occurring. The more effective the method is, and the more consistently the method is used, the less chance of a pregnancy. Nothing is 100%. So, when fertile people use less effective methods, it's just a matter of time before they're pregnant again.

Sondra: And it'll be sooner than later!

Counselor: Would you be willing to take another look at the methods you've tried?

Sondra: OK.

Counselor: The first pregnancy was a result of using rhythm, right? You thought you were at a safe time of the month.

Sondra: Yes.

Counselor: Were you surprised to learn how unreliable rhythm is?

Sondra: I knew there was a chance, but I didn't think it would happen to me.

Counselor: Back then you had no idea about how fertile you were, so you took a risk. Before I started working at Hope Clinic I never knew fertile women could ovulate twice in one month.

Sondra: I didn't know that.

Counselor: That's one of the many reasons rhythm is so unreliable for fertile women. The second pregnancy resulted from ...

Sondra: Going off birth control pills.

Counselor: Did your partner know you were off the Pill?

Sondra: Yes.

Counselor: Was he using condoms or using withdrawal during that time?

Sondra: No. We just thought it would still be in my system for a couple of months. My girlfriend went off the Pill and didn't get pregnant for three months.

Counselor: So it was a matter of not having the correct information.

Sondra: (Nodding).

Counselor: Then what was next? The IUD?

Sondra: Yes. Two of them in two years.

Counselor: That was a highly effective method and you had no pregnancies while you used it. But I understand there were infections and it had to be removed. You said you and your husband weren't getting along too well around that time, and he complained about the sponge you were using?

Sondra: That's right.

Counselor: It isn't easy to keep on using a method when the other person complains about it.

Sondra: I got tired of hearing his complaints, and it was hard to remove anyway.

Counselor: So it sounds like you both took a risk and went without it, and another pregnancy occurred.

Sondra: It was stupid.

Counselor: No, it wasn't stupid. It was a risk. You both took a risk with your body, and you were the one who lost out.

Sondra: (Looks sad).

Counselor: It's sad when we don't take as good care of ourselves as we could.

Sondra: (Sheds a tear, looking down).

Counselor: (After a pause). The best any of us can do when we let ourselves down is keep on learning about how to do things differently next time.

Sondra: (Sounding disgusted). I messed up two more times after that. I guess I didn't learn my lesson.

Counselor: What lesson?

Sondra: Not to have sex without using birth control.

Counselor: When people keep repeating the same thing over and over, it's not necessarily because they haven't learned the lesson, but that the whole lesson wasn't apparent to them. I think there may have been missing pieces to the puzzle. If you're willing to go along with me, I think I may have spotted a few of the missing pieces.

Sondra: Sure. What?

Counselor: I have two main observations from listening to your birth control history. Number one: Not having adequate information and assuming you're protected without checking it out. For example, assuming you were at a safe time of the month or that the Pill stayed in your bloodstream after you quit taking them. What I didn't hear was how you checked out your assumption to see if it was true.

Sondra: That's right. I didn't.

Counselor: In hindsight, how would you go about checking out an assumption about rhythm or how long the Pill stays in the bloodstream?

Sondra: Maybe ask my doctor?

Counselor: That certainly is one way. What is another way?

Sondra: The library?

Counselor: That's a possibility too. Another resource that is quick and up-to-date on contraception is the Planned Parenthood or Family Planning Clinic in your area.

Sondra: I have a friend who goes to Planned Parenthood, and I've been thinking about going there myself.

Counselor: I can give you their address and phone number before you leave my office today. Would you like to hear my second observation from listening to your birth control history?

Sondra: Yes.

Counselor: I noticed that sometimes you took good care of yourself and used very effective

125

contraception. Other times you took risks by not using anything at the time you conceived. You used the most effective birth control when you were married until you and your husband started having difficulties. And then when you weren't in a long-term relationship (your "one time fling" as you called it and your next boyfriend), that's when less effective methods or no method was used. I don't know if I'm on target, but I'm wondering if there is any connection between the nature of your relationships and your decisions about birth control?

Sondra: There could be. (Pauses). It's kind of awkward to talk about birth control with someone you don't know that well. And you don't exactly plan when it's (sex) going to happen. It's kind of a last-minute thing.

Counselor: So the embarrassment of bringing up contraception when you don't know if you're going to have sex with this person is an obstacle to preparing yourself for pregnancy-free sex.

Sondra: I guess so. Sounds silly for someone my age who's a mother of two.

Counselor: Feeling comfortable with your sexuality and being able to plan ahead for it doesn't necessarily come with age or with motherhood.

Sondra: True.

Counselor: Being comfortable with the idea of planning for sex comes with sorting out your values and making a decision about whether you think planning for sex is an OK thing to do.

Sondra: I don't think sex is wrong.

Counselor: Some people think sex isn't wrong as long as they're married, and others don't think there's anything wrong with having sex with a boyfriend. What do you think?

Sondra: Sex is OK either way as long as you love the person, and you don't have sex with just anybody.

Counselor: How would you classify the time you had sex one time, and how would you classify the time you had sex with the boyfriend who used condoms?

Sondra: The one time thing was stupid.

Counselor: Would you classify it as "wrong" in your set of values?

Sondra: Yes.

Counselor: What about the boyfriend after that?

Sondra: No, I don't think that was wrong.

Counselor: You both loved each other?

Sondra: I guess so. (Pause). No, not really. It was mostly physical. I knew I'd never want to marry him.

Counselor: Again, some people see nothing wrong with having sex with someone when it is mostly physical and not leading to marriage. Other people DO it but don't really believe it is right, once they think about it. Which way do you see it?

Sondra: (Thinking). I used to think it was wrong. But I'm not sure anymore. I don't know what I believe, really.

Counselor: This may be a missing piece of the puzzle you haven't examined up until now. When women aren't sure what they believe about having sex with men they aren't in love with, they often don't plan for it, and wind up using last-minute birth control, like condoms, rhythm or withdrawal. It is possible that once you give this question a lot of thought and decide what is best for you and then stick to your beliefs, you'll be less likely to take risks with birth control. Less risks, less pregnancies.

Sondra: (Seems reflective).

Counselor: It's nothing you need to decide right now, but exploring the answers within yourself may help you avoid another unwanted pregnancy.

THE RAPE SURVIVOR

Prevalence Of Pregnancy Resulting From Rape

We at Hope Clinic see approximately one to two women every **week** who are pregnant due to rape. If this number were multiplied by the number of all the abortion clinics in the country and was added to the number of rape survivors who carried to term, the total would be quite alarming. When people say "women don't get pregnant from rape," they clearly do not know what they are talking about.

Identifying The Rape Survivor

Clients fill out forms of demographic and medical information before the counseling session takes place. On one of our forms is the question, "Was this pregnancy a result of rape or forced intercourse?" First, the question lets her know she is not the only rape survivor seeking an abortion, and second, it lets the counselor know about her circumstances ahead of time. We chose to include the words, "forced intercourse," because so many women fail to define "forced intercourse by a boyfriend or ex-boyfriend" as rape. Many people still think rape is only perpetrated by strangers.

"When my boyfriend forced himself on me, I felt bad, but I didn't know it was rape," many women state. Rape occurs any time a male forces intercourse on a female against her will. It doesn't matter who the male is - boyfriend, husband, friend, uncle, minister, teacher, father, brother, Mom's boyfriend, stepdad, stepbrother, doctor, boss, priest, ex-boyfriend or ex-husband - the emotional effect can be equally disturbing. Sometimes sexual assault is perpetrated by a stranger in an alley or parking lot, but the majority of women who are raped have been violated by men they know in a place familiar to them. Women's emotional reactions to having been raped by either a stranger or someone familiar are strikingly similar.

Women who become pregnant from an act of rape are experiencing a double crisis. First, there is the degrading and frightening experience of being sexually violated. This experience often leaves women feeling dirty, defiled, grief-stricken, stupid, angry, scared, and robbed of all control of their body and their life. Then there is the aftershock of discovering the resulting pregnancy and having to make a major decision.

Reasons For Abortion

When rape survivors choose abortion, they usually give the following reasons. "I'm afraid I would hate the baby because I hate the man who did this to me. Having a baby I'd hate is not fair to the child or me." "This pregnancy is a constant reminder that this terrible thing happened to me, and that it isn't over! I want it gone so I can get on with my life." "How could I ever tell this child who and what its father was!" "I don't consider this a baby. It's like a cancer, and I want it out of me!"

Some women's feelings about the pregnancy are not as clear-cut as these, which makes the decision more difficult. More than one client has stated, "The decision was hard for me because this baby is a part of me, too, and I feel like I'm killing a part of me." Some clients anguish over the decision because of their beliefs about abortion: "I always said I'd never have an abortion unless I was raped. But I never thought I'd be raped. Now I feel bad about having an abortion because I still feel it's taking a life. But I don't want to go through this pregnancy because of whose it is. I don't want to go through nine months and then have to give it up, either!"

Even when rape survivors feel guilty about having an abortion, nearly all express a measure of relief afterwards. Many are eagerly anticipating feeling "back to normal" again. Every survivor of a trauma wants so much to feel NORMAL again. One of the ways you can help this client is to inform her about the "normal" symptoms of the rape trauma syndrome.

Symptoms Of Rape Trauma Syndrome

There is a strange truth about reacting to trauma: NOT feeling normal IS normal! When survivors know what the common emotional and behavioral symptoms of trauma are, they don't feel so "crazy" and "out of control." Give your client a list of the typical trauma symptoms. Hope Clinic counselors use a list we received from our local Rape and Sexual Abuse Counseling Center:

- fear
- anxiety
- moodiness
- irritability
- confusion
- inability to concentrate
- anger
- guilt, self-blame
- vulnerability
- shame or embarrassment

127

- denial of the assault
- blocking one's feelings
- a sense of powerlessness and helplessness
- obsession with details of the rape
- nightmares or night terrors
- distrust of others, particularly men resembling the rapist
- flashbacks - re-experiencing the rape as if it was occuring now
- concern about sexually transmitted disease
- concern about whom to tell
- nausea
- soreness and pain from the assault
- infections
- stomach upsets
- fatigue
- tension headaches
- sleep disturbances
- eating disturbances
- jumpiness, easily startled
- pregnancy
- menstrual cycle disrupted
- urinary or bowel problems

The list acts as a springboard from which she can talk about her own symptoms. It also gives her important knowledge that can decrease her anxiety and increase her feeling of control. People feel relieved when they know others have felt the same way they feel.

Feeling back in control is a major part of healing after surviving a sexual assault. For this reason if she views the abortion decision as an act of her own will and feels she is taking back the control of her body, the experience can be empowering. However, if she views herself as a victim who "had to have an abortion" because she was raped, the outcome will be far less favorable. Listen closely to the way she is viewing her decision.

Pre-Abortion Counseling Goals And Concerns

Counseling a rape survivor right before an abortion is not the same as rape counseling. The purpose of the counseling session is the same as for any client who seeks an abortion. However, it is important to acknowledge her circumstances and let her know you are there for her if she wants to talk about it. Leave it up to her how much or how little to tell you.

Although you don't need to know the whole story, you do need to ask if she feels protected from another assault by this person. She may have on-going contact with the perpetrator, such as a classmate or ex-husband. You can help her strategize ways to feel safe from him. Although there is no 100% safe place for the survivor of rape when the perpetrator is free and in close proximity, she could 1). get an order of protection; 2). change the locks on her door, if appropriate; 3). live with friends or family for awhile; 4). move to a new residence; 5). change classes or schools; or 6). change jobs. It certainly is unfair that the victim of a crime has to go to such lengths as to change jobs, schools, or residences, but sometimes safety requires drastic measures. Ask her first what she has already done for her safety, and then offer suggestions.

Another concern is whether she has told anyone what happened. If so, how did they react? If she has no one who is supportive, you will be the first person to offer the support she needs. You can also provide her with a counseling referral and a description of the services she can expect to receive. Some women are reluctant to contact rape crisis counselors for fear they'd try to talk her into taking the case to court. Most women I've counseled said they did not go to the hospital emergency room after the assault (where evidence is collected for court proceedings). They described wanting to be left alone to tend to their own wounds. Many take long hot baths immediately after being violated as a way of cleansing themselves emotionally and physically. Many also say they fear going to the police and assert, "I just wanted it to be over with." They need to know rape counselors will not try to make them do anything. They are there to listen, support, and help them heal.

At the time of an abortion the woman will be at least two to three months pregnant. Because of the time lapse from the time of the assault to the time she is seeking an abortion, she is usually in the stage of "trying to forget about it." In the counseling session, many survivors tell what happened in broad, general terms, and appear emotionally distant from the traumatic event. However, some cry and talk about recurring nightmares. Regardless of the client's present state of adjustment, let her know that healing from a trauma takes time, just like healing from a serious wound. Reassure her, "It's natural to want to hurry up and feel normal again. But there is no need to be impatient with yourself if some of the symptoms you thought were gone crop up again. They will eventually go away, but healing from a trauma doesn't usually progress in a straight line. It's more of a jagged line. People move forward and have setbacks." As time goes by, if she is taking care of herself, the setbacks will get fewer and farther between. Taking care of herself includes talking to a supportive listener about what happened, acknowledging her feelings and symptoms, and knowing they are all part of the post-trauma healing process. Taking care also means doing things that rebuild confidence in her safety, being tested for sexually transmitted diseases, including AIDS, and doing exactly what she is doing: making a decision about the pregnancy. Everyone heals at her own pace, and having the abortion behind her can be part of her healing process.

Women who have experienced sexual abuse or other trauma in their lives but who have never healed from it could greatly benefit from professional counseling. Even though some people show amazing resiliency, layers of trauma can wreak havoc if left unattended. Unless **she** brings up other traumatic life events, a pre-abortion counseling session is not the time to uncover her past. Simply give her a counseling referral and let her know, "Many women heal with or without counseling. But those who have chosen to talk to someone knowledgeable about emotional healing after sexual assault have said it was invaluable." Let her know it is strictly up to her IF and WHEN she feels like using the referral. She is in charge of her own healing.

Example Of Counseling The Rape Survivor Before Her Abortion

Christine, a 26-year-old nurse, looked nervous perched close to the edge of her chair with her coat and purse piled on her lap. I motioned to the chair beside her and invited her to lay her coat and purse on it. She murmured, "I'm OK" and chose to stay tucked beneath her belongings.

I told her I had reviewed the forms she filled out so I would know a little bit about her. I explained the purpose of the session and she scooted back in her chair, securing her coat and purse on her lap. "Where should we begin?" I asked, allowing her to take control. "I don't

know...**you** start," she instructed. When I suggested that I explain what would take place, she agreed.

As I began talking about the procedure itself, she asked, "Is it going to hurt?" "**Exactly** what I'd want to know!" I affirmed. I explained the range of feelings women describe and asked about her past experiences with uncomfortable medical procedures as a patient **and** as a nurse. She warmed up to the subject once she described herself in the role of L.P.N. As she talked, she gathered up her coat and purse and dumped them in a heap on the chair beside her. "Nurses are big babies when it comes to being a patient," she confided. I added, "Counselors aren't exactly Captain Courageous either!" We both laughed. Her face changed and she appeared apprehensive. "When you're a nurse, you're in control," she informed me, "but when you're a patient, you're at the doctor's mercy." Although we had not yet broached the subject of "forced intercourse" she had circled on her forms, I was struck by the way she had described being a patient. I thought, "She may as well be describing what it's like to be a victim of sexual assault." She went on to say she hated pap smears and was glad when they were over. I agreed wholeheartedly and then she said, "I wish men had to go through what we have to!" I joined in the fantasy with, "Can you imagine a man going through a pap smear or an abortion?!" She sneered, "They couldn't handle it! They'd probably pass out!" "Probably so," I concurred, "and as much as we hate it ourselves - at least we know how to endure." "Isn't that the truth!" she exclaimed. Her playful smile disappeared, and she stated, "I wish my ex-boyfriend had to go through what I'm going through!" She told me he was the one who "forced himself on her" after she had been "so stupid" to let him into her apartment. She said she "knew he was a jerk" and yet opened the door to him.

The session continued ...

Counselor: We all feel foolish sometimes for trusting people we suspect or know aren't worthy of our trust. If you could turn the clock back, what would you do differently?

Client: As soon as I knew who it was, I'd have told him to go away and leave me alone, and if he wouldn't go, I'd have told him I was calling the police. I would have called my brother, too, to make sure he didn't bother me.

Counselor: So what you'd do differently is follow your own better judgment and keep him away from you as much as possible.

Client (Sadly nods her head): After it was over, he left and I took a long hot bath ... as hot as I could stand it.

Counselor: Many of the women I've seen in similar circumstances have told me they took a long hot bath afterwards.

Client: Do you see many women like me?

Counselor: I see many more women who have become pregnant as a result of rape than anyone would guess. There's a lot of things about rape many people don't know. People think that rape only happens in dark parking lots by strangers, but most rapes occur in the woman's own home by someone she knows. Since some women are too embarrassed to tell anyone and seek support, I'm wondering if you told anyone?

Client: No, I felt too stupid at the time. Once I knew I was pregnant, though, I told my best friend. She's been great – she came with me today.

Counselor: Does she understand why you chose to have an abortion?

Client: Oh, yes. She knows I can't have this baby. I can barely take care of myself on my salary. She knows what I make because we work at the same job in the nursing home. Besides, I don't want a child I don't have any love for. I hate the father's guts, and I don't want his child. I don't want any ties to him whatsoever! I've felt so sick from this pregnancy, it's beginning to affect my job, too. I can't wait to be able to eat and get my energy back. I want to feel normal again.

Counselor: After the abortion, you certainly can look forward to feeling better. You'll be able to eat normally and the hormone-related fatigue will vanish as well.

Client: That's good!

Counselor: It's difficult to know when you'll really feel "normal" again because you were sexually assaulted, and there are ups and downs as you heal emotionally from the trauma.

Client: I guess so.

Counselor: When a man takes away the control of a woman's body and her life, it's no wonder women experience disturbing reactions. Let me show you a list of common reactions to having been sexually violated.

Client: (Looks thoughtfully at the list). I see myself in this list ... forgetful, irritable, and tired. Of course, the tiredness might be the pregnancy.

Counselor: That's part of the reason I showed you this list. Just in case the fatigue doesn't go away after the pregnancy hormones leave your body, I wanted you to know it is also a symptom of post-trauma stress. Wanting to feel normal is absolutely understandable, but feeling normal after a rape takes time. Many women get impatient with themselves when they have a setback after weeks of feeling OK. Healing from a trauma doesn't progress in a straight line. Healing moves in a jagged line, moving forward and then backward, forward and backward. You'll be adjusting to feeling safe again and regaining control in your life. Do you feel that choosing to end this pregnancy is one step in regaining that control?

Client: Yes, I do. If I couldn't have an abortion, I don't know what I'd do. I'd be so depressed, I might do something desperate. This way, I can get my life back on track. I don't want to feel pregnant anymore. Once this is over I can go back to work and start over. Maybe some people can get through a pregnancy and put their babies up for adoption, but I couldn't make it through the pregnancy!

Counselor: Was adoption something you considered?

Client: It crossed my mind, but I know I'd lose my job if I stayed so sick and couldn't work. I have to work to support myself. And I'm sick and tired of feeling sick. I want my own life back. I don't want to go through this pregnancy.

Counselor: So the pregnancy feels like something your ex-boyfriend forced on you, and getting an abortion would give you your life back?

Client: Yes, exactly.

Counselor: Then it sounds like you've given this a lot of thought from many different angles and that you're making a sound decision.

Client: I know it's the best decision for my life.

Counselor: Before we go on to talk about the abortion procedure and aftercare, I need to ask you if you feel safe from your ex-boyfriend?

Client: Yes. I moved to an apartment across the street from where my brother and his wife live. I told my brother that this guy was threatening me, and he and some of his friends went after him. I'm sure I won't be hearing from him again.

Counselor: Have you considered police protection?

Client: I don't want to involve the police unless I absolutely have to. I don't have any doubts that I'm safe from him now.

Counselor: I hear how certain you are that your brother and his friends were effective. If you would happen to need police protection, would you know how to get it?

Client: Yes. I know how to get an order of protection, if that's what you mean. I've done it before.

Counselor: OK, I just wanted to check that out with you. I'm glad you've taken steps to feel safe from him.

From there we went on to discuss the procedure, aftercare, and consent forms. She again brought up her fear of pain and fear of feeling out of control. I suggested we go back over the process and identify where and when she could make choices and be in charge. She discovered she could: 1). choose whether or not to take the muscle relaxer; 2). spend some time outside instead of waiting the whole time in the waiting room; 3). choose from a variety of relaxation strategies once in the procedure room; 4). choose whether or not to take the extra medication right before the abortion; 5). view herself as a member of team whose goal was to maximize her comfort and safety. She stated she had no other concerns about the abortion and was ready to sign the consent forms.

After her abortion, she was feeling fine when I visited her in the recovery room. Right before she left I gave her a counseling referral for future reference. "You may feel like using it later on," I suggested. "If you do, you've got the number to call." She put it in her purse and said she was glad the abortion was over.

THE CLIENT TERMINATING DUE TO FETAL INDICATIONS

People seeking abortions for fetal indications are usually married couples in their 30s and 40s who planned the pregnancy. Under the technology of 1994, many fetal abnormalities are not detectable until the pregnancy has advanced to the fifth or sixth month. Unfortunately this delay creates considerable grief for the couples and their families. After six months of looking forward to having this baby, people are given a diagnosis that compels them to make one of the most agonizing decisions they'll ever have to make.

They are faced with the question, "Do we carry to term, knowing our child will either die immediately after delivery or live with mental and physical suffering, or do we end the pregnancy?" Either choice results in mourning and grieving.

The literature reveals that couples make this decision within a few days of the diagnosis (Magyari, Wedehase, Ifft & Callanan, 1988). This is partly because there is so little time left before abortion is no longer an option.

Reasons For The Decision

Reasons for the decision directly relate to their love for their child and their other children. They may state they believe it is wrong to bring a baby into the world when it will suffer constantly and chronically with no hope of change. Even men and women who are special education teachers and who work with disabled children have stated, "I think it's better to end the pregnancy now than to bring our child into the world with so many strikes against him or her."

They may also state their limited financial resources would fail to cover the costs for the kind of care the child would need. This is a significant consideration especially for those who already have children for whom they must provide. They may explain, "We are responsibile for the children who are already **here**. It wouldn't be fair to them if we had to pour all our time, energy, and finances into the care of **this** child." Sometimes they bring up examples of what they've seen happen to relatives' families who have had severely disabled children.

Another reason may be a self-assessed inability to parent a severely disabled child. They do not believe they have the perseverence, patience, and fortitude required. Feelings of guilt, weakness, failure, and selfishness sometimes accompany this assessment, but as one woman stated, "I'd feel a lot guiltier if I lied to myself, had the baby, and then found out I couldn't cope with it. Now that would be unforgivable!"

One or both may also state they do not want to put themselves or their family members through the emotional consequences of carrying to term. In their estimation, "This is hard enough, but the grief and pain of seeing the baby suffer and die would be far worse."

Regardless of their reasons, the couples I have seen on the day of the abortion are feeling sad but certain of their decision.

Examples Of Fetal Abnormalities Detectable By Amniocentesis

Spina Bifida is a neural tube defect. During early embryonic development the vertebrae do not completely close around the spinal column. There can be wide variations in the severity of the defect. In its more serious form, the covering of the brain, spine, and spinal cord protrude outward through the skin in a small sac. Symptoms include paralysis of the lower limbs and both fecal and urinary incontinence. Severely affected infants may not survive. Exact causes are uncertain but genetic, environmental, and disease are all suspect.

Anencephaly is a lack of functioning brain tissue and sometimes the spinal cord. The fetal head and spine may be open because neural tissue, skin, and bone are missing. This is the result of a neural tube defect. Survival after birth is usually only a few hours. An excess of amniotic fluid is usually present during such a pregnancy and may assist in detection. Causes are uncertain but may be similar to those for Spina Bifida.

Hydrocephalus is the accumulation of cerebrospinal fluid inside the skull of the developing fetus where the brain should be. This may be caused by an overproduction of fluid or blockage of fluid flow within the fetal head. The fetus may develop a large head or the brain may collapse inward away from the skull. There is a thinning of the skull bones, prominent forehead and atrophy of the cerebral cortex. Severe hydrocephaly results in death.

Tay-Sachs Disease is an inherited degenerative neurological disorder predominantly found in Jews of Eastern European descent. Symptoms typically develop by seven months of age, and the disease is usually fatal by early childhood. The infant regresses mentally and physically with symptoms such as paralysis and blindness. Tay Sachs can be detected in utero by chorionic villus sampling, amniocentesis, and in potential parents via genetic analysis.

Cystic Fibrosis is a genetically transmitted disease of the endocrine glands. Symptoms include excess mucus secretions in the bronchi, pancreatic insufficiency, and heart disease. Prognosis is poor, and most will die by their teens or early twenties.

Niemann-Pick is a hereditary metabolic disorder. The infant's body lacks an enzyme necessary to prevent toxins in the body. The infant develops an enlarged liver and spleen, suffers progressive mental and physical deterioration, and failure to thrive. This disease is usually fatal by age three.

Down's Syndrome (Trisomy 21) results when there are three instead of two 21st chromosomes present in the genes. Symptoms include mild to severe mental retardation and heart defects. Persons with Down's may also have physical characteristics such as a flat nasal bridge and protruding tongue.

Huntington's Chorea is a hereditary disorder that causes progressive mental deterioration leading to dementia. Involuntary spasms of the face and limbs are also present. Onset usually occurs between ages 30 and 50.

Turner's Syndrome occurs in female fetuses where one X chromosome is missing. The child will lack ovarian development resulting in infertility and absence of sexual maturity. The child tends to be short in stature, have a webbed neck, and can be mentally retarded.

Klinefelter's Syndrome occurs in male fetuses that have an extra X chromosome. Characteristics include tall stature with disproportionately longer lower limbs, breast enlargement, small testicles, and no sperm production.

Tests To Determine Fetal Abnormalities

Amniocentesis is a procedure whereby amniotic fluid is removed from the uterus by a needle inserted through the abdomen and guided with the help of ultrasound. Fetal cells in the amniotic fluid can be examined for biochemical and chromosomal abnormalities. This process can only be performed in the second trimester.

Ultrasound is a process whereby sound waves are used to produce an image of the fetus on a monitor which is then printed on paper. The more advanced the pregnancy is, the more detectable the abnormalities will be.

Chorionic Villus Sampling is done in the first trimester. The chorion is the membrane surrounding the embryo during early pregnancy that functions as a primitive placenta. The cells of this tissue originate from the fetus and thus can be used for genetic analysis. Samples are taken through the cervix with the help of ultrasound to guide the instruments.

Fetoscopy uses fiber optics to see inside the uterus either through a small incision in the abdomen or through the cervix. Physical malformations can be seen at close range and fetal blood samples can be obtained.

As technology progresses, tests for fetal abnormalities will probably be able to be performed in the first trimester which will give couples the option of a first trimester abortion and more time to decide. As time goes by, some or all of the above tests may become obsolete. In addition, genetic engineering and surgery on the fetus in utero may become common practice in the future.

References For Fetal Abnormalities And Testing

Baker, J. & Allen, G (1982). The Study of Biology (4th ed.). Addison-Wesley Publishing Co.

Lui, D.T. (1991). A Practical Guide To Chorion Villus Sampling. NY: Oxford University Press.

Moore, K.L. (1977). The Developing Human: Clinically Oriented Embryology. (2nd ed). Philadelphia, PA: W.B. Saunders Co.

Thompson, J.S. & Thompson, M.W. (1980). Genetics in Medicine (3rd ed.). Philadelphia, PA: S.B. Saunders Co.

Common Feelings Of Clients

Research has shown that women who chose to undergo a fetal indications abortion may experience guilt, depression, grief, sadness, anger, and relief (Jones et al., 1984, Iles, 1989, and Lloyd & Laurence, 1985). Unlike the women who choose abortion for other reasons, women having fetal indications abortions seldom reported relief as the predominant post-abortion emotion (Iles, 1989). However, Jones et al. (1984) found that relief was the most prevalent feeling **immediately** after the abortion.

Guilt

Guilt may occur for a number of reasons. Guilt was found most often when a couple viewed the abortion as a rejection of a handicapped child, and when carrying to term would probably have resulted in a live birth (Iles, 1989). People who oppose abortion on moral grounds but feel abortion is best under the circumstances may feel guilty about "ending their child's life." However, some couples do not feel guilty about their decision or the abortion, but do feel guilty about not having produced a normal fetus.

Depression And Anxiety

In a study of 71 women undergoing an abortion for fetal indications, participants were followed up at one month, six months, and 13 months post-abortion. In the first month, levels of depression and anxiety were comparable to that found in psychiatric in-patients, but dropped back to normal at the six- and 13-month intervals. For those whose depression and anxiety were still high, the symptoms were related to concern over the outcome of a new pregnancy, failure to conceive again, or unresolved guilt (Iles, 1989).

In another study of 12 women who were interviewed three months to four years post-abortion,

133

two were still experiencing severe depression seven to 10 months after their abortion, while 25% were assessed as "doing fair" and 58% were "successfully recovered" (Donnai et al., 1981).

Grief

Grief, sadness, and loss appear to be the predominant emotions for couples choosing an abortion for fetal indications (Elder & Laurence, 1991, Iles, 1989, and Lloyd & Laurence, 1985). Researchers conducted interviews of 69 women in South Wales three to five years after their abortions. Eighty percent reported experiencing acute grief post-abortion and 75% reported having resolved the acute grief by six months post-abortion.

Poor resolution was associated with increasing maternal age and poor support from partners (Elder & Laurence, 1991). Lloyd and Laurence (1985) found that grief reactions from second trimester fetal indications abortions were as acute as that experienced after a stillborn. However, this study did not compare the length of time taken to resolve acute grief after a stillborn with the length of time taken to resolve acute grief after an abortion.

People grieve not only for the loss of a healthy baby but also for the loss of their hopes and dreams. The loss of the child is the primary loss, but secondary losses can be every bit as painful and need to be identified and grieved (Rando, 1989). For couples who already have a child or children, some of the secondary losses include: the completion of their family, a sibling for their only child or their children, the hope of a daughter if they already have a son, or a son if they already have a daughter.

If they don't have any children, secondary losses include the loss of parenthood, a family, an heir, a grandchild for Mom and Dad, and the future. Secondary losses for both parents and nonparents include losing their positive self-image, sense of normalcy in their lives, safety and order in the world, and their hopes and dreams for what their child would have become.

When grief is compounded by guilt, resolution takes longer and the acute symptoms may last longer (Rando, 1988). Due to the nature of the life crisis, guilt and grief inevitably intermingle

whether the couple decides to carry to term or choose abortion. There is often self-blame and a search for answers to the questions, "Why me?" "What did I do wrong?" The search for answers may also lead to blaming others and feeling angry.

Anger

The client or her partner may experience anger at God, each other, themselves, her doctor, the abortion clinic, and the world. They've been dealt a hard blow by Mother Nature and have every right to feel angry. Feeling scared and cornered by distressing and limited options can also create feelings of anger.

Relief

When a couple first finds out about their baby's diagnosis, they may feel trapped and worried that they may have no other option than to carry to term. This is especially true when their doctor informs them how few clinics in the country perform advanced second trimester abortions. When they discover there IS a place to go, and the medical care is professional and compassionate, they may feel enormously relieved.

Feelings On The Day Of The Abortion

Most couples appear sad and mournful but extremely resigned to what they feel is absolutely necessary. They usually have the full support of all their family members, their doctor, and even their employers, if they needed time away from work for the two- to four-day procedure. They usually appear solemn and frequently state they feel out of place in a waiting room full of young women seeking abortions for other reasons. They both seem focused on what is going to happen, what the possible complications might be, and whether there will be much pain for the woman or any pain for the fetus.

Recommendations For Sensitive Care Of Clients And Their Partners

When the client makes the appointment, she often reveals the nature of her situation, especially if her doctor wants a sample of tissue for genetic testing. At that time the person making the appointment should mark her chart clearly so all staff will be aware of her circumstances from the moment she walks through the door.

Most clients with fetal indications feel extremely out of place, and steps need to be taken to help them and their partners feel at ease. In a waiting room of mostly young women sitting next to their mothers or boyfriends, this couple stands out by virtue of their age and the maternity clothes she may be wearing. They may be scanning the room feeling bitterly alone, thinking theirs is the only unhealthy pregnancy in the room and the only one that was wanted. For these reasons, the less waiting before the counseling session takes place, the better. Feelings of alienation can be addressed in the session, and the rest of the waiting time can therefore be made more bearable.

Special efforts should be taken to involve the woman's partner (usually her husband) at every step of the process: the ultrasound, lab work, counseling, and recovery. The couple usually expresses a strong need to be together. She may also want her husband to be in the surgery room during the procedure. He may not really want to, but often feels an obligation to provide support to her any way he can. Hope Clinic does not permit anyone but staff and patients in the surgery room due to the state's regulations for licensed out-patient surgical centers. Even if the state regulations were not so stringent, we would still make only the rarest of exceptions out of respect for the partner's feelings. Every clinic has its own policy and every state has its regulations about permitting or prohibiting non-staff in the surgery rooms. Some clinics may permit the partner to be present on a case-by-case basis after consultation with the doctor and extensive preparation with the couple. In making this decision, care must be taken to consider the partner's feelings and beware of casting him in the role of support person for his wife. He, too, is grieving an enormous loss, and may have feelings of guilt, anxiety, and fear of the medical procedure. Sometimes the male partner is unable to identify his feelings or be able to express them, but observing his reactions during the description of the procedure can give you clues. A symbolic way he can be with her in the procedure room is by giving her a small object or love note she can take with her into the room.

The Counseling Session

Issues And Concerns

The first thing many couples talk about in the counseling session is how uncomfortable they feel because, unlike everyone else, they are not terminating a healthy pregnancy. Acknowledge the pain they probably feel when they see others having what they want - a healthy pregnancy - and yet choosing an abortion. Then find a connection between them and the others in the waiting room. Let them know how many other couples have chosen abortion in cases of fetal abnormality. Inform them that everyone in the waiting room wishes they didn't have to be there but feels strongly about the necessity of terminating the pregnancy. Usually the couple can identify with that description, and they move on to talk about themselves.

Ask them about the chain of events that occurred from the time of the testing to the time they made their decision. A lot has probably happened in a span of a few days. For most people the diagnosis comes as a shock. Frequently she has had a normal pregnancy with no indications of problems until a routine ultrasound or amniocentesis detected the anomaly. Most couples make the decision quickly, decisively, and with a great deal of heartache. They inform their families and usually receive their family's full support for the abortion decision.

For most people the decision comes down to this: they would rather spare their child a life of pain and misery rather than bring it into the world and watch it suffer. When you acknowledge the love and compassion you hear in their explanation, they usually breathe a sigh of relief that you understand.

Talking About Grieving

In the pre-abortion counseling session, it is important to discuss key concepts of grief and mourning with the couple.

1. Grieving a loss involves feelings of anger, guilt, sadness, and longing, and the ebb and tide of these feelings over time. Just when they start feeling better, something may trigger the same feelings all over again: the due date, the anniversary of the abortion, seeing babies and pregnant women, or baby commercials. They need to expect these normal setbacks and know that healing from a loss progresses two steps forward and one step back, like a jagged line.

2. Grieving takes time. Although friends and family will want them to feel better soon, there is no quick fix.

3. Men and women grieve differently and heal at different rates. Expecting each other to feel the same thing at the same time is setting themselves up for more heartache. A woman may become irritated with her partner if she doesn't perceive him to be as distraught as she is. A man may become impatient if his partner continues to feel grief-stricken and rebuff sexual advances. It's important for them to talk to each other, but it may be important for each of them to find someone else to talk to as well.

4. Family and friends may avoid talking about it because they don't know what to say. Or they may say things like, "You can always have another child," not realizing the couple became attached to THIS child and wanted THIS child. They mean to be comforting, but just don't seem to understand. Or they may say, "It was God's will." Nothing seems more senseless than to imagine a loving God willing suffering and pain to humankind. Going over the things people may say to them can be valuable preparation.

5. Some people feel comforted by having a memorial service to acknowledge the loss. It can be private, just for the two of them, or include close friends and family as well. Doing something symbolic like planting a tree in memory of the child can be meaningful.

Exploring Their Support System

Ask about their support system. Usually "everyone" knows she is expecting a baby, but only family and close friends know about the diagnosis and abortion. Talk about what they might tell acquaintances and co-workers. Some people want to avoid any potential conflicts by telling people she miscarried. Saying she had a miscarriage is a legitimate way of taking care of themselves. The last thing they need is moralizing from self-righteous people passing judgment on them for having an abortion. Most people will sympathize with a miscarriage of a wanted pregnancy, and that is the reaction they need and deserve from others. Some couples just assume everyone in the world will automatically sympathize with their having an abortion under their set of circumstances. Forewarn them some people will not be

at all supportive of an abortion, even under their dire circumstances. They need to consider this possibility to help them decide what they want to say to whom. Some people, however, feel strongly about telling people what really happened. They simply need to be prepared for the occasional cruel remark.

Friends and family may not be able to provide the kind of support one or both of them needs at this time (Jones et al., 1984). Counseling referrals may be an important source of support for them during the most acute phase of their grieving. The more guilt they express, the more likely they may need counseling afterwards. In addition, there are two booklets you can offer them that sensitively address the emotional issues of both the man and the woman: Minnick, M., Delp. K., and Ciotti, M. (1991), A Time To Decide, A Time To Heal, East Lansing, MI: Pineapple Press; Difficult Decisions, Centering Corporation, 1531 N. Saddle Creek, Omaha, NE 68104; and Lister M. and Lovell, S. (1991), Healing Together: For Couples Whose Baby Dies, Omaha, NE: Centering Corporation.

What To Tell Their Children

If they have other children who have been happily awaiting the arrival of their sibling, explore appropriate explanations of what happened to the baby. For small children and school-age children, telling them, "the baby died, and we're very sad," is probably sufficient. Let them know it is important to allow themselves and their children to express their feelings and grieve. The way they handle their grief will be a learning experience for their children. Their kids will also need reassurance that even though Mom and Dad are sad and upset, they will still take care of them. There are books that discuss ways to talk about the death of loved ones to small children, such as How To Talk To Children About Really Important Things by Charles Schaefer. It may be helpful and healing to include their children in whatever symbolic burial, blessing, or memorial they plan. For teenage children, the couple may decide to tell them the whole story.

Is It A Girl Or Boy?

Another issue is the sex of the baby. Do they know? Some people originally wanted the sex of the child to be a surprise at the time of birth. Others already have been planning specifically for a girl or a boy, and have selected a name. Some people still don't want to know the sex because they think they won't grieve as much that way. However, grief therapists find that grieving a specific loss is usually more helpful in the healing process than grieving something vague (Rando, 1988). Some people don't want to know if the child would have been a girl or a boy at the time of the abortion, but they have called back months or years later wanting to know (Iles, 1989). For this reason their doctor should have that information charted for future reference.

Research has found that memories of the baby can be important in the grieving process (Magyari et al., 1988). Offering the picture from the ultrasound is one way of providing them with a concrete memory. **If and only if the abortion is an induction procedure,** the couple can be given several options: having a photo of the baby after the abortion is completed, viewing the body, and/or holding it. One study found that 67% of the couples studied wanted the photo, 60% chose to view the body, and 40% chose to hold it (Magyari et al., 1988).

Tissue Samples For Genetic Tests

If their doctor has given them a kit for chromosome testing and transport, they usually bring this up in counseling as well as over the phone. The clinic's doctor and nurses need to know about the kit and follow the directions precisely. At the Hope Clinic, the Director of Nursing and the couple's counselor collaborate to make sure the tissue collection is done, packaged properly, and all paperwork for the lab is filled out correctly. This is a one-time opportunity for collecting a sample of fetal tissue for important tests for the couple's future pregnancies.

Most referring physicians have arranged for genetic counseling after the abortion. However, if they don't mention genetic counseling, strongly suggest they ask their doctor for a referral and consultation so they'll know their chances of conceiving a healthy baby in the future. Sometimes they feel so scared it will happen again they say they will never try again. However, people in this situation may feel one way at the time of the abortion, and change their minds as time goes by. A decision about sterilization is also strongly advised against until there has been adequate time to grieve and to be counseled about their chances for future anomalies.

Concerns About The Procedure

Concerns about safety and the possibility of sterility post-abortion is a major issue as is the intensity of pain she may experience. Another major concern is fear of fetal pain. In D&E and D&X procedures and in induction procedures that use Digoxin, it is extremely remote if not impossible for the fetus to feel pain. And even at the end of the second trimester, there is no conclusive evidence at this time that the development of the brain and nervous system is adequate for pain perception.

Recovery

Most abortion providers do not have private recovery rooms, as they must serve many patients. Hope Clinic and other second trimester providers may have ways of providing privacy during the recovery time, and many allow husbands to be with their wives during recovery, depending on state regulations and clinic policies. If not, the counselor can act as a messenger between them, passing handwritten notes, and letting him know how she is doing and when she will be discharged. Any extra service during recovery time is greatly needed and appreciated.

Post-Abortion

Couples who have chosen abortion due to fetal indications are some of the most grateful clients you will ever see. They express heartfelt gratitude for every bit of attention and care you give them during such a heartbreaking experience. From the letters we and other providers receive from these couples, it appears every staff member involved in their care is imprinted in their memory for a lifetime.

Example Of Fetal Indications Counseling Session

Mary and Joe, a married couple in their late thirties, explained on the phone they just received results from an amniocentesis and their doctor referred them to Hope Clinic for a second trimester abortion. When they arrived, Mary appeared tense, anxious, and curt to the receptionist. Joe seemed quiet, controlled, and attentive to his wife.

In the waiting room they sat closely together, giving the appearance of a human fortress. When it came time for counseling, both Mary and Joe were welcomed into the session.

Despite their apparent anxiety, they exuded an air of resignation. I started by telling them what I knew of their situation and assured them I and all the other Hope Clinic staff would do all we could to make their experience as comfortable and bearable as possible for the both of them. Mary and Joe murmured words of appreciation and he squeezed her hand as she spoke. "We just got the test results Friday and found out the baby has spina bifida. We talked about it all weekend. It's for the best..." Her voice trailed off and tears welled up in her eyes. Joe patted her hand and continued where she left off.

"The doctor said the baby's vertebrae is not completely closed around the spinal column, and the sonogram showed the spinal cord protruding through the skin. We had an amnio done, and it showed positive." Mary wiped tears off her glasses and Joe patted her knee. She sighed and he continued, "The baby would need an operation right away and might be paralyzed from the waist down. If it's severe enough, the baby may not live even after putting it through any number of operations. We don't want to see our child have to go through all that. This is hard enough on us!" He and Mary looked at each other. I felt moved by the depth of sorrow in their eyes and the tenderness in their touch. We all sat quietly.

Then she turned to me abruptly and asked, "What's this going to be like? Will it hurt?" Normalizing the pain of an abortion and comparing it to the pain of a miscarriage or premature birth tends to put the issue of pain into perspective and into the realm of acceptability. So I stated, "Most women at 24 weeks say there is some pain, but how much or how little is a very individual experience, and whether a woman has a miscarriage at 24 weeks or undergoes an abortion, there is bound to be some degree of pain."

From there I explained the entire abortion process and took care to use the term "baby" instead of the word "fetus" to stay closely in tune with their feelings. When I came to the part describing the evacuation of the uterus, tears came to Mary's eyes and Joe bowed his head. I let them know as soon as the amniotic fluid is removed, the baby is no longer living and does not feel any pain. Mary said tearfully, "I asked my doctor and he said it wouldn't come out whole." I answered, "That's true. The way our doctor does this procedure maximizes your safety and well-being. But there is another safe procedure called 'induction' in which the procedure is comparable to an induced miscarriage. We cannot perform that procedure at Hope Clinic, but I do know of a very reputable clinic in Wichita that can perform this procedure for you, if you'd feel more at ease knowing the baby was removed intact." Both Mary and Joe responded, "No, we're ready for this to be done today." Mary said, "We just didn't want the baby to feel anything. I feel better knowing it won't be in pain." They held hands, looked at each other, and Mary blotted her eyes.

I commented, "It's clear you love your baby very much. I'm wondering if your doctor told you if it was a boy or girl?" Mary answered through her tears, "It's a girl." "Have you chosen a name?" I inquired. Joe said, "Emily Lynn. We named her for Mary's great grandmother." "Emily Lynn is a beautiful name," I said, "And you've known and loved Emily for six months. She will always have a special place in your memory. Some couples decide to have a private memorial as a way to bless and honor the child's memory. Some people want to keep the sono picture. Catholics might decide to have a Mass designated in their child's name. Some people wait to do a memorial at the time the child would have been born. There's no right or wrong about it. I'm bringing it up because some couples have said a memorial was healing for them."

Mary said tentatively, "I'd already thought of it, but I didn't know what Joe or my parents would think." Joe responded, "I'll do anything that would help. I'm open." I commented, "You have a strong and loving relationship, and you both seem sensitive to each other. After a therapeutic abortion, it takes time to grieve the loss and make peace with yourself for whatever guilt, if any, you may feel." Mary spoke up, "I have been feeling guilty. Not just about ending my child's life but also about the abnormality. I know my doctor told me it was nothing I did, but I still can't help but think why did this happen?" Joe assured Mary it was not her fault. I interjected, "We all want to make sense of what seems to be senseless tragedies in our lives. And with time and thought, you can look for and find meaning in this. Joe may find one meaning and you may find another, and both may be valuable."

I pursued Mary's statement about ending her child's life. "What are some ways you will make peace with yourself about ending the child's life?" I asked. She said, "I don't know. I think by telling myself it had to be done or the child would have had a life of suffering." Joe agreed. Mary continued, "And I've got Joe to talk to." I stated, "Many women say it was healing for them to talk about their feelings to someone who really understood and to remember the reasons why they made the decision." I added, "For some people it's also very important they feel forgiven by God. Do you have a belief in God?" They both said yes and stated they believed in a forgiving, merciful God who knew their pain and would forgive them. They stated they were Catholic but did not ever go to confession and did not feel the need after this. I handed them the pamphlet, <u>How To Cope With Guilt</u> and a referral to Religious Coalition for Reproductive Choice if they needed pastoral counseling.

Joe then changed the subject and asked, "How long will it be tomorrow before I can see her in recovery?" I knew we were not short-staffed in the surgical area that day, so I told him we would set aside a special room so he could be with her immediately afterward and throughout recovery. I explained, "We're unable to provide private recovery for everyone, but we try to provide all the extras we can for our patients undergoing a fetal indications termination." They expressed gratitude and seemed relieved.

Mary then produced a plastic packet from her purse and said, "The doctor wants a tissue sample for the genetic lab." I assured her I'd make certain the doctor received the packet and that it would be transported properly.

They appeared more relaxed now and I asked if both families were aware of the situation. Mary responded right away. "Oh yes. They said whatever we decided, they'd support us. My parents are strict Catholics, but even they think this is for the best." I asked what people have said to comfort them. Joe said, "Well, her mother told her she can always try and have another one." I asked, "How did you feel hearing this?" He replied, "I know she was trying to console us. I've been trying to console myself the same way, saying we can try again. I have two kids by a previous marriage, but they're almost grown and live with their mother. Mary has an 18-year-old from a

former marriage, but we'd like to have one together." Mary agreed wholeheartedly.

I asked Mary how she felt when her mother told her she could always have another child. Mary said, "It irritated me. She meant well, but having another baby doesn't take away the loss of THIS baby." I agreed that when a loved one dies – whether they're 85 years old or 24 weeks into the pregnancy – they're irreplaceable. Joe commented, "I guess it's hard for people to know what to say. Hell, I don't even know what to tell other people about it. My boss knows. He let me off today and tomorrow, but my co-workers still think we're having a baby." Mary said two of her co-workers knew and they felt she was doing what was best. She stated, "I don't want to tell anybody else. It's none of their business, but I know they're going to wonder what happened."

We talked about the fact that not everyone would be sympathetic because some people don't believe abortion is justifiable in any circumstance. Joe and Mary decided they did not want to subject themselves to the possibility of cruel remarks, so they were going to tell co-workers and acquaintances they "lost the baby." Close friends and family already knew and were behind their decision 100%. Mary said her 18-year-old daughter was away at at college, but they had talked over the phone and her daughter told her, "I'm behind you no matter what!"

We went on to discuss sadness and loss and the grieving process. Although Joe and Mary seemed in tune with each other's feelings, I informed them that men and women do not always match each other in the intensity or expression of their grief. "Mary's experience of the loss involves her body as well as her mind and emotions," I said. "Men can certainly feel enormous loss, but they can't experience the same physical feeling of emptiness as women. Because of their total involvement, women may grieve longer and get irritated with their husbands for 'getting over it' so soon."

Joe took ahold of Mary's hand and said, "If I could go through everything with you, I would." She smiled, grabbed a tissue, and cracked, "Would you get up on the table for me?" Without skipping a beat, he looked at me and said, "You see how she ribs me? I'm trying to be a nice guy and she's trying to get me up on that table!" She laughed for the first time. He grabbed her hand and said,

139

"Mary's a survivor. She'll make it. We've been through other hard times. We'll make it through this one." She agreed.

I agreed they both seemed capable of "making it through" and gave them the booklet, Difficult Decisions and How To Cope Successfully After An Abortion. "These booklets may be helpful not only to you but also to your family. Difficult Decisions is for couples faced with the tragic news of a serious fetal anomaly. It addresses their feelings, the difficulty of the decision facing them, how to care for each other, and prepares them for what other people may say to them." We finished the session by discussing their next visit to her doctor and the genetics counselor, and I gave them a counseling referral in the event they felt the need for additional counseling.

THE ANGRY ANTI-ABORTION CLIENT

Why Abortion Opponents Choose To Have An Abortion

Every abortion clinic across the nation sees its share of women who vehemently oppose abortion both politically and religiously who then come face to face with a situation in which they choose an abortion for themselves. An incredulous news reporter once asked me, "Why would a person who is strongly against abortion have one?" The answer is simple: for the same reasons that anyone else chooses to have an abortion.

Once these women are pregnant – or, in the men's case – once they become the partner in an unplanned pregnancy, the **reality** of a pregnancy may be vastly different than the **idea** of it. For instance, the idea of someone carrying to term and placing her baby for adoption may sound noble and appealing, as long as it's happening to someone else. The idea of canceling or postponing one's college education due to childbirth and childrearing may not seem like such a big deal until it's **your** educational goals at risk. Many people choose an abortion because financially they cannot afford to provide for a child (or another child). Financial hardship may sound like a small price to pay for the privilege of giving life until you're the one who has to stop and think what comes AFTER giving life?!

People who hold strong beliefs about **anything** don't necessarily follow their beliefs; but when they act in opposition to their beliefs, guilt, anger, fear, and shame may result. Anti-abortion clients certainly may feel all of these emotions and have a variety of ways of showing their distress. Some have called and requested special treatment, such as performing their abortion on a Sunday or at night so none of their fellow protesters will see them. Many abortion providers have accommodated these requests for special privacy measures, and many have rued it afterwards. There are many true stories of protesters who got right back on the picket line the very next week once their own clandestine abortion was behind them. Giving special treatment to an anti-abortion activist does a disservice to other patients, the staff, and to the client herself. While done in the spirit of compassion, sneaking her in and providing special treatment creates an unreal quality to the experience and better enables her to pretend it never happened. In the name of fairness, mental health, and quality care, providers need to decline taking part in these charades.

The client I want to discuss here is the woman who is vehemently opposed to abortion but is seeking one herself and behaves angrily and aggressively toward staff and fellow clients. This is the woman who may drive up in a car with the message, "Adoption Not Abortion!" or "It's a Baby Not a Choice!" plastered on the back bumper. She is the one who tells you she has condemned and ostracized friends or family members who have chosen to have an abortion and labeled them murderers. She may have marched on Washington, D.C. to protest legal abortion, wielded placards and picketed clinics, or preached against abortion to her Sunday school students. She may be the leader of her pro-life church group or a volunteer at her local anti-abortion pregnancy test center. This is the person who has invested enormous emotional energy in the rigorous condemnation of everyone and anyone connected with providing or obtaining an abortion. And now she finds herself rubbing elbows with people she considers "the untouchables." Although there are some fake patients the antis "plant" to invade and disrupt a clinic, this patient is genuinely pregnant and seeking an abortion.

Anti-Abortion Client Reactions On The Day Of The Abortion

On the day of her appointment she is typically agitated, demanding, mistrustful, and above all, volatile. Any fear, shame, and guilt she most likely feels are tucked firmly away behind a layer of razor sharp hostility. She targets staff members and fellow patients alike with hurtful barbs, insults, accusations, and expressions of contempt.

Within a matter of minutes she wreaks havoc at the front desk and in the waiting room by provoking everyone around her. For example, one woman I'll call Patty marched into the clinic and loudly scolded the receptionist, "It's your fault I'm late! You gave me lousy directions on the phone!" Then Patty proceeded to offend the patients sitting around her in the waiting room. She was overheard by a staff member jeering to her girlfriend, "Look at all these people – doesn't anybody know how to use birth control!" and "I hear sometimes they leave part of the baby inside you." A counselor was promptly called to take Patty into counseling. The sooner this client is taken into a private office and attended to, the better it is for everyone.

Your Objectives

Your objectives with this client are to:

1. Remain professional even though she will push you to the edge.

2. Match her energy and power as you express empathy for the difficulty of her position.

3. If she rebuffs all attempts of yours to connect with her, set firm limits on her verbal abuse toward you and other patients and staff.

4. If she ignores the limitations, decline her as a patient. It is a disservice to the other patients to subject them to her disruption and abuse. It also depletes the staff of the energy they need to attend to all the other patients.

Example Of A Counseling Session With An Anti-Abortion Client

When Patty was called into the counseling office, she glared and asked sarcastically, "Oh, is this the **counseling** I have to go through?" Once inside my office she sat down and snapped, "I want you to know I don't believe in abortion, and this is nothing but a slaughterhouse! It makes me sick just to sit here and look around!"

Counselor: "I can see it disgusts you to be in an abortion clinic because you believe we're slaughtering babies!"

Client: "It's not just what I believe. Everybody KNOWS that's what you're doing here."

Counselor: "Then tell me, why are you here?"

Client: "I have NO choice! It's something I HAVE to do!"

Counselor: "I want you to know right now you are free to leave any time."

Client: "I know this is what I have to do. I just have no other choice."

Counselor: "What made you rule out the choice of adoption?"

Client: "I can't go through nine months and all that pain of childbirth and then give it up!"

Counselor: "Can you tell me why you feel so strongly you could not give it up?"

Client: "I already have one child, and I know what it's like feeling movement and then going through childbirth. I know I couldn't part with it after all that!"

Counselor: "Many women do not want to go through nine months and then give their child to adoptive parents. What made you rule out the choice of keeping the child?"

Client: "I can't. That's all there is to it. Look, I just want to get this over with. Aren't there some little papers I have to sign?"

Counselor: "Our clinic believes in taking the time to assess the patient's physical and emotional well-being before and after an abortion and to ensure informed consent. If you want to be rushed through and treated like a number, you're in the wrong place."

Client: "Well, I didn't know it was going to take so long. Nobody told me I'd have to go through all this."

Counselor: "You're saying no one told you to expect to be here a total of four hours?" (The secretaries always prepare the clients at the time they make the appointment to expect a four-hour stay at the clinic.)

Client: "Hell no! I've got to go to work in two hours!" she exclaimed.

Counselor: "Maybe you better reschedule on a day when you have enough time."

Client: "This is a f---ing bunch of bull! You people don't know what the f--k you're doing. Do you expect me to sit out there with all those trashy women all that time?"

Counselor: "I don't deserve to be cursed at, and I will ask you to leave if you continue using abusive language."

Client: (Gets the message but changes the subject) "How can your doctor kill babies all day long?"

Counselor: (Switches the focus back on the client) "Because he doesn't believe it's killing, but you do. Why do you want him to kill your baby?"

Client (Looking startled and then becoming teary): "The father in this pregnancy is a son-of-a-bitch."

At this juncture, the client dropped her fierce facade and became receptive to discussing her lack of support, rejection from boyfriend, religious beliefs, her political activism against abortion, and lack of coping skills. The counselor told her she needed to return home and seek additional counseling before the doctor would provide an abortion for her because she was at high risk for a poor emotional outcome.

Client: "I have to have the abortion today! You can't send me home! I'll be just fine afterwards!"

Counselor: "I know there's a part of you that does not want to be pregnant. But there's another strong part of you that does not want to participate in what you believe to be killing a child. That part needs to be respected and attended to. We will not consider performing an abortion for you unless you seek additional counseling before the abortion."

Client: "But we drove two hours today! I can't take off work again, and I don't have anyone to drive me back here! I've got to have it today!"

Counselor: "I know you are angry and feel inconvenienced, but I am not going to participate in anything I believe will be harmful to you."

The client reluctantly took the referral and never returned.

What Happens After The Abortion?

The angry anti-abortion client who bullies her way through the abortion clinic process and continues to lash out in all directions usually leaves mad. She is also usually unreceptive to and contemptuous of a counseling referral. We can do our best to point people in the direction of beneficial resources, but we can't make them help themselves. What we can do is decide not to participate in providing them with an abortion. What happens when you do provide an angry anti-abortion client with an abortion?

One woman who worked in a free, anti-abortion pregnancy test center came to Hope Clinic angry but became receptive to talking about her sadness and guilt during counseling. After her abortion she wrote me a letter and told me, "I am grateful for what you all did for me. When I first walked through your door I was mad at myself and scared. I know now that everything about abortion I ever told the girls who came to me at Birthright was false. I've decided to make up for any harm I've caused by writing to my legislators urging them to keep abortion legal. I never thought I'd ever need your services, but I did, and I don't regret the abortion. I just regret I got pregnant."

On the other hand, the angry client who clings to her rage instead of dealing with her feelings of shame and guilt is very unlikely to change her views. This client may become so guilt-ridden and filled with shame and rage, her abortion experience can fuel the fire of her zealotry against legal abortion. Those who were previously involved in anti-abortion activities may intensify their activism as an act of repentance and try to prevent other women from choosing abortion. Some have joined groups such as W.E.B.A. (Women Exploited By Abortion) and claimed they didn't know what they were doing when they had the abortion. They blame the doctor and clinic staff for "not telling me I was killing a baby."

When I interviewed women years after their abortions, one woman told me she atoned for her "sin" by deliberately getting pregnant again, going to a Christian home for single mothers, and placing the baby for adoption. She said she had gone on radio talk shows to speak against abortion at the urging of the pro-life organization to which she belonged. Although she had stated she had a strict Catholic upbringing and "knew abortion was killing," she also told me she didn't know what she was doing at the time of the abortion. "I thought I was just getting unpregnant," she said, "and the doctor didn't tell me I was killing a baby."

Some women who said they professed strong moral opposition to abortion and angry feelings at the time of the abortion described severe negative reactions afterwards. They also stated they wished they had sought therapy a lot sooner than they had. Almost all who had finally sought counseling said they benefited from it.

Are Abortion Clinics Obligated To Provide Abortions To Angry Anti-Abortion Clients?

A few abortion providers hold the philosophy that they are obligated to serve any woman requesting an abortion because they believe it is her right. These providers believe it is wrong to place more weight on their judgment than on hers and to deny her access to their services because of her angry behavior and moral beliefs. However, abortion providers have the right and the responsibility to refuse service to people who are offensive and abusive to other patients and to staff, and who may be at high risk for physical or emotional complications. These angry clients may also be more likely to involve the clinic in a lengthy and costly legal suit **regardless** of whether there are any grounds.

THE INCEST SURVIVOR

As you might expect, the client whose pregnancy is a result of incest is often a young teen under the age of 15. When incest is the known cause of the pregnancy, the adolescent's mother, grandparent, or legal guardian almost always accompanies her to the clinic. Sometimes charges have been filed and the county sheriff must transport the fetal tissue to a lab where bloodwork can be done to determine paternity for the court proceedings.

Issues And Concerns

Since major issues for incest survivors include shame, mistrust, and secretiveness, there are bound to be occasions when clients convincingly fabricate a story about a boyfriend and never reveal the truth. A few times such clients have called weeks afterwards to tell us the real story and seek help. I have no doubt there are other incest survivors whom we never know about. Some may deny the reality to themselves as well. This is especially true if they have sought help from their mother or other family member and been told they are imagining things. Denial runs rampant in incestuous families.

When incest is the known cause of the pregnancy, the young woman has usually been in contact with a case worker or sexual abuse counselor. If not, she needs a referral and information about what counseling can offer her. Healing from sexual abuse is a process that takes time and professional care. To become familiar with treatment for incest survivors, I recommend Adele Mayer's excellent treatment manual, Incest.

During the pre-abortion session, the counselor needs to let the client know she can choose to tell as much or as little as she wants about what has happened. Usually the client is quiet and compliant, and **that's** OK. The counselor can reinforce her courage, strength, and ability to heal. The client also needs to be given as much control over the abortion experience as possible. Control has been denied her by the perpetrator, and she may not be accustomed to exercising her own will. Nonetheless, restoring control in her life will be part of the healing process. The counselor can ask her whether she wants the person accompanying her to join them in the session when explaining the procedure and aftercare. If the clinic has both female or male physicians, she needs to be able to choose whoever would make her more comfortable. When in the procedure room, the counselor needs to ask her if she would like her hand held. Any additional relaxing medications the client can have need to be offered. The counselor should also inform the medical staff about the client's circumstances.

Sometimes the only way a young incest survivor can tolerate an abortion procedure is with a general anesthetic. It will be important to know where to refer for an abortion under general. A good indication of her ability to tolerate the abortion is if she can tolerate a pelvic exam.

Example Of Counseling An Incest Survivor

Tanya, age 14, appeared quiet and shy. At the time of the appointment, her mother had explained the situation to us and told us a sonogram revealed she was 15 weeks pregnant. She also stated their sheriff would need to transport the fetal tissue for paternity testing. Arrangements were made with our Director.

On the day of her abortion, Tanya was seen alone first. Tanya stated she wanted the abortion herself because "the baby's my stepfather's, and I don't want it." She also stated she felt too young to become a parent and did not want to go through the pregnancy with everyone at school knowing, so adoption was out of the question. She asserted that what she wanted was to go to school like other kids her age.

She said she told her mother what happened once she had missed her third period, since she was used to missing periods. Fortunately, her mother believed her and had her step-father arrested. Tanya and her mother were in counseling, and had talked about her pregnancy options. Tanya told me her counselor was supportive of her decision to have an abortion, and she had an appointment to see her counselor the following Wednesday.

Tanya said she expected to feel "much better" emotionally after the abortion. She denied feeling sadness or guilt about having an abortion, and expected no regret afterwards. Because sexual abuse often leads to depression, I asked about symptoms, and she confirmed that she had been feeling depressed "most of the time" because of her step-father. The pregnancy had made her feel even more depressed, she said, and at times she wished she were dead. However, she did not have a suicide plan or method and felt the counseling she was receiving was beneficial.

Her main concern was fear of the procedure. I asked if she would like her mother to join her to hear about the procedure and aftercare, and Tanya said yes. When her mother joined the counseling session, she seemed very supportive. She said counseling was helping them both, and she was just sorry she hadn't known what was going on before this happened. She blamed herself, and we talked about her love for her daughter and sadness about not having been able to protect her. We also discussed the steps they were both taking to heal from the trauma and the strength of their relationship.

Tanya's mother asked if she could be present for any part of the procedure, and I explained why she couldn't (state regulations). Tanya looked apprehensive, and her mother began to reassure her she'd be OK. I told her I would introduce her to the nurse who would be with her, and I offered to be with her as well. She and her mother seemed comforted by this suggestion. Tanya proved a very cooperative patient both days. By the second day she was familiar with me, the nurse, and the doctor. She was still scared, but not as petrified as the day before. After everything was over and she was discharged from recovery, both she and her mother seemed greatly relieved and grateful.

THE CLIENT WITH A MENTAL ILLNESS OR MOOD DISORDER

Issues And Concerns

A literature review on psychological sequelae after an abortion reveals that women who have a mental illness or poor psychological functioning have a higher incidence of poor coping after an abortion (Payne, Kravitz, Notman, and Anderson, 1976, David, Rasmussen, & Holst, 1981, Dagg, 1991, and Major & Cozzarelli, 1992). Hope Clinic's experience has found the incidence of poor coping to be higher among those women with mental illnesses who are not compliant in taking their prescribed medications for their illness than for those who are in compliance. In consulting with various psychiatrists in the St. Louis area, we have discovered that hormonal and chemical changes occuring in the body after an abortion are partly responsible for the symptoms of poor coping in this population.

Before we instituted our protocol for clients with mental illness, I had counseled a 24-year-old woman who seemed perfectly lucid and appropriate at the time of our counseling session. She stated she did not want to bring a child into a life of poverty, and couldn't take care of the two children she had. She told me she had been unable to provide for her children, and they were made wards of the state. She did not want to have another child that would have to be taken from her. She stated she had no moral qualms about abortion and anticipated no regret. Three days later she became psychotic. She had gone off her antipsychotic drugs a few days before the abortion without her doctor's knowledge. She had not revealed this information to me at the time. Fortunately, I had spoken to her mother at the time of the abortion who told me her daughter's children had been made wards of the state due to her daughter's neglect. Her mother seemed supportive and in total agreement with her daughter's decision. She, too, did not mention her daughter's mental condition. However, she was the one who made the phone call to me two days after the abortion. She told me her daughter called to tell her she was hearing voices "from the dead baby" and was threatening suicide. Her mother then explained her daughter was manic-depressive and had been hospitalized in the past for hallucinations. I urged her mother to take her to the psychiatric hospital for admission and to call me if her daughter was unwilling to go. A few hours later, her mother called to tell me her daughter was in the hospital and back on her medications. Two weeks later her mother informed me her daughter was fine, and once back on the medications no longer hallucinated. Her daughter told her and the psychiatrist she felt the abortion was the best decision.

Hope Clinic's Protocol For Screening Clients For Mental Illness

When making their appointments, clients are asked if they have ever been prescribed antidepressants or "nerve pills." This way we have been able to screen many of our clients on the phone before they arrive at the clinic. These calls are routed to a counselor, and the counselor asks her the following questions.

1. Have you ever been diagnosed with depression, manic-depression, schizophrenia or other mental illness or disorder?

2. Have you ever been hospitalized for the illness/disorder? How long ago? How long were you in the hospital?

3. Were you prescribed medication to manage the disorder? How long have you been taking it?

4. Is the doctor who gives you the prescription for your medications a psychiatrist?

5. Are you presently taking your medication? If YES, good! We then instruct her to keep taking it as usual, including the day of the abortion. If not, when and why did she quit? Is her doctor aware of this?

6. When was the most recent time you saw your therapist or the doctor who gives you the prescription? How often do you see him/her?

7. Did you talk to either of them about the pregnancy and abortion decision? If not, why not? If yes, were they supportive?

Using This Information For Our Clients' Welfare

After the screening process, if she has a mental illness and has quit her medication without consulting her psychiatrist, has been hospitalized in the past, and does not see a counselor, she is considered high risk for poor coping. This is especially so if she has any other risk factors for poor coping. We will ask her to bring us a letter from her psychiatrist or therapist stating the following:

1. She has discussed the pregnancy and abortion decision with him or her.

2. She has made an appointment to see him or her again after the abortion.

We want her to bring this letter with her on the day of her abortion. It must be in her chart BEFORE we perform her abortion. We have found if we wait to receive it after the abortion, the client does not comply in seeking the kind of emotional help she needs. We will give her a referral if she no longer has a therapist or psychiatrist, and we will help facilitate making an appointment for her if she has any difficulty doing so herself. The client who balks at seeing a therapist or psychiatrist and demonstrates noncompliance with managing her illness is potentially a very high risk for not only poor coping but also failing to follow post-abortion aftercare.

If the woman is presently in an inpatient treatment facility for her disorder, we want her to bring a similar letter from her psychiatrist or therapist.

If she states she is taking her medication, sees a therapist, has good support for her decision, and does not have any complicating factors, we will NOT require a letter from her therapist. She is demonstrating the desire and ability to manage her illness. We may simply ask her to sign a consent form that states she agrees to continue taking her medication after the abortion and will make a follow-up appointment with her therapist.

By following this plan of action, Hope Clinic has concrete evidence that the client has taken steps to take care of her emotional well-being after the abortion, and that we did everything we could to link her with appropriate resources and support. Some women have told us they would have never carried through with seeking help if we had not required them to do so.

Sometimes there are extenuating circumstances, and we waive the requirement of receiving the letter prior to the abortion. However, in those cases the client must sign a consent form that states she agrees to consult her psychiatrist or therapist soon after the abortion and to start taking her prescribed medication no later than the day after the abortion. It also allows Hope Clinic to exchange information with her therapist or psychiatrist. We may also request that we talk to the support person who came with her to the clinic to reinforce the importance of her following through with the agreed-upon plan of action.

ADOLESCENTS AND PARENTS

Adolescents' Reactions to a Pregnancy

When adolescents find out they are pregnant, they may experience any of the following:

1. Fear – of what to do, of parents' finding out, of parents' reactions, of what her boyfriend and others might think.

2. Denial – of the pregnancy test results, the symptoms, the pregnancy itself.

3. Guilt – from having sex or from not using birth control.

4. Hope – of getting out of school, having a direction in her life, getting married and leaving her parents' house, OR of staying at home and continuing to depend on parents.

5. Safe – from having to go to college or get a job, and from moving out on her own.

6. Joy – of having a baby of her own, giving her boyfriend a child, becoming a mother, and receiving attention.

7. Anger – toward her boyfriend or herself for getting pregnant.

8. Satisfaction – of feeling grown up, knowing she's fertile, or maybe satisfaction of using the pregnancy as a way to get back at her parents or boyfriend.

Sometimes at the time of the pregnancy test, the adolescent client wants to stay and hear about her options, but often she is thinking about whom she is going to tell as soon as she leaves the clinic. If the boyfriend is still in the picture, she usually wants to tell him and talk about what to do. She may already know how he'll react, or she may not have a clue. Here are some of the most common male reactions to a teenage girlfriend's pregnancy.

Boyfriend's Reactions

1. Fear – of what to do, of what she'll decide, of his or her parents, of his girlfriend expecting marriage or financial assistance, of failing in his responsibility to her, or of a negative outcome.

2. Denial – of the pregnancy, his paternity, or his responsibility towards her.

3. Guilt – that he got her pregnant, that they didn't use birth control.

4. Anger – toward himself for not taking precautions, or toward her if he thinks she got pregnant on purpose.

5. Satisfaction – of feeling grown up and able to father a child.

6. Hope – of keeping his girlfriend, of proving his manhood.

7. Joy – of having a family of his own.

As discussed in the chapter on significant others, the male partner's reaction can greatly affect both the woman's decision and her feelings about the decision. While some young women are eager to know what their partner thinks about the pregnancy, others fear the worst and choose not to tell, especially if they've already severed the relationship. Almost all women, especially adolescents, want and need to tell **someone** they're pregnant and receive help and support. If support is not forthcoming from their boyfriend, then most adolescents turn to a parent. The younger the adolescent, the more likely it is she will involve a parent.

Parents' Emotional Reactions To Their Teenager's Pregnancy

Parents' reactions vary from family to family and run the whole gamut from fury to delight. Behaviors can include crying, shouting, hitting, withdrawing, throwing the teen out of the house, or supporting, comforting, hugging, and helping with decision-making. Some parents – usually mothers – are happy and want their teenage daughter to have the baby and let them raise it as their own. Some parents pressure their daughter into carrying to term and relinquishing the baby for adoption as a punishment. Others engage in physical and emotional abuse as they vent their rage. Many parents, however, try their best to support their daughter in whatever she decides to do about the pregnancy.

Most of the parents at Hope Clinic have described a combination of the following emotions and issues.

1. **Disappointment**: It is understandable that parents might feel disappointed when their teenage daughter gets pregnant. Parents usually want their children to finish school, get married, and have a home and financial stability before they take on the responsibility of parenthood. They might also feel disappointed that their child disobeyed their moral teaching not to have sex before marriage.

2. **Failure**: Parents often feel responsible for the actions of their children, and when their children "fail," they feel they, too, have failed. They may feel like a **total** failure as a parent, a role they have taken very seriously. If they actively tried to prevent the pregnancy by offering to take her to get contraceptives or by preaching abstinence,

they may feel defeated. They may chide themselves, saying, "There must have been something else I should have done!" And if they have always viewed their daughter as "the perfect child," they may experience her "fall from grace" as a reflection of their failure as parents.

3. **Sadness**: Some parents feel sad because their daughter's pregnancy signifies she is no longer their little girl. Parents may feel sad that their daughter has to learn about life the hard way and go through emotional and/or physical pain. A daughter's predicament may trigger painful feelings from her mother's own past - when she got pregnant as a teenager, for instance. Mothers who experienced the same thing often want a better life for their daughter without the struggle and heartache they went through. And even if they believe abortion is the best alternative for their daughter's life, they may also feel sadness about losing a potential grandchild.

4. **Anger**: Many parents feel angry for a number of reasons. They may feel their daughter betrayed their trust by being sexually active. They may feel disrespected because all their preaching against premarital sex and getting pregnant went unheeded. Some feel vexed at having to spend money and time on "her mistake." The pregnancy may further disrupt a family that is already having problems. Besides feeling angry at her, parents may feel angry with themselves if they think they have failed to parent her "right."

5. **Rejection**: When a teenager rejects the parents' moral teachings, the parents often perceive this as a personal rejection. Their feeling of rejection may intensify if their daughter refuses their advice about what to do about the pregnancy.

6. **Fear**: Parents who are accustomed to controlling and limiting their children's behavior to socialize or protect them may feel scared once their teenagers are no longer compliant. They may not know what to do and consequently feel powerless. This fear may be expressed in angry, punitive, and controlling behavior, such as putting a ban on dating, boyfriends, late hours, using the car, etc. Of course, this strategy usually ends in on-going power struggles, rebellion, hurt, and bitterness.

7. **Shame**: Usually parents are heavily emotionally invested in the behavior of their children.

If their children perform well and receive social, academic, or professional rewards, they feel proud. If their children fail in some way, they may feel embarrassed, ashamed, or somehow at fault. If parents believe teenage sex and pregnancy is shameful, they, too, may share the shame of their daughter's pregnancy. People who are particularly affected by what other people think of them and their families may be deeply shamed by their daughter's pregnancy.

8. **Guilt**: Parents may feel guilty that they were unable to prevent the "mistake" from happening. They may feel guilty for not being what they think are the perfect parents. If they have always been against abortion and now are supporting their daughter's decision to have one, guilt may result. They may feel hypocritical, especially if they have been vocal about their belief against abortion in the past, perhaps politically active in the anti-abortion movement, or involved in "pro-life" activities at church. If they don't support their daughter's decision and refuse to have anything to do with it, they may also feel guilty they let her down.

9. **Love For Their Daughter and Support For The Abortion Decision**: Most parents who accompany their daughters to the abortion clinic are supportive because: 1). they want their daughter to enjoy her teen years - dating and going out with friends - without the responsibility of parenting a child; 2). they want their daughter to finish her education; 3). they don't want her to marry so young; 4). they don't want her to struggle as a single parent; 5). they don't have the financial ability to help her raise the child adequately; 6). they know they would wind up raising the child and do not want to; and 7). they didn't want her to go through the same hardships they did as teenage parents.

Because adolescents know that parents sometimes react intensely to a teenage pregnancy, some teens are afraid to tell their parents about their pregnancy. In some states an adolescent can choose whether or not to tell her parents. Other states have passed Parental Involvement Laws that require an adolescent to reveal her pregnancy to one or both her parents.

Parental Involvement Laws And Their Impact On Adolescents

Some states require anyone under age 18 to tell her parents about her pregnancy before she can obtain an abortion (Henshaw & Kost, 1992). Some laws require consent from one or both parents, even if the parents are divorced or have been estranged from their daughter for years. Other states mandate that parents be notified but do not require consent. As of this writing there are still some states where minors can obtain abortion services without either parental consent or notification. Hope Clinic is located in Illinois where neither consent nor notification has been necessary. As time goes by, however, more and more states enact laws restricting adolescents' access to abortion.

Motives Underlying Parental Involvement Laws

Ostensibly the purpose of parental consent laws is to promote family communication and parental involvement in minors' decisions about their pregnancies. However, studies on the effects of parental consent laws show that positive family communication does not necessarily occur when it's forced; in fact, parents' knowledge of a teenage pregnancy can create damaging consequences to the family (ACLU, 1986, Henshaw & Kost, 1992). On the surface, parental consent laws can appear benign to the average legislator and to the population at large who believe parents SHOULD know what their teenagers are doing. Some think such laws will act as a deterrent to teenagers' sexual activity; others seek to involve parents because the adolescent is seeking a medical procedure with the possibility of complications. However, judges and counselors who have dealt with minors seeking abortions have concluded these laws erect another unnecessary barrier to abortion (ACLU, 1986).

The real aim of the proponents of parental consent laws appears to be limiting access to abortion for at least one segment of the population (ACLU, 1986). From 1973 to 1986 all parental consent laws were drafted by anti-abortion activists and introduced into legislatures by anti-abortion legislators. Social service professionals and medical organizations have opposed these laws and supported the ethic of confidentiality for all women, including adolescents (American Medical Association, 1992, ACLU, 1986).

Dysfunctional Families and Abusive Situations

Those of us in the counseling and medical professions have encountered too many dysfunctional families and abusive parents to believe such laws are beneficial to many adolescents. In one study of 1,519 teenagers seeking an abortion, 24% chose not to tell their parents for fear of physical abuse or being kicked out of their home (Henshaw & Kost, 1992). In the same study 3% of the teens who told their parents voluntarily were in fact abused or kicked out of their home.

My client, a 16-year-old I'll call Cindy, was one of the significant numbers of adolescents who did not want to tell her parents because she feared abuse. She lived in Missouri but came to Illinois for her abortion because of Missouri's parental consent law. She came with her 18-year-old boyfriend and his mother. She recounted what she had witnessed two years before when her older sister got pregnant. "My mother came into our room one night and threw off her covers. She started slapping her in the face and punching her in the stomach again and again. They were both screaming and my mother was hollering and calling her a whore. Then she kicked her out of the house. I heard my sister begging to be let back in. It was horrible. I don't ever want that to happen to me." Her boyfriend's mother told me, "Her mother is an alcoholic. When things get too bad over at her house I let Cindy stay with us. I'm afraid what would happen to her if her mother knew about this."

Another one of my young clients whom I'll call Angela, described the extreme emotional abuse and abandonment her sister had undergone at the hands of her parents because of a pregnancy. Her family was "strict Italian Catholic." She said she vividly remembered the December night when her pregnant, 17-year-old sister ran out of the house crying, and her father furiously threw all her clothes at her in the front yard, screaming "I only have ONE daughter now!" She recalled Christmas Day when her father ceremoniously dumped all her sister's wrapped Christmas presents into a large trash bag and ordered Angela and her little brother to watch as he dumped it in the trash. Since that day Angela has been told repeatedly by her father she is his only daughter and his only hope. She has been striving for perfection ever since – getting straight A's, fastidiously cleaning her room, going to Church –

and hiding unacceptable behavior. "My parents don't even know I have a boyfriend much less that I'm pregnant!" she cried.

Mary Jo, a 17-year-old client, found out the hard way what her parents would do if they knew she was pregnant. She hadn't told them, but her mother found her pregnancy test receipt in her purse. When her mother angrily confronted her, she denied it. That night her mother told her stepfather. "He threw me on the floor and kicked me in the stomach with his pointy-toe cowboy boots and told me that's what sluts get for messing around," she said.

The Judicial Bypass

Proponents of parental consent laws point to court bypass options written into many of these laws as an answer to teens in danger of abuse. However, the prospect of having to go to court, stand before a judge, and reveal her pregnancy and family secrets is frightening. The bypass process imposes a significant and intimidating obstacle for adolescents seeking an abortion. Research on the emotional consequences of undergoing court bypass procedures showed this experience was more stressful to adolescents than the abortion itself (Donovan, 1983).

Six state court judges who heard nearly 90% of the bypass petitions in Minnesota testified in the case, Hodgson v. Minnesota. Judge Gerald Martin stated he thought the minors found the whole court bypass process "a very nervewracking experience." Judge Garrity, who had heard bypass petitions in Massachusetts, testified that the parental consent laws and bypass procedures "just gives these kids a rough time. I can't think it accomplishes a darn thing." He perceived the court process as absolutely traumatic for minors (ACLU, 1986). Even after undergoing the stress of the court process, the adolescent is not guaranteed her petition will be granted. The success of the judicial bypass depends upon the attitudes of the judges. And while some judges grant most or all requests for exemptions from telling parents, others grant none at all (Schoenberg, 1992).

Abortion providers must know exactly what their state's law says and means. If there is a judicial bypass written into the law, the provider needs to find out all the legal steps an adolescent must take to utilize that option. Then, the director of the clinic needs to make a decision if and how to help adolescents through the red tape of the court process. In some clinics patient fees may need to increase to cover the cost of staff time taken in 1). discussing the court process with the adolescent over the phone; 2). helping to make arrangements with legal counsel; and 3). accompanying her on the day of the court proceeding to decrease fear and expedite the process. Other clinics seek volunteers in the community who are willing to help expedite this process. A staff member is still needed to organize the volunteer effort and make arrangements with the minors and the volunteers. For more information on how to accommodate the requirements of a parental involvement law, write to The National Abortion Federation, 1436 U Street, Washington, DC 10009 for *A Guide for Abortion Providers: Parental Involvement Laws.*

Some Adolescents Voluntarily Choose To Tell Parents

In a study of 1,519 adolescents choosing an abortion in a state with no parental consent laws, 45% of the teens had voluntarily told at least one parent (Henshaw & Kost, 1992). Of the teens who were 14 years old or younger, 55% told their parents voluntarily, and by the time of the abortion, 90% of the parents knew about the pregnancy. The younger the minor, the more likely their parents were told. Other factors that increased the probability the adolescent had told parents were 1). if she felt she could discuss her feelings in general with her father; 2). if she felt she could discuss sexual issues with her mother; 3.) if she lived with only one parent; and 4). if she was unemployed or not attending school.

Why Some Adolescents Choose Not To Tell Parents

Daughters who chose not to tell their parents in this study were more likely to be older than 16 years of age, white, employed, Catholic, and living with neither or both parents.

The most frequently reported reason (73%) for not telling parents was "didn't want to hurt or disappoint parent." Fear of parents' anger was the second most reported reason (55%). Tied for third place was "didn't want parents to know I was having sex," and "thought parent would make me stop seeing my boyfriend." Other rea-

sons given for not telling included, "parent has too much stress already," "didn't need parent to help me decide what to do," "it would cause problems between parents," "parents would make me leave home," "I'd be punished," "parent would make me continue the pregnancy," "fear I'd be beaten," and "parent would make me have an abortion."

When Daughters Don't Tell But Parents Find Out

When parents found out about the pregnancy in ways other than the daughter telling them, the consequences were worse than when the daughter told them herself (Henshaw & Kost, 1992). Worse consequences included increased stress and problems between parents, and less support, less understanding, and more punishment for the daughter. Parents who found out were also three times more likely to stop their daughter from seeing her boyfriend, and were two times more likely to pressure her into having an abortion. Longer delays in decision-making occurred when parents found out about the pregnancy. The authors of the study suggested these negative consequences may explain why the daughter chose not to tell her parents, or it may be a reflection of the parents' disappointment in their daughter's failure to tell them herself.

Alternatives to Telling Parents

Keep in mind when exploring her fears about telling parents there may be viable alternatives, such as the judicial bypass written into some state laws and the possibility of referring her to a clinic in another state without parental involvement laws.

Adolescents' Reactions to Parental Involvement Laws

When someone calls to make an appointment, they should be told about the state law and if they should bring identification and proof of age. Requirements vary, depending on each state law. Adolescents who had hoped to avoid involving their parents may react initially with distress, fear, or anger and may start crying or pleading for an exception to be made in their case. They may also ask, "Is there any place I can go where I don't have to tell my parents?" In any case, the staff member taking the call needs to listen to their fears and explore the probability of their fears coming true.

One of the most common initial responses may be, "My parents will kill me!" In the vast majority of cases, what they mean is "they'll be very angry." However, some parents are capable of doing serious bodily harm. When Spring Adams, a 13-year-old from Fruitland, Idaho became pregnant by her abusive father, telling him about the pregnancy proved fatal. Her father shot her to death with a .30 caliber rifle while she lay sleeping (ACLU Reproductive Freedom Project, 1991). A 16-year-old client of mine and her 19-year-old boyfriend both feared for their lives. Although she was not faced with a parental consent law in Illinois, there was the danger of her father becoming homicidal if he found out she was pregnant. Her mother came with her daughter and boyfriend and confirmed her daughter's fears her father would shoot to kill. Her mother had long been abused by him, and he had already been in prison for violent crimes. Recently he had been released and was back at home. The boyfriend was so nervous he couldn't stop sweating and trembling and could barely talk. So, before dismissing the statement, "my parents would kill me," ask what she means.

Fear Of Abuse

1. Tell me what you mean when you say "they'd kill you."

2. Describe how your mother acts when she is angry and upset. (Specifically ask about any history of hitting, punching, kicking, yelling, threatening her verbally or with a gun).

3. Describe how your father acts when he is angry and upset. Ask for the same specifics as above.

4. If she IS describing abusive behavior, empathize and validate her fears. Then let her know you are required by law to report child abuse. Has the abuse ever been reported in the past? What happened?

5. Discuss the judicial bypass and/or refer to a clinic with no parental involvement laws.

Fear Of Causing Severe Health Crisis To An Ailing Parent

Sometimes an adolescent's parent or custodial grandparent is recovering from a heart attack, "nervous breakdown," or cancer treatment, and she is afraid the news of her pregnancy will cause extreme stress and a serious relapse.

1. Validate her concern for her parent's well-being.

2. If the law requires only one parent's involvement, ask how the other parent would react. Would her other parent be likely to agree it would be best to avoid telling the ailing parent? I once spoke to a client who said she was "Daddy's girl," and he was recovering from heart surgery. She was afraid for his health and she said if her mother ever found out she was pregnant, she'd deliberately tell her father to cause a rift between the two of them. She stated, "Then, if he died, my mother would blame me for it. That's the way she is. She's been blaming her own sister for their father's death for years. She's always telling me I'm just like my aunt. This would be final proof to her."

3. Explain the judicial bypass process or refer her to a clinic in a state without parental involvement laws.

Fear Of Disappointing And Hurting Parents

Fear of disappointing parents can be a powerful deterrent to telling them. The shame underlying this fear can lead to desperate measures if the teen sees no way out. The case of Becky Bell attests to the lengths a teen will go to protect her parents and her relationship with them. Becky was a minor from Indiana where parental consent is a prerequisite for an abortion. Rather than tell her parents, Becky died from a self-induced or illegal abortion (the whole truth has never been uncovered). Right before she died of a uterine infection from a septic abortion, she gave her mother a special friendship bracelet. Her parents have traveled nationwide, speaking publicly and decrying parental consent laws (Sharpe, 1990).

1. When exploring the adolescent's statement, "They'll be disappointed," ask if she thinks they will flatly reject her, or if their disappointment will simply make them feel sad for a time. If the adolescent concludes her parent's disappointment would be temporary, helping her differentiate between rejection and temporary disappointment

can make telling them much less catastrophic.

On the other hand, if she feels certain they will permanently reject her, the judicial bypass or referral may be appropriate. One 16-year-old client described how her father hatefully rejected both her brothers when they impregnated their girlfriends while still in high school. She stated, "He kicked them out and told them he hated them. He has never talked to either of them since. My older brother lives in Chicago now. The other one is in Tennessee. My mother does whatever my father tells her, but I can tell she wishes it were different. He watches our phone bill so he knows we're not calling my brothers without him knowing. I'm his only daughter, so I know it would be 10 times worse for me and my mother if he knew I was pregnant."

2. Are there other things she has done that disappointed her parents? Do they still love her?

3. Has she ever been disappointed by something her parents have or haven't done? Does she still love them?

4. What do her parents want for her future? How will those dreams for her affect their reactions to her decision? If she wants to keep the baby, how might they react? If she wants an abortion, how might they react?

Fear Of Her Parents' Forcing Her To Carry To Term

1. What makes her think her parents would force her to have the baby? One 18-year-old client stated she got pregnant at age 15 and wanted an abortion, but her religious mother talked her into having the baby. Once the baby was born, her mother took the baby and is raising it as her own. "I had to move out of the house and live with my grandparents. I wasn't allowed to see my own son for a whole year after he was born. He thinks my parents are his parents. He calls me 'Sissy.' I'll never go through that again!" Other clients have described carrying to term in the past and being pressured into placing the baby for adoption as a punishment for getting pregnant.

2. Even when parents have professed anti-abortion beliefs in the past, many support their own daughter having an abortion if they believe she's not ready for parenthood.

3. What are her beliefs about abortion?

4. If her parents are religious, there may be a friend of the family or pastor who is willing to mediate between her and her parents. I have seen a baptist minister who came with both the mother and her daughter to Hope Clinic for moral support. He told me, "I'm here because they need me. In I Corinthians 13:13 Paul said, 'And now abide faith, hope, love, these three; but the greatest of these is love.' I try to show my congregation love above all."

5. How strongly does she feel abortion is preferable to adoption or keeping the baby? When parents have been supportive and helped their daughter raise the child, some teen mothers have been able to continue their education and achieve their goals.

Fear Of Anger

1. Describe how your mother acts when she's angry (check for abusive behaviors). What will she probably say to you in this situation? What will she probably do?

2. Describe how your father acts when he's angry (same as above).

3. Do you have any sisters who got pregnant in their teens? What happened? How did your mother react? How did your father react?

4. Some girls have found it helpful to have another adult present when telling their parents. When another adult is in the room, parents are less likely to lose control. Would you feel more comfortable having someone with you? (If yes), whom could she tell who'd be willing to be with her?

5. Timing is important. A quiet, relaxed time of day provides a better atmosphere than when parents are feeling rushed, hungry, distracted, or upset by something else.

6. You don't have to tell them both together. Which parent would you prefer to tell first?

7. Imagine the whole scene realistically from beginning to end so you won't get stuck imagining only the scary part. After their initial reaction, most parents get down to business and help their

daughter decide what to do. Imagine yourself surviving their angry reactions and then getting on with problem-solving.

8. Rehearsing the scene beforehand can help decrease your fear because it gives you a sense of control. You and I can run through it now. I'll be you. Whose part do you want to play? Your Mom or your Dad? I want you to say what you think they'd say if they were at their worst.

Helping Her Tell Her Mother Or Father (Rehearsing The Scene)

Counselor (As Daughter): "Mom, is this an OK time to talk to you?"

Client (As her Mother): "Yes. Why?"

Counselor: "I have something to tell you, but I'm really scared and upset with myself. It's hard to talk about it."

Client: "What is it?"

Counselor: "I did a pregnancy test on myself and it was positive."

Client: "What?! Oh my God!"

Counselor: "I feel so stupid and so sorry."

Client: "I can't believe it! How could you do such a thing!"

Counselor: "I can't believe it either. I feel so awful."

Client: "I thought you knew better!"

Counselor: "I'm disappointed with myself, too. I'm so mad at myself. I can't believe I made such a terrible mistake!"

Client: "Imagine how I feel! I guess everything I ever taught you meant nothing."

Counselor: "You might think that, but it's not true. If I could erase what I did, I would."

Client: "It's too bad you didn't think about it before you did it. Now look at the mess you're in!"

Counselor: "That's why I got up the nerve to

tell you. I knew you'd be furious, but no matter what I do, I'll need your help."

Client: "Well, leave me alone right now. I need time by myself."

The counselor stops and asks the client, "Then what would you do if she told you to leave?"

Client (As herself): "I'd go to my room."

Counselor: "How long do you think it would take before she was ready to talk?"

Client: "Probably a few days. I hate it when she gives me the silent treatment."

Counselor: "What do you do for yourself when you have to endure the silent treatment?"

Client: "I call up my best friend, and I stay out of my Mom's way. Sometimes I clean up around the house to try and make it up to her."

Counselor: "And in a few days it's over and she talks to you?"

Client: "Yes."

Counselor: "So you think this is pretty much how it will go when you tell her?"

Client: "Yes."

Counselor: "It sounds like even though it's scary and unpleasant, you have a way of enduring it, as you have done in the past."

Mothers And Daughters

The parent most pregnant teenagers turn to is their mother (Henshaw & Kost, 1992). Many more mothers accompany their daughters to Hope Clinic than fathers. Some mothers are extremely supportive and offer their unconditional acceptance and support no matter what their daughter decides. Others try to pressure their daughter into doing what they believe is best and disregard her feelings. And when their persuasion fails, some mothers reject their daughters either by withdrawing love or in extreme cases turning them out of the house.

Supportive Mothers

Even when Mother's initial reaction is crying, shouting, criticizing, or stony silence, most mothers rally around their daughter and allow her to make her own decision. Some daughters are astonished at their mother's unconditional support. They have stated, "She was upset at first, but she really helped me. I know now I can go to her for anything." Mothers have offered financial and emotional support with whatever decision is made. Once the abortion is decided upon, mothers have given their daughters financial help, transportation to the clinic, and most of all, a shoulder to lean on when their boyfriend deserted them. Sometimes mothers decide to share their own long-hidden secret: they, too, had an abortion. For many pregnant teenage daughters the most cherished gift they can receive from their mothers is the gift of love and acceptance when they are feeling ashamed.

Supportive mothers who come to the clinic want to know if their daughter will be safe, cared for, and able to have children later on. They also want to know about aftercare so they can be helpful afterwards. Supportive mothers show concern for their daughter's emotional and physical well-being.

Unsupportive Mothers

Sometimes unsupportive mothers also bring their daughters to the clinic. However, unlike mothers who come with their daughters to provide moral suport, these mothers have other motives. Some are pressuring their daughters to end the pregnancy because they do not want to be stuck raising their grandchild. Other mothers drop off their frightened 13-year-olds and leave them by themselves until four hours later. When asked where their mother went, they answer in soft, shy voices, "Shopping" or "She said she had other things to do."

Just as some women can become desperate when they feel trapped by a pregnancy, some mothers commit acts of desperation when **they** feel trapped by their daughter's pregnancy. A mother may turn a deaf ear to her daughter's feelings and drag her in against her will, insisting she have an abortion. When it becomes known the abortion must be the woman's own free choice no matter how young she is, some of these mothers explode in rage. I remember one mother snarling,

"I'll take her home and throw her down some steps and abort it myself!" Fortunately, she was calmer and more rational by the time she left counseling. Some mothers throw fits of hysteria, wailing, sobbing, threatening, and pleading. One mother feigned a heart attack, wheezing and clutching her heart, and pouring 10 bottles of pills out of her purse. Another mother slid down a wall onto the floor faking a faint. Some are experts at manipulation; others are genuinely at their wits' end and need professional help. The daughter's pregnancy may be the proverbial straw that breaks the camel's back.

Mother-Daughter Power Struggles

Before the pregnancy ever occurred, Mother and Daughter may have already been entangled in a succession of moves and countermoves to establish control. Mother has set limits around dating and curfew, for example, and Daughter has tested the boundaries. The tighter Mother has pulled in the reins, the harder Daughter has pushed in the opposite direction. Mother battles for control; Daughter battles for independence. When Daughter gets pregnant, the combat zone becomes her very body. The challenge becomes, "Who gets to decide what to do with it?"

At times the daughter states "At first I wanted to keep the pregnancy, but it was only because my mother told me I had to have an abortion. I didn't want to do what she told me to. I still don't want her to think I'm doing this because she told me to." In some families the only way daughters break away from their mothers is through a pregnancy. Achieving independence comes only through achieving the state of motherhood oneself. Even if the daughter ends the pregnancy and does not become a mother, the emotional effect may be the same. She has exercised her own will over her body and life and made a major decision on her own.

Some daughters sit down and immediately begin the counseling session by stating, "My mother is making me do this!" When they find out their mother cannot make them have an abortion, some teens appear triumphant. Others back down on their accusation and stammer explanations why it's really their own decision. Sometimes it is necessary for the counselor to talk to both the daughter and her mother to help them listen to and be heard by each other.

Helping Mothers And Daughters Communicate

A Counseling Scenario With An Angry Daughter and Mother

When a coercive mother and her daughter are in the counseling session together, the mother usually tries to get the counselor to join her in criticizing her daughter. For instance, the mother might turn to the counselor and say, "She thinks raising a baby will be easy as pie! A lot she knows at her age!" The counselor might make a general statement and then make a suggestion to enhance communication, such as, "People judge a situation to the best of their ability. I don't know if either of you is able to understand the other's viewpoint and feelings, but I want to give you both an opportunity to talk and be heard." Then the counselor turns to the daughter and invites her to talk, but suggests she talk to HER (the counselor), not her mother. This tactic diffuses some of the anger and hostility. The daughter and mother will speak differently to a third party than they would to each other, even in each other's presence. The counselor is listening to their tone as well as the content of what is expressed. Once their tone and content are devoid of derision, the counselor will invite them to deliver the message directly to each other.

For example, the counselor turns to the daughter in the above scenario and says, "Julie, if your mother were to listen to you, what would you like to say? For now, say it to ME, not to her." The counselor sits between them and draws her chair a little closer to Julie.

Julie (Says defensively): "I don't want the abortion!"

Counselor: "Help me understand that. Say it to me, not to your mother."

Julie: "I don't want to kill the baby."

Counselor: "One reason is that you don't want to kill the baby. You talked about some other reasons, too. Would you share those reasons with me again?"

Julie: "Joe (boyfriend) wants the baby, too, and he said I can move in with him and his Mom."

Mom, interrupting: "Oh, that's ridiculous!"

Counselor immediately quiets Mom: "Just a moment. I just want to hear from Julie right now. I'll make sure you have your turn."

Counselor turns back to Julie: "When Joe said you could move in with him and his Mom, did you both talk to his Mom?"

Julie: "Yes. She wants me to have the baby, too, and said I could live with them."

Counselor: "And that seems to be an option."

Julie: "Yes."

Counselor: "So you'd have to move away from your family to do that?"

Julie: "Yes."

Counselor: "And your mother doesn't think that would be a good idea?"

Julie: "I don't know what she thinks!"

Counselor: "Ask her what she thinks."

Julie (Turning to Mom, but not looking at her): "What do you think?"

Mom (In a hostile tone of voice): "You know that boy is NOT going to take care of you or that baby!"

Counselor (Draws chair close to Mom): "I'd like you to say it to her in a tone and manner so that she might hear it. I know you are a gentle person and you are in a very difficult situation. I want your daughter to hear your concern and I want to help you say it in a way that she can really hear your meaning. Tell her your concern again - gently."

Mom: "I don't want you to end up like me. You know how hard it has been for us...after your Dad left us. I want more for you than what what I had."

Counselor: "Are you worried about your daughter?"

Mom: "Yes!"

Counselor: "Tell her how worried you are."

Mom (In a caring tone of voice): "I'm very worried about you."

Counselor: "Thank you. You said that so well. Do you love your daughter?"

Mom (Starts to cry): "Of course I do. I wouldn't care about what she did if I didn't love her."

Counselor: "What has your daughter meant to you in your life?"

Mom (Dabbing her eyes): "Everything. She means the world to me."

Counselor: "She's very special to you. Tell me more."

Mom: "It has been her and me all these years. I don't know what I'd do without her."

Counselor: "Are you afraid you'll lose her?"

Mom (Crying): "Yes, and I'm afraid she'll lose what she could have in her life if she has this baby."

Counselor (Turns her chair to Julie): "Talk to me. Don't talk to her. What did you hear your Mom say?"

Julie: "That she loves me."

The dialogue continues in this vein until they both feel heard. They may not come to an agreement about the pregnancy, but they have had an opportunity to reconnect emotionally in a meaningful way. The counselor may end the session by complimenting them on their ability to communicate under stressful circumstances and giving them a referral for further counseling.

Fathers And Daughters

A father often doesn't know about his daughter's pregnancy because she chooses not to tell him (Henshaw & Kost, 1992). Admitting sexual activity to her mother is hard enough. And even when she tells her mother, both Mother and Daughter often agree not to tell Dad because they fear he'd be angry, hurt, or suffer more stress than he is able to bear (Henshaw & Kost, 1992). Sometimes the daughter is scared that her father would physically hurt her or her boyfriend and refuse to

let her see her boyfriend again.

If a client states both her parents know about the pregnancy, ask about each parent's reaction. When asked, "What was your father's reaction?" many patients reply, "I let Mom tell him. I don't know how he reacted. Mom said he was upset, but he's been pretty quiet around me. We don't talk much as it is, so nothing has changed really." However, some clients state their dad made them feel better about their decision to have an abortion. The client might explain, "My dad and I both want me to get through college and make something of myself first before I become a parent. He thinks abortion is best, too." Occasionally the daughter chooses to tell her dad and not her mom. In these cases the client usually describes her relationship with her mother as "strained" and her father as "close." More than one caring dad has accompanied his daughter to the abortion clinic because they both feared Mom would be too upset or would be against the abortion due to her religious convictions.

A Word About Step-Parents

In cases where parents are divorced and remarried, the daughter may choose to tell some, all, or none of her parent figures. Whom she tells seems to depend upon the closeness of the relationship. For instance, she may confide in her stepmother rather than her biological mother if she feels more comfortable talking to Stepmom. Many a step-parent has accompanied his or her stepdaughter to the abortion clinic and provided a lot of love and support. And, if the teenager lives with a step-parent who is abusive to her, she can be just as negatively impacted by his or her mistreatment as she would be by her biological parent.

Counseling The Parents

We can help parents or step-parents sort out their feelings and provide them with an empathic listener. Because they don't want anyone else to know their daughter got pregnant, they often have not confided in anyone else. Sometimes Mom has borne the burden alone. Just giving the parent an opportunity to talk and be listened to can be an enormous relief. And once the parent feels supported, she or he can be a stronger support for the daughter. The following are typical statements parents make in counseling that can be used as a springboard for meaningful discussion.

Parents' Counseling Issues

1. **"I thought she knew better!"** When parents feel disappointed in their daughter, they may need a gentle reminder that their daughter probably feels disappointed in herself, whether she shows it or not. She is probably feeling ashamed and sad, knowing she let them down. It may help them to think back to a time when they disappointed their own parents and remember how they felt and what they needed from their parents.

2. **"I feel sorry she has to learn her lesson the hard way."** When parents feel sad witnessing their daughter's pain, it reflects their loving concern for her. Can they recall a time in their life when pain became an effective teacher? Both they and their daughter can view painful mistakes as something important from which they can learn.

3. **"Sure, she makes a mess of it and now I have to bail her out of trouble! She should have listened to me in the first place!"** Parents have a right to feel angry and express their anger as long as it doesn't result in physical or emotional abuse. Name-calling and excessive criticism doesn't teach or prevent future mistakes. Letting their daughter know why they're angry without belittling her is critical. To whom can they vent and release all the hurtful things they want to say? Letting it all out to a third party can help them identify what they are angry about and restore their composure. When communicating to their daughter, it helps if they start out with the word, "I" instead of "you." (e.g., "I feel angry that you didn't take better care of yourself," instead of "You should have known better!"). They need to focus on their own feelings instead of criticizing hers. And again, can they recall a time when they didn't listen to their own parents and fell flat on their face? How did they feel? What could their parents have said to them that would have been helpful?

4. **"She doesn't care what I think is right or wrong. She does whatever she pleases!"** Because their daughter seems to have adopted a different set of values doesn't mean she is rejecting them. And it doesn't mean she rejects everything they taught her. Are there some things they believe or do differently now than when they were growing up? Does this difference of opinion mean they reject their parents?

5. **"Here I trusted her and look what happened! I shouldn't have been so trusting!"** Parents often feel betrayed if their adolescent is having sex "behind their back." They also feel compelled to put more constraints on their daughter's comings and goings. The two big issues of control and protection may become a primary concern to the parents after an abortion and a primary source of resentment to the adolescent.

A common strategy some parents may employ to reestablish control after an abortion is to prevent their daughter from seeing her boyfriend. The assumption is if she doesn't have access to him, or if she only sees him in the daytime, then sex won't happen. A gentle reminder that sex can happen anywhere anytime, and that forbidden fruit is even more tempting may shed light on their solution. They need to ask themselves, "What is the desired end result I'm seeking?" The desired result may be, "I don't want her to get hurt again," or "I don't want her to get pregnant again," or "I don't want her to have sex, period!" One of the hardest tasks of parenting a teenager is letting go. Parents are used to protecting and shielding their young children from harm. However, as children grow older and go through their teens, they must take over the task of taking care of themselves. Taking care includes protecting themselves from harm and making moral decisions. Making moral decisions isn't always easy, even for mature adults. The best we can all do is learn from our mistakes.

Parents also may not realize that women who are fortunate enough to have their boyfriend's support before and after an abortion fare much better psychologically than those who don't have his support. Caring for their daughter may need to include allowing her the continued presence of a caring partner. Taking away an important source of support may do more harm than good. Sometimes the daughter doesn't want to see him as much as she did before and is willing to go along with this strategy. But, this is one area in which there needs to be some negotiation.

6. **"I don't want her to get pregnant again, but I'm afraid if I let her have birth control, she'll think I'm giving her a free license to have sex."** Many parents don't want their teenagers having sex, but want to be realistic about the probability

it's going to happen again. They want a way to convey their disapproval of teen sex while at the same time leaving room for her to use contraception IF she is going to have sex anyway. They can simply state, "I still do not approve of sex at your age, but what I want more than anything is for you to take care of yourself and use birth control if you ARE going to be sexually active. Parents do not need to be the ones to take her to the clinic and pay for contraception. Engaging in adult activities may require that she and her boyfriend make adult decisions such as arranging transportation to the clinic and a way to cover the costs. Some parents need the reassurance that when a girl goes on the Pill, it doesn't mean she is going to say yes to any guy who comes along. Women don't become promiscuous just because they are protected from pregnancy.

7. **"I tried to instill morals in my kids. I guess I failed."** Parents who see their daughter's pregnancy as a sign of their failure as a parent may become depressed. This is especially problematic for those whose primary identity is being a mother or father. They will probably readily agree that no human being can control another person's every move - including their child's. And if they cannot control their every move, they cannot be responsible for their every action. Children are not puppets. Parents may certainly have influence over their children's beliefs and behavior, but they are not responsible for their children's achievements or their failures.

8. **"I've always believed abortion was wrong, and now here I am helping my own daughter have one!"** Parents may need to reevaluate their belief that abortion is "wrong." They may reach a new conclusion that bringing a child into the world when the mother can't take care of it physically, emotionally, or financially is "more wrong" than abortion. They may also decide trying to pressure someone into going through nine months of pregnancy and then give the baby away is "more wrong" than abortion. There are many reasons why good people have abortions, and why other good people support them through that process.

If they still conclude abortion is morally wrong, they may feel caught in a bind: Do they support their daughter in her time of need even if she wants to have an abortion, or do they desert her and wash their hands of the abortion? Some

parents find a compromise. They tell their daughter where they stand on the moral issue of abortion and reassure her they'll love her no matter what. Some parents even provide transportation and money if she has no one else to help her, despite their beliefs. Nonetheless, they may still feel guilty. What do they need from themselves and from God (if they believe in God) to feel forgiven? What does their faith teach them is necessary for God's forgiveness? They may need to speak to an understanding minister, rabbi, or priest about the subject of God's forgiveness. Some people feel confident in God's ability to forgive them, but can't seem to forgive themselves. Talking to a good friend, counselor, or pastoral minister may help them out of the rut of self-condemnation.

Pre-Abortion Counseling With The Adolescent

Emotional Reactions In Counseling

Adolescents usually communicate more openly when seen individually without parents in the counseling session. If the parent is in the room, the young woman usually clams up and lets her parent do all the talking. An occasional "yes" or "no" may be all she manages to say. When the counselor sees her alone, she will usually disclose more about her feelings and situation. It may be helpful, however, to talk with her mother or whoever accompanied her and inform them of the abortion procedure and aftercare instructions.

It is reasonable that the adolescent may be cautious, even mistrustful of you. She probably views you as an authority figure. She may feel you are going to side with her mother if there is a conflict. It is important to let her know you are there to meet her needs. As with any other client, but perhaps even more so with the adolescent, you need to empathize with her and let her know you are not judging her. Teenagers also feel very strongly about their privacy, so she may need reassurance that everything discussed is strictly confidential.

The younger the adolescent, the more likely she will be quiet and nervous in counseling. Communicating with adults is not a young teen's forte. Prolonged silences, averted eyes, and mumbled answers are not uncommon reactions for the teens 14 and under. Using humor, self disclosure, and informal chatting can help break the ice. Sometimes she is simply overwhelmed by fear. This is probably the first time she has been asked to speak for herself when in a medical setting. There is the usual fear of the unknown, fear of doctors, fear of pelvic exams, fear of pain, fear of being judged, fear of talking about sexual matters with a strange adult, fear for her safety, fear of being recognized by someone she knows, fear she'll be sick afterwards or that her body will be damaged and sterility will result. Fear can immobilize. So, approach the subject of fear as a normal reaction and work through each one with her.

When describing the procedure to a young teen, you might want to ask if she'd like her mother (or whoever brought her) to join you. If she is agreeable and her mother is supportive, the time spent describing the process can serve to put her at ease. Often her mother interjects reassurances or gentle humor when her daughter shows signs of fear. If her mother is effective, then you can join her style of comforting. If she is ineffective and in fact detrimental to her daughter's well-being, modeling other behaviors can help both of them.

Exploring Her Decision

Sometimes when you ask an adolescent, "How did you come to the decision to have an abortion?" the response is, "My Mom is making me." After you explain she cannot be forced to have an abortion by her Mom or anyone else, she often recapitulates and says, "Well, I want the abortion, too. I don't want to get married and I'm only 15. I know I'd love the baby if I had it, but I want to finish school." It is crucial that she acknowledges her own reasons for having the abortion. They might be the same reasons as her mother's or they might be different. Sometimes the young woman points out the pressure she has been feeling from her parents. They are SO anxious for her to have an abortion, she feels pushed rather than supported. Help her sort out her own feelings and separate them from those of her parents. The point is, it's her life, her pregnancy, and her decision.

One 16-year-old confided, "At first when I knew they wanted me to have an abortion, I decided to have the baby just so they wouldn't think I was doing what they wanted. Then I thought how stupid that was. I really didn't want

the responsibility of having a kid yet. It still makes me sick that they think I'm doing what they want." I told her, "Well, YOU know the truth, and I know the truth. Besides, it was smart of you to untangle it all and do what was best for you, despite the fact your parents wanted the same thing." She laughed.

Sometimes the adolescent genuinely feels trapped by her home life and sighs, "There's no choice but to have an abortion!" She might describe her home situation as "Impossible! My parents said I couldn't live at home if I had the baby, and they refuse to sign for me to get married." Or she may recognize that her family is under a financial burden as it is, and another mouth to feed would be disastrous. Although the situation may be a bleak one, you need to point out she DOES have a choice. Sometimes those choices boil down to these unpleasant facts:

1. She could carry the pregnancy to term and live at home with her parents, but may have to endure daily ridicule, criticism, and unhappiness. Once the baby is born, they could change their feelings and accept both her and the baby, or they might reject the child, too.

2. She could move in with her boyfriend, his family, friends or relatives or go to a residence for single mothers, have the baby, and place it for adoption. Most adolescents and their parents do not really want her to leave home. Living in a residence away from home without friends or family often seems dismal and scary. But the fact remains it IS an option, and some teens have chosen that option.

3. She could end this pregnancy and make plans for her future independence and a time when she COULD support herself and a baby without her parents. She would need to explore her ability to cope with this decision and put her energy toward building her future.

The ultimate question is: Which option does she think she could emotionally handle better than all the other options? Sometimes the process of elimination is easier - going from the hardest to the next difficult, and so on. When it comes down to the last two choices - which are usually living at home and keeping the baby versus having an abortion - she needs to think: 1). How will she probably feel and how will she cope with those feelings?; 2). How will her parents and family probably feel?; and 3). How might their feelings affect her, and how will she cope?

Sometimes an adolescent decides to have an abortion because she feels she could deal with her post-abortion emotions better than she could withstand her home life while carrying to term. In other words, she would rather keep her relationship with her family as is than to have the baby under upsetting conditions. And that is a choice. Try to identify the values behind the choice and reflect them back to her. "So what you're saying is that you'd rather live at home without the kind of disruption you described than to go through with the pregnancy and have the baby." She will probably agree with your summary or edit and elaborate on what you've said. Ask her if she needs any more time or counseling apart from your facility before she makes a final decision. Remind her once the decision is made and the abortion behind her, she cannot undo it. Ask about possible regret and discuss the negative effects on her if she blames her parents for her decision afterwards.

On the other hand, if the daughter concludes she does really want to have the baby and definitely does not want an abortion, then it's time to talk to whoever brought her. Usually it's her mother. Mom is usually operating from "the cold facts," with little thought of the daughter's emotions. The daughter is often viewing the pregnancy from an emotional standpoint with little thought of the reality of raising the child at her age. The mother who has dragged her unwilling daughter in for an abortion usually cites financial problems, need for education, and freedom for seeing friends and dating as logical reasons for terminating the pregnancy. The daughter may be thinking about having the baby of the one she loves. You may need to help them open their eyes to the other's perspective, giving both validity. The mother needs to realize the consequences of pressuring her daughter to have an abortion are very different from pressuring her into having other kinds of medical procedures such as a bad tooth pulled.

Sometimes the daughter believes her boyfriend will come through for her, and the mother believes he'll desert her. Advise both to get together with the boyfriend and his parents to discuss the situation. The mother and daughter need to hear what everyone involved is willing and not willing to do for her and the baby. Without this joint consultation, the mother and daughter will probably continue to struggle in a private tug of war, battling about their assumptions.

Sometimes a mother is convinced her daughter will get over an abortion within a matter of days after the abortion. Adolescents who feel in charge of their decision can cope well immediately after an abortion. But anyone who feels badgered into it cannot be expected to feel fine. When the abortion experience is the ultimate in a series of power plays between her and her mother, and the daughter perceives she has lost, she may become depressed, despondent, angry, and defiant.

If the daughter is adamant about having the baby and the mother feels defeated, then Mom may become depressed, despondent, and angry. If they have been playing a lot of other "I win - you lose" games, the pregnancy may represent the ultimate power conflict. You need to realize you can only do so much in the short time you have to work with them. They could use a referral for family counseling to help resolve bitter feelings as the pregnancy progresses.

Adolescents' Post-Abortion Emotions And Coping

Years of Hope Clinic experience has shown the most common immediate post-abortion feeling is relief. The tense, frightened, teary-eyed adolescent before the abortion often becomes relaxed, smiling and talkative once she is finished and ready to go home. However, there are situations that set the stage for emotional distress after an adolescent's abortion. Some studies have concluded that adolescents as a group are not negatively affected by having an abortion, and in fact benefit from it (Melton, 1986; Osofsky & Osofsky, 1972; Rosenthal & Rothchild, 1975; Zabin, 1989). Other studies have revealed that some adolescents do suffer psychological distress, just as some adult women do (Margolis, et al., 1971, Cvejic, et al., 1977, Campbell, Franco, & Jurs, 1988, Perez-Reyes, & Falk, 1973, Wallerstein, Kurtz, & BarDin, 1972, Franz & Reardon, 1992).

One study by Franz & Reardon (1992) researched post-abortion reactions of adolescents who were seeking help from a group called WEBA (Women Exploited By Abortion) at the time of the study. They discovered post-abortion psychological distress in adolescents if: 1). the adolescent perceived herself to be pressured into the abortion; 2). having and keeping the baby was her first choice, but her situation led her to decide to end the pregnancy; 3). she felt abortion was and is killing a baby; 4). she felt rushed to make the decision; and/or 5). she perceived herself as not fully informed at the time of the abortion. In addition to these factors found in Franz & Reardon's study, any of the characteristics of poor copers described in Chapter 13 applies both to adolescents and adults.

I have also discovered that adolescents who express emotional difficulty after an abortion may be grappling with the following issues:

1. Feeling abandoned by the boyfriend if he either rejected her or has withdrawn from her.

2. Feeling bitter toward her parents who may have pressured her to terminate the pregnancy. Feeling a lack of independence and control over her own life.

3. Feeling imprisoned at home by parents who are either overprotecting or punishing her for having had sex.

4. Feeling alone with no one to talk to.

5. Feeling disillusioned. She may still be fantasizing that having the baby would have worked out somehow, especially if she saw the pregnancy as a way out of a bad home situation.

6. Feeling bitter toward men and angry with herself for giving in to sexual pressure.

7. Feeling ashamed (e. g., for having sex, having an abortion, disappointing her parents).

Contraceptive Decision-Making Post-Abortion

After an abortion, an adolescent is sometimes reluctant to think about using birth control. She may be ambivalent about continuing sexual activity, never having been sure about it in the first place. She needs encouragement to take the time to think privately about her values and what she wants from her relationship with her boyfriend. Counselors can point out her ability to make decisions about this area of her life, having just made a major life decision. She can decide what she wants to do instead of letting things happen to her. I will never forget the look on one patient's face when I said, "As women, we can't afford to wait for our prince to come and wake us up, and then take care of us. We need to wake up before he gets here, and take care of ourselves." In the time it took me to utter the words, her expression went from startled to disappointed to resigned. There was a pause, and I admit I felt as though I had just told a little kid there was no Santa Claus. She broke the silence and said, "How true."

Sometimes an adolescent will say she has "learned her lesson" and will not have sex anymore until marriage. She may be making that statement because she assumes it may please you. She needs to hear from you that any decision she makes is OK - abstaining or using birth control - as long as it is what SHE feels is best.

Sometimes stating the obvious can bring people back to the reality of the need for contraception: "This pregnancy has proven you are fertile, and barring any major complication, you will continue to be fertile after the abortion." There is so much misinformation spread by the anti-abortion forces about infertility after an abortion that it is probably worth stating routinely. While most people get a chuckle out of that proclamation, some say, "I was wondering about that." The latter is true particularly for patients who have had multiple abortions.

It is equally important to check out the status of the relationship. Is the boyfriend still involved? If so, have they talked about future abstinence or sexual activity? Does she know what he wants? How important is it to her that she please him? Some young women would rather give in to his desire for sex and make him happy than do what they really want. Others have the strength of will to assert their needs and risk disappointing him. Still others have no desire for sex right after an abortion experience, but change their own minds as time goes by. Referring them to a Planned Parenthood or Family Planning Clinic and giving them "The Birth Control Guide At A Glance" and the Hope Clinic booklet, I'll Never Have Sex Again may be helpful.

161

Chapter Nineteen

Birth Control

One of the best ways to learn about all methods of contraception is to read the book, Contraceptive Technology. It can be ordered by writing to Irvington Publishers, 195 McGregor Street, Manchester, NH 03102. For the most up-to-date information, I highly recommend the monthly publication, Contraceptive Technology Update, which can be purchased from American Health Consultants, Inc., 3525 Piedmont Road, Building Six, Suite 400, Atlanta, GA 30305.

Exploring the client's birth control history during the counseling session enables you to help her decide on effective contraception strategies for the future. Abortion providers have amassed a body of knowledge about people's common fears, misconceptions, and misuse of birth control. We can also attest to pure method failure for every contraceptive, including male and female sterilization, and combinations of methods. I have even seen one example of a combined vasectomy and tubal failure!

COMMON PROBLEMS AND MISCONCEPTIONS ABOUT BIRTH CONTROL

The Pill

1. "I can't remember it."
One of the biggest problems people have is remembering to take a pill every day at the same time. Knowing what to do about missed pills is just as big of a problem. When you hear about the hectic schedules women juggle - taking care of children, working different shifts, and going to school full time - you'll wonder how they remember their pills at all. Exploring memory tips is important. Some women decide to set their alarm clocks for the same time every day. Some buy alarm watches and keep their pills in their purse. Many connect pill-taking with another activity they engage in, like meal time. Whatever time she chooses, ask her if she will be able to remember it on weekends as well as on weekdays.

School and work schedules change as time goes by, so women also need to know how to switch times without jeopardizing their protection. They are told to finish one package first, and when they start a new package, they can take it at the new time of day.

2. "I thought it would stay in my bloodstream for a while after I went off."
After having taken the Pill for months or years, people think it stays in their system for months and continues to protect them. Just because Aunt Martha didn't get pregnant for three months after quitting the Pill, she thinks everyone has a three-month "grace period." This happens so frequently, every woman who starts using the Pill should be warned about this myth. A simple explanation

will help enhance her understanding: Each pill has enough hormone to prevent ovulation and will last in the bloodstream for about 24-28 hours (some of the stronger pills last longer, but we've got to keep it simple). Once a woman has taken her last pill, 28 hours later there may not be enough hormone left to keep her from ovulating. She could ovulate any time, any day after quitting her pill. She needs to use another contraceptive immediately if she doesn't want to get pregnant. What method would she choose?

3. "I missed two pills, and I made them up, but we didn't use any backup methods. We didn't think it was necessary."

Knowing what to do about missed pills is complicated enough, with all the varieties of instructions (Williams-Dean & Potter, 1992). However, even when people know what to do about it, they often fail to abstain from intercourse or use back-up methods for the prescribed amount of time after missed pills. They either assume it will stay in their bloodstream a long time, or they feel awkward with barrier methods. Both men and women get accustomed to the spontaneity afforded by the Pill. I suggest every pill user learn to use and keep a supply of spermicides and condoms on hand just in case of missed pills or expired prescriptions.

4. "I ran out of my prescription and we started using something else" (condoms, withdrawal, rhythm, spermicides).

People don't always realize pharmacies and clinics will not refill an expired prescription. She needs to ask how long her prescription will last and then mark her calendar to make an appointment at least one month ahead of the time it expires.

Another strategy for missing pills, quitting the Pill, and running out of prescriptions is to suggest switching methods.

5. "I quit the Pill because of side effects."

Nausea, headaches, irregular bleeding, weight gain, irritability, or depressed mood seem to be the side effects most responsible for women quitting the Pill. Many women have no idea there are many different brands and that they may react differently to different dosages and chemical compositions of the two hormones. Many people think all pills are alike, so they don't consult their doctor. Then again, sometimes they complain,

but their doctor doesn't take them seriously. So they quit.

6. "I quit because I was on it for five years and I thought I should give my body a rest."

Every woman going on the Pill needs to know the latest long-term research on the Pill. So many women are afraid it will build up in their system and do some kind of harm. To date the only known long-term condition a minority of women may experience is benign liver tumors (Contraceptive Technology, 1990-92). Possible links between long-term pill use and breast cancer is still under study and so far inconclusive (Clinical Consensus In Obstetrics and Gynecology, 1990). Most of my clients have never heard of the potential protective effects of the Pill against ovarian and endometrial cancer (Contraceptive Technology Update, Nov. 1992). We need to keep abreast of the results of more long-term research as time goes by. As of this writing, if the woman has no contraindications, she can stay on the Pill safely all the way up to the age of menopause (Thoren, 1993).

The Sponge

1. Removing the sponge is problematic for many women. Instructing her to squat and push with the same muscles as those she uses to have a bowel movement helps to remove it if she can't find the loop. As she is pushing, she needs to get ahold of it with her fingers and slowly pull it out. Demonstrating other spermicides in case she has trouble with the sponge gives her a "plan B" in case "plan A" doesn't work.

2. Many women don't know the sponge has been found less effective for those women who have had a baby than for those who have never given birth vaginally (Contraceptive Technology, 1990-92).

3. Allergic reactions such as burning and itching cause discontinued use. Other spermicides with less percentage of Nonoxynol 9 or other methods may be the answer.

Other Spermicides

1. Burning and itching are problems for some women.

2. Dislike of the "messiness" is another reason

for discontinued use. The sponge seems less messy to women than suppositories, creams, or foams.

3. Disruption of spontaneity can cause discontinued use.

Implants

1. Irregular bleeding is not tolerable to some women. One client kept using tampons throughout the month and wound up with vaginal dryness, irritation, and infection, and then had the implants removed. Instructing them to use pantyliners instead of tampons for light spotting may help.

Depo Provera Shot

1. Irregular bleeding may not be tolerable, especially if they are athletes, dancers, or have other occupations where bleeding is a nuisance or an interference.

2. Some women worry they're pregnant when they miss periods.

3. They may fail to go back in three months for another shot and think it will last indefinitely in their bloodstream.

The IUD

1. She may be unaware of the fact that her body expelled it.

2. After it was removed, no decision was made about another method.

The Diaphragm

1. The woman may feel lower back or pelvic discomfort and take it out before six hours has elapsed from the time of intercourse.
She may need a refitting or a different method.

2. She keeps getting bladder infections. She needs to urinate after having intercourse, so the diaphragm is not pressing on a full bladder. She may be prone to bladder infections and need another method.

3. She only uses the diaphragm when she thinks she is ovulating.

Condoms

1. Itching, burning, or chafing may cause the woman to want her partner to discontinue use. Switching brands and type of lubricant may help. If it has Nonoxynol 9, she may be allergic to that chemical.

2. If he keeps his penis inside her vagina too long after intercourse, the condom can slip off. Once the penis gets soft, semen can spill out of the loosened condom. He needs to withdraw from her vagina before his penis gets soft, and he needs to hold the condom on to his penis as he withdraws.

3. He may rub his penis on the outside of her vagina without the condom on and some sperm may leak out. He must have the condom on before his penis comes near even the outside of her vagina. Women can get pregnant without penetration.

4. He may have intercourse without the condom, pull out, put the condom on, and resume intercourse and ejaculate. Some ejaculate may have already been expelled.

Vasectomy

1. He didn't get the post-operative sperm check and they went ahead and had intercourse.

2. He may want no more children but is afraid of surgery, the local anesthetic, doctors, pain, prostate cancer, and complications. He thinks it may decrease sex drive and cause impotence and the inability to ejaculate. He keeps putting it off, and she gets pregnant using less effective methods.

Tubal Sterilization

She wants no more children but is afraid of a tubal because she fears general anesthesia, surgery, and doctors. She thinks it requires hospitalization and lengthy recovery and equates it to a hysterectomy. Two other prevalent myths are "it makes you fat" and "it brings on menopause." She keeps putting it off and gets pregnant using less effective methods.

Birth Control Guide At A Glance

I designed the "Birth Control Guide At A Glance" to help undecided clients weigh the pros and cons in choosing a method. We encourage the woman to show it to her partner and discuss it together. For those who say they prefer to abstain, we give it to them explaining that if and when they change their minds and do become sexually involved, they'll know what methods are available. The Birth Control Guide can be purchased by writing to The Hope Clinic.

Abstinence

The client may resist the idea of using contraception because she says she is not going to have sex any more. Explore this option and help her do some reality testing.

Some women broke up with their boyfriend or finalized a divorce before they discovered the pregnancy. Unless a new partner has entered the picture, she probably doesn't need birth control at this time and will say so. Other women, especially adolescents, are still involved with their partners but nevertheless vow to abstain. It is important for you to know whether she has just entered a new relationship or whether she has broken up, is separated, or divorced. The probability of her abstaining may partly depend upon the status of her relationship with the partner as well as her present feelings. It is your role to shed light upon the situation without disbelieving her intentions.

When The Partner Is Still In The Picture

Often it is the teenager who says she will abstain because she has learned her lesson and will never let "it" happen again. An appropriate reply might be, "I can imagine how you feel, after all you've been through recently. After an abortion some people want to swear off sex forever. But as time goes by - maybe weeks, months, or years - people change. And we all have a right to change our minds. It may be especially hard to continue to abstain if your boyfriend doesn't feel the same way you do. Have you talked with him about it?" She may answer, "Not exactly, but I intend to," or "Yes, we talked it over, and we both agreed not to do anything again until we get married." Or she may admit, "We talked it over and he's not happy about it, but that's too bad."

In any case, she needs encouragement to communicate with him. For abstinence to be effective, his cooperation is necessary. Having both parties present during this counseling session can be beneficial; however, if he is unavailable, you can still pose some questions to her. Does she sometimes feel pressured by him sexually? Is he a "sweet-talker?" Does he pout? Does he get angry if she doesn't give in? What if two months from now they find themselves in a situation where they're alone, feeling warm toward each other, and one thing starts leading to the next? Before they know it, they're heading for the point of no return! Sometimes this is exactly how this pregnancy occurred. Discuss what they could do if they did wind up in that situation:

1. As soon as they realized what was happening, they could decide to leave and go somewhere with a less romantic atmosphere.

2. If they often found themselves getting aroused and fighting the urge to have sex, they'd need to reconsider what they want and talk about it.

3. If they decided to resume a sexual relationship, they'd need to wait until she was protected. They need to know now that if she chose the Pill, she would have to make a doctor's appointment, then wait for her period to start before she could begin taking the Pill. THEN the Pill would not become effective until at least two weeks later. That could be a total of two months, and many people get pregnant during that waiting time. Inform them of other methods that are readily available, such as spermicides and condoms. This "prepare for the future" approach lets her know:
   a. That you understand her present feelings about not wanting sex, and that it's OK!
   b. That you're not going to push her into using birth control immediately.
   c. That she and her partner might change their minds and resume sexual activity, and that's OK if it's a mutual choice.
   d. That when the time comes, even if it's two years down the road, they can be prepared and prevent pregnancy.
   e. That to prevent pregnancy, she must communicate with her partner about her needs and wants and have information on a readily available method.

When She Is Not Currently Sexually Involved

It is reasonable to agree that she does not need birth control at this time. It is helpful to paint a picture of how a new sexual relationship evolves. "People don't usually plan or discuss when they'll have intercourse together for the first time. It CAN be done, but it usually doesn't happen that way. Nevertheless, most people can tell where the relationship is heading. When, where, and how the first intercourse might occur is usually left up to fate. Then comes that fateful night when they're alone together, feeling intimate, and it becomes obvious to both of them what's going to happen if somebody doesn't stop the action. Many men just assume the woman is protected by the Pill or other hormonal contraceptive, and so they don't think there's a need to stop. It's up to the woman to tell him that she is unprotected. It's either break the mood or wind up pregnant again."

Ask her what method she would choose if and when she feels it is time to protect herself. Whatever method she mentions, give her some information about how long it would take to obtain it and work effectively.

The Divorced Or Separated Woman

Often this woman is feeling ashamed because she thinks she should have known better and swears, "It won't happen again - it was just one of those things." She needs to know that if she is not expecting sexual activity, she may leave herself unprotected and get caught off guard. Some divorced women haven't used birth control for years because their husbands have had vasectomies. If she does not want any more children, she may be interested in a tubal sterilization just in case she chooses to become sexually involved in the future.

The woman who is separated may still be ambivalent about whether to focus on getting back together with her husband or continue another relationship. She may need counseling to help her clarify what she wants. Sometimes this client is telling herself she shouldn't be having sex with another man, but her feelings and desires are telling herself something different. If she isn't honest with herself and doesn't make a conscious decision, she may wind up pregnant again.

The Booklet, _I'll Never Have Sex Again_

I have written this booklet to give to clients who say they're swearing off sex forever and therefore don't want birth control. The booklet helps them identify specific sources of anxiety that create ambivalence or fear of sex and explains how these fears can lead to unprotected sex and pregnancy. It provides useful information to women who are super-fertile, fed up with contraceptives, and afraid of another pregnancy. It also discusses fear of trusting men after being betrayed and rejected. The booklet offers ways to get needs met without placing oneself in jeopardy of an unplanned pregnancy. Copies may be obtained by writing to The Hope Clinic.

Chapter Twenty

Second Trimester Abortion

REASONS FOR SECOND TRIMESTER ABORTION

Only 10% of all abortions in the United States are second trimester abortions (between 13 and 24 weeks of pregnancy), and fewer than 1% occur after 20 weeks (National Abortion Federation, 1990). While second trimester abortions occur much less frequently than first trimester abortions, many people wonder why it occurs at all. The most common reactions people express about women seeking second trimester abortions are anger and disbelief. "Why would anyone wait so long?!" As counselors and nurses, we need to know why. Through understanding, we will be better able to deliver compassionate, quality care to these clients.

First, some women have experienced no pregnancy symptoms or weight gain until they are beyond their fourth month. Some of these women continue to have menstrual periods. Others attribute the lack of periods to their usual, irregular cycles or to stress. Some of these women are genuinely unaware they are pregnant and are shocked to discover the pregnancy, much less the length of pregnancy! I have found that counseling this type of second trimester client can closely resemble a first trimester counseling session in its emotional content. While this client expresses shock that she is in the second trimester of preg-

nancy, she is usually in the early part of the second trimester. Like a first trimester client, she has recently discovered the pregnancy. Her decision-making process often matches that of a first trimester client.

Other clients have been operating under the powerful influence of denial for months on end. These individuals demonstrate a remarkable ability to ignore and deny the reality of the pregnancy, despite all the telltale signs. For them, the truth is too painful to face. Sometimes the woman has been bombarded with a series of life crises all within a short period of time, and the pregnancy is more than she can bear. The woman becomes unable to handle any more traumas, and so unconsciously clicks on the defense mechanism of denial. One client, mother of three, recently divorced, and even more recently fired from a job, had also just lost her mother. She had managed to deny a pregnancy until she was five months. "Everything hit me at once. I thought I was coping - trying to contend with each blow as it came, but I guess this was one too many!" She said it frightened her to think she was capable of blocking out something so obvious. Women suffering from multiple losses, traumas, or unresolved grief sometimes cope with an unwanted pregnancy by denying its existence. They are often still squeezing into their size five jeans. They sometimes rationalize that blood from unreleased periods has simply "backed up" and bloated their abdomen or that they've simply gained a few pounds from overeating. They have continued to behave as though they were not pregnant, even managing to engage in activities they never could do during past pregnancies. "I've gone all this time exercising regularly, when my last two pregnancies tired me out completely!" one client exclaimed.

If this client expresses concern about her ability to block out an event as major as a pregnancy, address the issue of denial. Let her know this is a common way people avoid facing a trauma, and that she is not "weird." If people don't acknowledge that a trauma exists, they don't have to deal with it - at least not at the moment. However, the problem does not vanish, but remains to be dealt with.

What may be frightening is that people do not always consciously decide to use denial; it happens without their knowing it. The client may be afraid she is unknowingly using denial in other parts of her life, and it may be true. Let her know that people resort to denial when deep down they believe they cannot cope with the problem. She can instead choose to believe that she IS a good problem-solver, and that she CAN cope. Point out that she has managed to confront this pregnancy, make decisions about it, and act upon those decisions. She can also reach out to other people for support when life's problems feel overwhelming. When we believe in our ability to problem-solve and know we can ask people for emotional support, any burden becomes lighter and more manageable. This is one way we can take care of ourselves consciously and need not rely upon denial to protect us.

The next type of second trimester client is probably the most common. This is the teenager who is very uninformed about her body and reproduction. In addition, she has felt scared, ashamed, and alone as the months have gone by. The boyfriend is usually no longer in her life and wasn't there for her at the time she first suspected the pregnancy. Often she keeps her "awful secret" to herself. She vacillates between consciously worrying about a possible pregnancy and unconsciously repressing such thoughts. She may tell herself to carry on and forget about it, and believes it will go away on its own. She tries to fool herself into believing it doesn't exist. But part of her persists in suspecting it does. She usually

arrives at the clinic in the late second trimester or beyond, wearing either big baggy clothes or still squeezing into her jeans in an attempt to conceal the truth. This client actively hides any signs and verbally denies she's pregnant to friends and family if they happen to ask. All too often her parents have colluded with her in denying the reality by not noticing it or confronting her. One 16-year-old sat before me, abdomen protruding with a seven-month pregnancy beneath an oversized T-shirt, stating that neither parent had questioned her appearance. I asked, "Do you presently live with your parents? Do you come into contact with each other?" When she replied yes to both questions, I asked if her parents had so much as questioned her weight gain. "My mom just said I shouldn't eat so much," she answered. As it turned out, her family frequently "didn't talk about problems." Sadly enough, many dysfunctional families deal with every problem by sweeping them under the rug, and the children learn to ignore problems and hope they go away. Pregnancy is just one of those problems.

Other clients delay seeking an abortion because of repeated negative pregnancy tests and because of doctors whose pelvic exams are several weeks off target. They therefore assume they have more time to gather money and transportation for the abortion than they actually have. Most of the time this is an honest error on the doctor's part. However, some doctors deliberately withhold the results of positive pregnancy tests on young, unmarried women in the hope that the patient will be "too far" or too poor to obtain a second trimester abortion. These physicians are purportedly staunch "right-to-life" crusaders, and yet their behavior denies these women prenatal care if they decide to carry to term!

Some clients wind up in their second trimester because of the time it has taken to collect enough money for the procedure. Each time they thought they had enough, the pregnancy progressed into a new fee bracket. Back and forth they go running from clinic to clinic, until they find a clinic that performs advanced second trimester procedures. Paradoxically, the client who is initially unable to get a few hundred dollars for a first trimester abortion winds up collecting five times the amount months later. Sometimes the money issue is complicated by the client's feeling of ambivalence about the pregnancy.

Ambivalence about the pregnancy is a common reason for a delayed abortion. A woman may want the baby but is unsure about her financial ability to raise the child. Sometimes she is doubting her emotional and physical readiness for parenthood as well as her financial capabilities. She may be half-hoping that something will change in her life to enable her to care for the child once it's born. Sometimes she is waiting for her male partner to come through for her. "I thought that if he knew I was serious about keeping the baby, he'd change his mind and help me out. Instead, he left town."

Teenagers may want the baby and deliberately hide the fact from parents, hoping that by the time they're "showing," it will be too late for an abortion. But when Mom and Dad find out, and she is "within the limit," parents sometimes persuade her that she cannot raise a child herself; and they have neither the means nor the desire to raise the child for her. This is usually an unhappy client whose scheme has backfired. She often feels defeated and stuck with no place to turn. If her boyfriend's parents won't take her in, if she refuses to consider a home for single mothers, declines adoption, and living with relatives is not an option, then she has painted herself into a corner. She is likely to view her parents as ogres and may seem blind to the part she played in creating the mess. Ask her, "What did you really want by getting pregnant?" Did she want independence? Someone to love? A home and family other than the one she has? Point out that there are other ways to achieve these goals that won't be as likely to backfire as getting pregnant. Even if the client seems sure of the abortion decision, she and her family would probably benefit from counseling both pre- and post-abortion. A referral for family therapy after the abortion is in order to head off depression, running away, or other acting-out behavior on the daughter's part, and possible punitive or helpless behavior on the parent's part.

Some second trimester clients have deliberated long and hard due to moral conflicts about abortion. They may have been leaning toward abortion ever since they discovered the pregnancy, but have been struggling with guilt feelings. They may be reassuring themselves, "Somehow I'll find a way to cope and have this baby." But as the pregnancy progresses and becomes more real, their ability to reassure themselves wanes. The reality and the enormity of the re-

sponsibility hits, and they realize they can't cope after all. This client usually is suffering from a loss of self-esteem, guilt, shame, and a sense of defeat. She needs skillful pre-abortion counseling and a referral for on-going counseling as well. A pro-choice pastoral minister may also be an excellent resource for her. Find out from your state's Religious Coalition for Reproductive Choice about those who are willing and able to take these referrals.

Another scenario is the woman who had originally planned the pregnancy, but by some dark twist of fate, has found herself in a distressing situation midway through the pregnancy. For instance, one client sadly explained that her 36-year-old husband was convalescing from a major heart attack, and both their finances and her attention were being consumed. "He is disabled, and I have to work to help make ends meet. I have a four-year-old and now a husband I have to constantly attend to. I'd collapse from exhaustion if I had a newborn on top of it!" she explained.

Another client and her husband had planned the pregnancy, and at 17 weeks she was rushed to the emergency room for severe abdominal pains and fever. "I was shocked to learn I had gonorrhea and had to be treated before it got any worse. I confronted my husband in tears, and he confessed he was having an affair and KNEW he had contracted gonorrhea. He had been treated in another state, so I wouldn't find out! I thought I was in a nightmare. I have another young child and only a part-time job. I'm now separated and living with my sister and her two kids. There is so much hurt and uncertainty about the future that I can't see continuing this pregnancy. I'm scared of what the disease did to the baby, as well as my fear of what the future holds for me and my son."

One woman's house had burned down, and she suddenly had no place to live. She had three children and was holding down two jobs. Her boyfriend was unemployed and had been living with them.

Another woman's young husband was killed in a car accident, and she was adamant she could not cope with a second baby all by herself. She had just moved with her two-year old across the country to be back with her parents.

The women who originally intended on carrying to term are usually suffering from multiple losses and may need help in sorting them out and in accepting the need to grieve. Some of the advanced second trimester patients are those who have just received test results showing severe fetal abnormalities. These pregnancies are usually planned and wanted, and the patients and their partners are deeply grieving.

Finally, many women are not aware of the existence of any distinctions between a first and second trimester abortion. They may not even know that abortion is legal, much less the differences in trimesters, procedures, and fees. Consequently they are faced with a number of rude awakenings.

All of the above-mentioned reasons why women delay seeking an abortion are among those I have encountered repeatedly. I imagine there are about as many reasons for the delay as there are individuals. Everyone is different, and that is why our counseling approach needs to reflect those differences.

DESCRIPTION OF SECOND TRIMESTER PROCEDURES

Dilation and Evacuation Procedure (D & E)

The Procedure And Aftercare

A D&E procedure is a two-step process which takes place over a period of two or three days, depending on the doctor's preference. The Hope Clinic uses a two-day procedure from 15 - 24 weeks LMP. The first part of the procedure is designed to open or "dilate" the cervix, and the second part removes the contents of the uterus.

On the first day the patient undergoes a sonogram. A sonogram is painless, much like an x-ray, and measures fetal size by means of sound waves. After her sonogram, the patient sees a counselor who will discuss her decision with her, making sure the decision is firm. Once the process has begun on the first day, the woman **must** return the next day and go through with the entire procedure. After counseling, she will undergo a five-minute procedure in which the doctor inserts several osmotic dilators into the cervix. An osmotic dilator is natural (Laminaria) or man-made material (Dilapan, Lamicel) that soaks up mois-

ture from the cervix and expands. When it expands, it pushes the cervix open and thus dilates the cervix. This is a gradual, gentle process that takes hours to produce adequate dilation. Laminaria is dried, compressed, sterile seaweed that resembles a slender twig and is about two and a half inches in length. Each Laminaria expands to about twice its width. Dilapan and Lamicel work similarly. The doctor determines how many osmotic dilators to insert, depending on the gestational size of the pregnancy and the tightness of the woman's cervix. The insertion only takes a few minutes and can cause strong cramping. After the dilators are in place, the doctor places a small vaginal packing of betadine-soaked gauze against the cervix to add an antiseptic moisture that helps the dilators expand.

The woman needs no recovery time after this part of the abortion. She can get dressed and return home or to a nearby hotel with the person who brought her. We advise our patients to stay close to the clinic - within a 45-minute drive. We also advise that someone stay with her overnight in case of an emergency. Miscarriage and hemorrhaging **may** occur overnight if her cervix dilates faster than usual. Although unlikely, it **can happen.** The client is given her prescriptions for antibiotics and pain pills, and is asked if she understands all the aftercare instructions. These instructions will vary among clinics.

1. Do not eat or drink anything after midnight except a small amount of water.

2. Use sanitary pads ONLY. NO tampons.

3. You may take a bath or shower.

4. Do NOT have sexual intercourse or place anything in the vagina for the next two weeks.

5. Under NO circumstances should you attempt to remove the Laminaria (Dilapan or Lamicel) yourself.

6. Do NOT engage in strenuous activity such as bike riding, running, aerobics, etc.

7. Stay with a responsible adult overnight.

8. Stay overnight within a 45-minute drive from the clinic.

9. Do NOT drive yourself, in case any of the medications make you drowsy.

10. Start your antibiotics tonight, take as directed, and finish the bottle.

11. You will probably experience cramping overnight due to the cervical dilation. Use the pain pills as directed, if you need pain relief.

12. You MUST return tomorrow to complete the abortion process. It is important to finish the abortion the next day because once the Laminaria is inserted, the abortion has begun. If you would change your mind and leave without having the Laminaria/Dilapan/Lamicel removed, within a few days miscarriage and hemorrhaging could result as well as a serious pelvic infection, possibly causing shock and death if left untreated. The consequences are serious and could be fatal.

13. Call our 24-hour number immediately if:
    a. You begin soaking more than two pads per hour with bright red blood.

    b. You experience severe cramps or pain that is unrelieved by the pain pills.

    c. The gauze and dilators fall out.

These are all signs of a possible miscarriage.

How do most patients feel overnight?
Most of our patients report intermittent cramping overnight, no bleeding whatsoever, and no problems. Occasionally the cramps are bothersome enough to cause restless sleep. Most patients say they are anxious to get the rest of the procedure over with.

The second part of the procedure:
On the second day the patient will experience an abortion procedure similar to a first trimester vacuum aspiration. The second day's procedure usually takes between seven to 15 minutes, depending on the length of pregnancy. Every doctor works at his/her own pace. First, the patient will receive an I.V. mixture of a muscle relaxer, pain reliever, and medication to prevent hemorrhaging. The doctor begins the procedure by removing the gauze and osmotic dilators. They slip out easily and painlessly. A local anesthetic is administered to the cervix. Finally, the uterus is evacuated by a combination of vacuum aspira-

tion and forceps. The more advanced the pregnancy, the more painful the cramping (usually).

After the abortion, the patient is escorted to the recovery room where she will spend at least one hour. During this time the nurse takes her vital signs, monitors her I.V., and periodically checks her bleeding. Before she is discharged, she will receive one more prescription to continue prevention of hemorrhaging.

Second trimester abortion aftercare:
She will need a post-abortion exam two to three weeks after her abortion. The aftercare will vary from one facility to the next, but she will probably be instructed to abstain from having intercourse, douching, using tampons, and swimming for two to three weeks to prevent infection. She may be told to resume normal activities when she feels like it, but no heavy lifting or strenuous exercise for one week. Bleeding may last anywhere from a few days to two weeks. Patients may receive any of the following kinds of post-op medications to: prevent infection, contract the uterus, dry up the milk in the breasts, and decrease and relieve cramps.

Induction or Instillation Procedures

An induction procedure is not generally used unless the patient is past 19 weeks. In this method, a substance that causes uterine contractions, such as prostaglandins, is injected into the amniotic sac to bring on labor and subsequent expulsion of the fetus. It can be thought of as an induced miscarriage.

Osmotic Dilation with Induction Procedure

The purpose of the combined use of osmotic dilator and induction is to reduce the time the woman spends in labor by dilating the cervix prior to the induction. The entire process takes between two to four days, and the patient will either stay overnight in a hospital, hotel, or at home, depending on geographic distance from the clinic. On the first day, after a preliminary sonogram and pelvic exam, Laminaria or other osmotic dilators are inserted into the cervix. Using sonography to locate the fetus, the doctor inserts a long spinal needle into the patient's abdomen and injects Digoxin into the fetus or the amniotic sac. This action stops the fetal heart and thus prevents a live birth. On the following day more osmotic dilators are inserted to continue dilating the cervix.

On the third day the doctor inserts a long spinal needle into the patient's abdomen to draw out amniotic fluid and replace this fluid with prostaglandins, a substance that causes contractions. This process creates pressure and some discomfort, but most women say it sounds more painful than it is.

After the prostaglandins start contractions of the uterus, it usually takes anywhere from five to eight hours to complete the miscarriage. Most clinics make sure the woman is assisted during this time by caring staff, so she won't be alone once the fetus is expelled. She may be given relaxation or pain medications to help relieve the pain. Though not routinely done, the doctor may need to use the vacuum aspirator and curette to completely clean all the tissue from the uterus.

Induction procedures used to be done using saline solution, but saline abortions are outdated, having a higher complication rate and having largely been replaced by prostaglandins procedures. As time goes by, abortion procedures change and improve to increase patient safety and comfort.

Induction procedures are safer than D&E procedures for late second trimester abortions under the following conditions: when the patient has had a C-Section within the year, the patient is obese, she has a twin pregnancy, or her cervix is stenotic (very tight).

D & X (Dilation And Extraction)

Dilation and Extraction (D&X) was first described at the September 1992 National Abortion Federation conference on risk management. The physician uses osmotic dilators to dilate the cervix over a period of one to five days for adequate dilation, and then the physician extracts an intact fetus without the woman undergoing labor. This procedure was developed to spare the woman the pain of labor while being able to remove the fetus intact. Having an intact fetus can be very beneficial in cases of fetal abnormalities. Viewing or holding the body may help couples who are undergoing a grieving process. It can reinforce their decision and help them say their goodbyes. As of

this writing, D&X procedures are not prevalent, and those doctors who perform them do so mostly for fetal indications abortions.

On the first day of the procedure the physician inserts osmotic dilators into the cervix. This dilation process is repeated on a second, third, fourth, or fifth day before the final extraction of the fetus is attempted. The softness or tightness of the cervix and the length of pregnancy will determine how many days of dilation is necessary before the extraction occurs. At the time of the extraction, the doctor ensures there is no live birth by locating and cutting the umbilical cord. Then the fetus is removed manually and with forceps.

SAFETY AND RISKS OF SECOND TRIMESTER ABORTION

The following information has been taken from the article, "The Safety of Mid-trimester Abortion," in the Medical Digest (Grimes and David, 1987), and the book, Abortion Practice (Hern, 1990).

Most of the legitimate information on the comparative safety of abortion is derived from the results of the largest study in the world, "The Joint Program for the Study of Abortion." It was conducted by the Center for Disease Control from 1975 to 1978 in the United States at 13 facilities that provided detailed reports on 84,000 midtrimester procedures. Even though this data is 16 years old at the time of this writing, it is still the largest reliable study of abortion complications to date.

"**Serious complication rate**" was defined as the number of women per 100 abortions who sustained one or more of these three complications: 1). infection; 2). hemorrhage requiring blood transfusion; and 3). any complication requiring surgery such as laparoscopy, laparotomy, hysterotomy, or hysterectomy.

Dilation And Evacuation Urea-Prostaglandins

In comparing the safety of 9,572 D&E and 2,805 urea-prostaglandins F2a (instillation or induction) abortions, the serious complication rate for D&E was 0.5 per 100 abortions. For urea-prostaglandins, 1.0 per 100 abortions. Those complications occurring significantly more frequently with urea-prostaglandins included hemorrhage, fever, retained tissue, failed abortion, endometritis, and cervical injury needing repair. However, the frequency of uterine perforation and subsequent surgery was five times higher with D&E than with urea-prostaglandins.

With D&E, complication rates increase as the pregnancy advances in gestational age.

Urea-Prostaglandlins v. Saline Instillation

Comparing 4,778 saline abortions with 2,805 urea-prostaglandin abortions, the urea-prostaglandin method was two times safer than the saline - a highly significant difference. The serious complication rate for urea-prostaglandins was 1.0 per 100,000, and 2.2 per 100,000 for saline. Saline abortion resulted in more frequent incidence of hemorrhage requiring transfusion.

Coagulopathy Or "D.I.C."

Coagulopathy or Disseminated Introvascular Coagulation (D.I.C.) is the occurrence of hemorrhage NOT due to any abortion-related complication. Rather, hemorrhaging occurs because the woman's body is unable to produce enough of the clotting factor in her blood. This condition is not predictable beforehand. A recent study of 16,000 abortions at an abortion provider in Los Angeles that uses both D&E and saline instillation estimated the rate of coagulopathy to be 191 per 100,000 D&E abortions and 658 per 100,000 saline abortions.

Effects Of Second Trimester Abortion On Subsequent Pregnancy Outcome

There is limited available information on subsequent pregnancies carried to term after instillation abortions. The available information indicates no significant increase in premature births or low birth weight.

With D&E abortions, successful later pregnancy outcomes seem to depend upon the way in which the cervix was dilated. If the cervix was dilated manually, using rigid dilators, to a diameter of 16 mm or more, women had a 2.5 higher risk of subsequent low birth weight deliveries than for women whose cervices had been dilated with Laminaria or other synthetic osmotic dilators,

such as Dilapan or Lamicel (Hogue & Peterson, 1984).

Risk Of Death

D&E abortions carry the lowest risk, with three deaths per 100,000 at 13 to 15 weeks gestation; nine deaths per 100,000 between 16 to 20 weeks; and 12 per 100,000 after 21 weeks. The total risk of death with D&E per 100,000 is 4.9. The risk of death in childbirth is 6.6 per 100,000. Second trimester D&E abortion is safer than childbirth if it is performed before 21 weeks and similar to childbirth after 21 weeks when underreporting of deaths due to childbirth is taken into account. (Grimes, 1984).

Instillation abortion carries a risk of 5.5 deaths per 100,000 at 13 to 15 weeks gestation, 12.0 per 100,000 at 16 to 20 weeks, and 13.3 per 100,000 after 20 weeks. The total overall risk of death from instillation abortions is 9.6 per 100,000. This is two times greater than the 4.9 per 100,000 for D&E abortions. However, after 21 weeks, the death to case ratio from D&E or instillation is about the same.

Saline procedures carry the highest risk of death of all the second trimester methods, with the overall rate of 11.6 per 100,000.

Causes Of Death

The causes of death from D&E differ from the causes from instillation. For D&E, infection (usually related to retained tissue) and hemorrhage (usually but not always related to uterine perforation) caused 70% of all D&E related deaths from 1972 to 1981.

For instillation abortion, amniotic fluid embolism was the leading cause of death followed by infection, and hemorrhage.

Amniotic Fluid Embolism

Amniotic fluid embolism is a complication associated with second trimester instillation abortions. It is related to gestational age and to the amount of amniotic fluid that enters the woman's circulation. It is neither preventable nor predictable. Between 1972 and 1987 only one death from amniotic embolism occurred with a D&E procedure, while 18 deaths occurred from this cause with instillation abortions.

175

During the time abortion has been legal in the United States, the safety of both first and second trimester abortion procedures has improved dramatically. This trend is due largely to physicians' increasing experience and skill, their discovery and sharing of improved techniques at various gestational ages, the obsolescence of abdominal surgical abortion procedures (hysterotomy), improved abortifacients such as urea-prostaglandins, and use of osmotic dilators such as Laminaria, Dilapan, or Lamicel.

During the 1980s President Ronald Reagan's Administration took an anti-abortion stance that led to the repression and disassembly of the Abortion Surveillance section of the Center for Disease Control. Abortion Surveillance had collected, analyzed, and reported morbidity and mortality statistics on abortion procedures from all across the United States. For this reason there are little or no U.S. statistics on the subject from 1981 – 1992.

THE DIFFERENCE BETWEEN FIRST AND SECOND TRIMESTER COUNSELING

When Hope Clinic started doing second trimester abortions in 1982 I wondered what, if any, differences there would be in counseling first and second trimester patients. As time went by, I discovered there are indeed some important areas to address.

Importance Of Returning To Complete The Procedure

Because the procedure is a two-day process, safety necessitates the patient return on the second day to complete the abortion. Most people faithfully comply with our instructions for a safe procedure. There are factors that increase the chances the patient may fail to follow through and thus put herself at risk of serious consequences.

Reasons Why The Patient May Fail To Return To Complete The Procedure

1. Ambivalence about the decision in a second trimester patient can result in her changing her mind overnight and wanting the osmotic dilator removed so she can carry to term. If she changes her mind, she runs the risk of having damaged the fetus by having taken the antibiotics and pain pills overnight. In addition, the introduction of the dilator into the cervix could cause a serious infection that, if left untreated, could cause blood poisoning. Any dilation that has occurred could cause a miscarriage that may lead to hemorrhaging and maternal and fetal death. It is possible for the pregnancy to continue uninterrupted without complications if the patient has the dilators removed, but she is increasing the risks.

2. If the patient intends on staying overnight with an unsupportive and unhappy parent or partner, and she feels guilty, sad, or ambivalent about the abortion, she increases her risk of changing her mind overnight. Even when the patient is not staying with unsupportive people overnight, she sometimes phones them, reveals what she is doing, and lets herself be talked into changing her mind. Sometimes the parent or partner arrives on the scene in the middle of the night to "save" her from going through with the abortion and succeeds in jeopardizing her health and life when she asks the doctor to remove the dilators. Even riskier is the occasion in which the parent or partner takes her back home **without** having the dilators removed. In this instance the patient fails to come back the next day and may vanish without a trace. Unless she immediately sees a doctor to have the dilators removed, she is at risk for possible pelvic infection, blood poisoning, miscarriage, hemorrhaging, shock, and death. All these risks are explained to her in the counseling session, and she signs consent forms that state she understands the possible consequences.

Fortunately, the vast majority of people do not put themselves in jeopardy when they have had a thorough explanation of possible complications. But because in rare instances these things have happened, the counselor needs to impress upon the patient how important it is to return the next day to complete the abortion. In addition, the counselor would be remiss if she did not explore the following:

a. How sure is the patient about her decision? Who knows about the abortion?

b. If her parents or partner do not know about the abortion, what does she think they would do if they found out tonight?

c. How possible is it for this to happen?

d. What would she do?

e. Does she understand the consequences if she fails to complete the procedure once it has begun?

3. If the patient's male partner is abusive and he is the one staying with her, he may rape or beat her overnight or refuse to let her return to finish the procedure. All of these possiblities have occasionally happened at clinics that provide second trimester procedures. When any of these occur, the woman is at risk of major life-threatening complications, including uterine perforation, infection, blood poisoning, hemorrhage, shock, and death.

At Hope Clinic we want our patients to stay overnight with someone supportive and do not want to take risks with batterers. We will help her contact someone she knows is responsible and who will stay with her overnight. In the counseling session, we find out if her partner forces her to have sex. If so, we help her plan a safety strategy to avoid him for at least two weeks post-abortion. She may not be receptive to making a permanent break away from him, but may be accustomed to breaking away temporarily and agree to do so.

Other Differences Between First And Second Trimester Counseling Issues

Lack Of Support By Male Partner

There are far more second trimester than first trimester patients who do not have the support of their male partner. For many second trimester patients, their relationship with the male partner was superficial and short-lived. He stopped seeing her prior to her discovering the pregnancy. For those who were involved in a meaningful relationship, they often break up before she finds out she is pregnant, or he abandons her once she informs him. Frequently, second trimester patients don't tell their estranged partners about the pregnancy and keep the secret to themselves, not knowing who to tell or what to do. They explain their ex-boyfriend wouldn't care, already has another girlfriend, or is long gone. Most second trimester patients need supportive others to compensate for the lack of male partner support. They may finally confide in a girlfriend or sister. In the case of a teenager, her mother is usually the one who confronts her and takes her to the doctor where they both find out the truth.

Denial

A greater proportion of second trimester patients than first trimester patients use denial as a way to cope with life's problems. The pregnancy is just one more problem they feel they can't face. People who generally use denial often come from dysfunctional families. Many teenagers in their second trimester have parents who blinded themselves to their daughter's pregnancy symptoms and denied the obvious.

Fetal Movement

Feeling fetal movement generally starts to occur between four to five months. Women who deny and repress feelings in their attempt to fend off problems usually cut themselves off from feeling fetal movement. Most second trimester clients do not bring up this subject. When a client does bring it up, you need to let her know some women are very much affected by feeling movement, and others are not. Then ask how she feels about it. The client often responds, "I feel sad (or guilty) because I know it's alive and tomorrow it won't be." Acknowledge her feelings and explore her expectations for coping after the abortion. Some women state they feel "empty" and need to grieve the loss after the abortion. It is important they also keep in mind the reasons they felt the abortion was their best option. Depending on the client's expectations for coping, she may need to reconsider other options or utilize a counseling referral.

Deceived By Their Bodies

Some patients feel deceived by their bodies if they never experienced any symptoms of pregnancy, including a continuation of periods while pregnant. They express bewilderment, feeling stupid and duped by their own bodies. They may need reassurance that other women have also experienced no symptoms whatsoever until their sixth or seventh month.

Fetal Indications

Second trimester patients may be married couples mourning the loss of a wanted, planned pregnancy to which they have grown very attached but which they decided to end due to fetal indications.

Adolescents' Baby Fantasy

Second trimester patients may be immature adolescents who enjoyed the fantasy of having a baby but not the reality. Once the reality of the financial responsibility hits and personal sacrifices of parenting become apparent, they decide to end the pregnancy. They may be mourning the loss of a wanted pregnancy to which they have grown attached and the loss of all the accompanying hopes and dreams. The fantasy usually lasts as long as the boyfriend is still around and her parents don't know about the pregnancy. Once the partner gets scared and changes his mind or her parents find out, the bubble may burst.

What Does It Look Like?

Second trimester patients seldom ask the question, "What does it look like?" In fact, many more first trimester clients ask this question than second trimester clients. Perhaps the latter suspect what it looks like and don't want to know the details. Some clients have explained, "It doesn't matter what it looks like because my situation won't change, and my decision won't change."

If she asks, "What does it look like?" you may want to ask her what she imagines it to look like. How big does she think it is? First trimester clients usually think it's much bigger than the reality, and second trimester clients usually think it's smaller than it really is. It is preferable she face the truth BEFORE going through the abortion than finding out afterwards. If she knows beforehand, she has the opportunity to change her mind if the truth is too painful. Even if she does not change her decision, she has the opportunity to discuss her feelings and expectations for coping. Sometimes the client asks about fetal development and after she receives the answer, exclaims, "Oh, I wish you hadn't told me ... now I feel worse!" A counselor might reply, "There must have been a reason you asked for this information. Tell me how it affects you." The majority of women states it does not affect their decision, but it increases their guilt and/or sadness. Exploring their support and coping strategies is important.

Viewing Fetal Tissue

Far fewer second trimester clients than first trimester clients ask to see the fetal tissue after the abortion, and most first trimester clients do NOT ask to see it. However, whether or not the client is allowed to view the fetal tissue after the abortion is a policy that varies from clinic to clinic. One philosophy holds that the patient has the absolute right to view it; another philosophy maintains that only those patients who can handle it emo-

tionally will ask; yet another philosophy affirms that patients who are self-punishing will ask to see it for that purpose. Some clinics carefully screen the patients before granting the request; others have no screening process; and still others have a blanket policy not to show the fetal tissue. If a clinic decides to show the tissue, there needs to be some discussion with the client beforehand regarding her expectations and feelings; and screening the clients who engage in self-punishing behaviors is important. There are other more constructive ways for the client to cope with guilt than making herself view the fetal remains. Giving the highest quality emotional and medical care in an atmosphere of dignity and compassion should always be the guiding force behind our policies.

Ambivalence Or Regret

It is vital that you find out if a second trimester client is SURE of her decision or if she fears true regret. If she leaves your office, starts the procedure, and then the next morning calls to say she changed her mind and is leaving without completing the abortion, she is in danger. Any second trimester client who demonstrates ambivalence or who fears regret should be sent home with a counseling referral. She needs to be told about any fee changes with the passage of time. But it is inadvisable to hurry up and compromise her safety just so she can have a cheaper abortion. You are responsible for using your best judgment for her well-being.

THE SECOND TRIMESTER COUNSELING SESSION

You will want to help the client explore what lies behind her delay in seeking an abortion.

Of course, it would be offensive to ask (even nicely), "Why did you wait so long?" Instead, there are a series of questions that help piece the puzzle of the past months together for both of you. These questions are not meant as an interrogation. They are meant as a way to tailor the counseling session to meet her individual needs. For example, the woman who just found out she was pregnant at 15 weeks may be genuinely shocked, especially if she had no symptoms and continued having periods. She may have different issues from the woman who delayed the abortion due to severe moral conflicts or whose husband died suddenly. The counselor will be active-listening, clarifying, and giving support.

Exploring Why The Client Is In Her Second Trimester

A 17-year-old young woman dutifully followed me to my office, sat down crossing her ankles, and waited for me to speak. I explained the purpose of the session and chatted with her to put her at ease. Once she seemed more relaxed, I asked:

About what month was it that you first suspected you might be pregnant?

Client: (After a pause) Right before spring break in March.

Counselor: What gave you the clue?

Client: I missed my period.

Counselor: What did you tell yourself when you thought, "I might be pregnant?"

Client: I told myself it wasn't really anything. Just a missed period.

Counselor: You were hoping you weren't pregnant and that it was nothing more than a missed period.

Client: Yeah.

Counselor: Did you tell anybody at that time about your suspicions?

Client: No.

Counselor: When the next month went by, and you missed another period, did you tell anyone?

Client: Yes. My boyfriend.

Counselor: What did he say?

Client: He said it probably wasn't anything and not to worry.

Counselor: What did you tell yourself then?

Client: I guess I just put it out of my mind. I didn't want to think about it.

Counselor: It was hard to face that you might be pregnant, so you pushed it out of your mind.

Client: Yes. I guess I just couldn't face it. I didn't want to have to face my Mom.

Counselor: It's scary to be in high school and pregnant and have to tell your Mom. (After a pause) What happened in May?

Client: My boyfriend started going out with somebody else. We sort of broke up. I told myself my missed periods were probably just stress.

Counselor: It would be very stressful to see your boyfriend going out with someone else. Breaking up is very upsetting. Did you talk to any friends about the break-up with your boyfriend?

Client: Yeah, but not about anything else.

Counselor: I know you've told me you pushed the possibility of a pregnancy out of your mind, but sometimes when women do that, they still have moments when they think of what they would do if they really were pregnant. Was there any time when you thought you might have the baby?

Client: No, I never did. I kept hoping I wasn't pregnant.

Counselor: What happened that led you to get a pregnancy test?

Client: My Mom noticed that I hadn't been having periods, and last week she took me to the doctor to find out what was wrong. He told us I was pregnant.

Counselor: You said back in March one of the things you dreaded facing was your Mom finding out you were pregnant. How did you feel when it happened?

Client: Bad. It wasn't a shock or anything for me, but my Mom was shocked. She took it better than I thought, though. I wish I had told her earlier.

Counselor: There are always things in our lives we don't want to face. Sometimes we tell ourselves we CAN'T face it and so try to ignore it.

Client: That's what I did.

Counselor: What have you learned from this experience?

Client: That I can talk to my Mom about anything. And that some problems don't go away. They just get worse.

Counselor: It's good to know your Mom will come through for you, and it's very useful to know some problems get worse the longer you ignore them. What do you think you'll do the next time you miss a period?

Client: Get a pregnancy test right away.

Counselor: That would be a good idea. There's something else I've observed about you in this situation. You WERE able to face the very thing you dreaded the most. It did feel bad, just as you feared, but you lived through it.

Client: And it wasn't as bad as I thought.

COUNSELING THE CLIENT WHO IS TOO FAR ALONG IN THE PREGNANCY FOR AN ABORTION AT YOUR CLINIC

Counseling Objectives

When you must break the bad news to a client that she is too far along in the pregnancy for your facility to provide an abortion for her, it is helpful to keep the purpose of the session in mind: 1). To talk REALITY to someone who probably has not been facing reality (especially if she is beyond 24 weeks); 2). To convey that taking control is both possible and necessary; and 3). To help her organize the steps she needs to follow in order to TAKE ACTION.

Client Reactions

When you first see the client after her sonogram, she will probably appear either distraught or numb. You have either confirmed her worst fears or given her a shock if she has had periods all along. There still may be an angry or tearful display of denial that she "just can't be that far along!" Sometimes the client has suspected the length of her pregnancy and calmly resigns herself to continuing the pregnancy. This is espe-

cially true for the teenager who successfully concealed the pregnancy until it was too late for the abortion her parents wanted her to have.

But the client who denied the pregnancy and repressed the signs and symptoms will probably appear shocked. Having to face the awful truth can shatter her defenses and thus, she becomes angry and makes one last desperate attempt to deny the truth. She may argue the accuracy of the sonogram, explaining why she can't possibly be that far along. She needs understanding that it's hard to be told you can't have something you want because you're "too late." She also needs a firm but patient explanation that a sonogram measures size, not time, and the measurement today showed the size of the fetus to be equal to the size of a ___ week fetus. It is the size that determines what kind of abortion procedure to use, and some doctors cannot provide the kind of procedure she needs. She needs to be referred to a doctor who can perform the right kind of procedure for her safety. She may still argue that she doesn't care what kind of procedure your doctor uses and will try to persuade you to "make the doctor do it anyway." A firm, unwaivering statement that your doctor will not do anything to jeopardize a patient's safety is necessary to deter her from any further pleading. Then redirect the topic to the options that remain open to her.

If she seems too distraught to pay any attention, you can ask if she would like the person who came with her to join her in your office. If she says yes, let them have some time alone after you have explained briefly the nature of the problem to the support person. If she does not want to include whoever came with her, ask if she wants some time alone to collect her thoughts. Rejoin her after a few minutes. Usually when you return she will seem more composed. Help her plan what to do next.

If she does not have a support person and appears very upset, and rejects any options other than "having the abortion here and now," switch gears from problem-solving to active listening. Asking, "Can you tell me a little about your situation to help me understand?" will probably open communication. After listening and supporting her, you may want to explore what prevented her from seeking an abortion sooner. Making a general statement such as, "It's not uncommon for someone in the situation you described to find it too painful to face the pregnancy at first," can let her know she is not the only one in her predicament. You could continue, "In fact, some women suspected the pregnancy much sooner, but found it too unbearable to admit. Can you tell me how it was for you?" As she speaks, you may want to find out what month she first suspected the pregnancy. Your understanding and empathy for her inability to face the truth can help assuage her shame and anger.

If She Is Still Eligible For An Abortion At Another Clinic

At this point she may be more open to hearing about her options. This may be a good time to ask if she'd like her support person to join her. This person may need to know that she is unable to have an abortion at your facility and why. Then you need to go over her remaining options. If she is within the limits of another clinic, offer the referral to her with a brief description of the following: 1). the kind of procedure used at the referral clinic and how many days it takes for the completion of the process, 2). the safety of second trimester abortion, 3). the reputation of the referral (the more you know, the better), 4). the cost and necessary transportation, and 5). how much time she has before her length of pregnancy is too far for an abortion at this clinic or anywhere.

Money and Transportation Obstacles

The cost and/or transportation often pose immediate obstacles, especially if she is still thinking she "can't" tell anybody. Explore who else would probably be willing to lend her money, if she could muster the courage to tell them. What feelings would she experience when telling this person? How would he/she probably react? What might be the positive results of telling him/her? What might be the negative consequences? Is being able to have an abortion worth whatever negative consequences arise from telling this person?

Sometimes people complain adamantly, "There's NO WAY ... 1). I can get that much money!, 2). I could ever tell anybody, 3). I could get off work that many days, and 4). I could find the transportation." And yet these same people find ways to accomplish all four "impossibilities." Most of the time they find solutions when they confide in someone who helps them think of workable solutions.

For those people who tell you, "I guess I'll have to go through with the pregnancy," they need to know they still have two options: adoption and parenthood. They certainly don't have to make a decision then and there, but equipping them with appropriate referrals and information will help them in their decision-making.

Too Far For An Abortion

Abortions performed past 24 weeks are RARE. After checking with the National Abortion Federation, I have found no abortion facility in the United States that will provide an abortion past 34 weeks, and those procedures are done only in cases of life endangerment or severe fetal anomalies. The FEW abortion clinics in the country that provide abortions past 24 weeks usually draw the line at 27 LMP weeks if there are no extreme extenuating health circumstances. Most second trimester abortion providers have seen the occasional client who says she is five months pregnant and in reality is practically ready to deliver. Sometimes the client has gone into labor while having her sonogram or while talking to the counselor.

The client who is past 27 weeks is faced with the stark reality that she will be having a baby in a few months, weeks, or days. You will need to convey to the client and her support person that: 1). abortion in the third trimester is *not* an option without extreme health problems or documented fetal indications and 2). there are two options remaining: carrying to term and keeping the baby or carrying to term and placing the baby for adoption.

If The Client Threatens To Self-Abort

Sometimes the client is so angry (at herself and at being told she can't have what she wants) that she exclaims, "Then I'll just abort it myself!" Her threat may be an expression of anger or even an attempt to make you give her the abortion she wants, no matter what! But it may be something she seriously considers doing out of desperation. At the moment she may not care that self-abortion is dangerous. She needs to know 1). most self-abortions don't work and 2). the woman is the one who usually winds up damaged. Let her know many women in her situation are scared and mad at themselves and others who are not there for them. Despite her fear and anger, she can take charge and make a plan of action about what to do next, and you will help her. Ask if you can bring in her support person so she has someone to help her take the next step once she leaves your office.

If The Client Threatens Suicide

A few women become so desperate that they tell you, "If I can't have an abortion, I'll kill myself!" Some may be saying that to manipulate you into giving them the abortion, and others may really see no other way out of the dilemma. It's better to err on the side of caution and take her seriously. Let her know you hear how scared and angry she is. She may need some time to cry. Be with her.

Assessment Of The Risk Of Suicide

Tell her you know that some people threaten suicide because they feel so overwhelmed, while others have been seriously thinking about suicide even before they arrived at the clinic. Ask the following:

1. Have you thought about ending your life before?

2. Have you ever attempted it?

3. (If yes) How long ago?

4. What did you do? (take pills, cut wrists, use a gun?)

5. Did you call someone after you did it?

6. Did someone find you? What happened?

7. Were you hospitalized? How long?

8. Did you see a psychiatrist? Counselor?

9. Were you prescribed antidepressants?

10. How long did you continue seeing the psychiatrist or counselor? How long did you continue taking the medication?

11. Looking back, how did you feel when you realized you were still alive?

If she has never attempted suicide before, then ask:

1. Have you been thinking about taking your life before today?

2. (If yes) Did you have a plan for how you would do it?

3. Did you have the means to do it? (a loaded gun, pills, etc.)

4. What made you decide not to?

Danger Signs Of High Risk (Bongar, 1992, and Maris, 1992)

1. Any previous suicide attempt. This increases the chance for another, successful attempt. The more recent the attempt, the higher the risk.

2. Verbal statements like "I just want to die. Everybody would be better off without me. Nothing matters anymore," indicate risk.

3. Putting their affairs in order and giving away possessions.

4. Personality and behavior changes. Depression lifts and the person seems happy and relieved, or they start taking risks, or they become isolative and uncommunicative.

5. Diagnosed or undiagnosed depression. The person has classic symptoms of depression but has never received treatment; the person has quit seeing her therapist and has quit her prescribed antidepressants without the doctor's knowledge.

6. She has a concrete plan for carrying out the suicide, and it is lethal.

7. The method for committing suicide is available to her.

After Making The Assessment

Let her know you need to bring in the person who came with her, and they need to know she is thinking about suicide. Your goal is to link her up with people who care about her and with professional help. Together with her and the support person, you can create a plan of action, with concrete steps for them to take once they leave your office. If she is at risk of suicide and willing to be admitted to the hospital, then your doctor can admit her. Hope Clinic counselors have a working relationship with our county's Mental Health and Crisis Counseling Coordinator. The Coordinator is willing to assist us in getting a patient evaluated and admitted.

The client's support person is crucial in helping her get the assistance she needs. This person may be very helpful in soothing her if she is sobbing uncontrollably and/or refusing to be admitted. Sometimes giving them a few minutes to be alone together is beneficial.

If it turns out the patient is not high risk for suicide, and has become calmed, then she may be receptive to hearing about the options available to her and the next step she needs to take. For example, the next step may be to tell one of her significant others who doesn't know she's pregnant. Her support person can help her decide who needs to be told next. This may be one of her parents. You need to build in measures of safety in the plan to help reduce her fears. Her friend can reassure her he/she will go with her when she tells this person. If she needs counseling, her friend can go with her. You can make the initial call to the counseling services, and let her finish making the appointment, so she has had some part in taking control. When people feel overwhelmed, they feel out of control, and they need help in getting back in control. You and her support person are helping her put one foot in front of the other, but she is the one who does the walking.

The Client's Options

Keeping the Baby

When a client is told she is no longer eligible for an abortion, the most common reaction is tears. Many explain that they haven't the financial resources necessary to raise a child, even though they may want the baby. If the client's main concern is financial inability to pay doctor bills and provide for a child, would she consider receiving state or federal aid? Has she known anyone receiving this assistance? If she is even slightly interested, she needs a referral to her state's Department of Public Aid so she can make an appointment to determine her eligibility.

If she thinks she will probably keep the baby, she needs to contact a doctor. She may need a referral and encouragement to make an appointment as soon as possible. Depending on her situation, she may also need referrals to various social services and family counseling, especially if she is an adolescent who fears parental rejection.

Telling parents she is pregnant and will deliver soon is sometimes the worst dilemma for the adolescent. If the consequences of telling her parents sound severe, provide a referral for crisis counseling and help her make a safety plan. What friend or relative would probably allow her to live with them on a temporary basis? Are there any emergency youth shelters in her area or residences for pregnant teens? If she expects physical abuse and is a minor, you need to ask if her parents have ever been visited by a caseworker from Department of Children and Family Services. If yes, she needs to contact that caseworker and ask for his or her involvement. If no, she needs the number to call in case of physical abuse. If she admits to current or recent past abuse, she needs to know you are obligated by law to report child abuse, and let her know what will probably happen within the next few days. If she seems very much alone, explore possible support people in her life who can help intervene with her parents. Help her make a simple list of what she needs to do next once she leaves your office. Let her know you are concerned and want to hear from her. Is there any phone number at which you could reach her? If a support person has accompanied her to the clinic, it may be helpful to enlist their continued support and include them in the next plan of action, with the client's permission.

Adoption Referral

If she is not at all interested in keeping the child, she needs to know that if she places it for adoption with a reputable adoption agency, then she will not have to pay the doctor or hospital bills. However, if she changes her mind and decides to keep the baby after the birth, then she must assume the responsibility for those costs. Often an adoption agency will arrange for the woman to receive Public Aid, if possible, from the beginning. They have learned that all too often the woman who intended on placing the baby in an adoptive home takes the baby home herself once it is born.

When referring her to adoption agencies, make sure she has several referrals and encourage her to call more than one. She needs to ask questions of each agency to see which agency will best meet her needs. Will they cover all her medical expenses? If she needs to continue her high school education and will be kicked out of her school (some church-affiliated schools do), will they help her continue her education? Will she be able to participate in choosing the adoptive parents for her child? Do they offer open or closed files? Which does she prefer? Do they offer on-going counseling before, during and after the birth? Will she be able to know how the child is doing as time goes by?

Counselors' Reactions

Common Feelings

Some clients are so distraught or stunned at the time of receiving the bad news that they are unable to think and process information. The support person becomes indispensable at this time. Counselors are used to being allies and able helpers, but under these circumstances they become bearers of bad tidings. The counselor's ability to help is greatly diminished because the client's length of pregnancy severely limits available options. The client still wants what the counselor cannot offer: an abortion.

Seldom is there closure at the end of the session because the client and her support person so often leave disappointed, downhearted, and anxious about the future. She may feel doomed and unable to see how things will work out. Neither may feel satisfied or resolved.

Counselors can feel sad, powerless, and unable to let go of lingering thoughts about the client after she leaves. They may have nagging worries about her well-being as the day goes by. There are a number of ways a counselor can let go and restore equanimity.

Letting Go Of Clients' Plights

1. Talking to someone on staff who understands the feelings you're experiencing can be cathartic. Sometimes it helps to tell the story of what happened and how you felt more than once before you go home.

2. If you find yourself continuing to think about it after your catharsis, you can employ thought-stopping and comforting self-talk. For example, if you catch yourself thinking, "What a terrible situ-

ation that poor thing is in! It's going to be awful when she gets home!" you can stop the negative thinking and switch gears. You can instead think, "Nobody knows what's going to happen, so I don't have to assume the worst. Sometimes what we think is the worst thing that can happen to us turns out to have meaning for us as time goes by."

3. Keep in mind even though people may seem extremely upset and helpless at one point in time, once they have time to think, they'll come up with what they need for what they want OR they'll cope. "Where there's a will, there's a way."

4. Focus on what you CAN do for clients instead of what you CAN'T do. You can only work with what they give you to work with. It is not your fault she came to the clinic with a 30-week pregnancy. Whom did you see today that you could and did help?

5. Think about a real life story that seemed disastrous but turned out well. A rape survivor I saw once told me when she was raped at 15 and was too far for an abortion, she thought her life had ended. Then she thought, "I'll place the child for adoption." After the birth she chose to keep the baby boy. At the age of 36 she could look back and tell me that her son was the most caring, loving child, and he was the one who got her through some hard times in her life. "I don't know what I'd do without him," she asserted. You never know!

6. Silently affirm that she will take the right action for her life. If you believe in God, entrust her care to God.

Chapter Twenty-One

Post-Abortion

HOW WOMEN FEEL IMMEDIATELY AFTER RECOVERY

After the recovery time (an hour or less) women usually feel relieved and ready to go home. They may have some cramping, and they almost always feel hungry. After recovery they are sometimes still groggy from any muscle relaxers and pain relievers they received. They may simply be tired from a long day. Other times they haven't had much sleep the night before due to nervous anticipation, and they are feeling sleepy. Some women are alert, relaxed, and ready to leave.

POST-ABORTION COUNSELING AFTER RECOVERY

Most women don't need counseling right after their abortion or in the future. Those who do need it usually show signs of emotional distress in the recovery room, such as despondence, continuous crying, or angry outbursts. A patient may be feeling angry that her boyfriend didn't have to go through the same ordeal as she did. Anger can be triggered if she experienced more pain than what she expected. Sometimes she is angry at herself but displaces the anger onto the medical staff. In this case nothing they do for her is "good enough."

Crying during recovery can mean she is feeling 1). relieved and is releasing tension, 2). physically uncomfortable due to the cramping, 3). emotionally out of control due to the drugs that were used to relieve pain and anxiety, 4). guilty, or 5). sad. Once she has identified the source of the tears and conveyed it to you, you will be able to comfort her appropriately. The woman who feels guilty is often comforted by going back over the reasons why she felt the abortion was necessary. Reviewing strategies for coping with guilt and planning what to do for herself the rest of the day is also helpful.

When she reveals her tears are tears of sorrow, empathy may be all that she needs. Having her restate why she felt the abortion was necessary often has a calming effect. Sometimes she wants a few private moments with her boyfriend or husband. A few minutes with him is usually all it takes for her to regain composure and feel ready to go.

If the woman states, "I don't know why I'm crying, but I can't seem to stop," it is probably due to the medications or the drop in estrogen. Reassure her that other people have been affected the same way - crying involuntarily - by the drugs that were used to relieve pain and tension. It simply takes time for the drug to wear off.

When tears are caused by physical discomfort, her signs of distress disappear as soon as the discomfort subsides. By the time she is ready to

185

leave, she is usually feeling fine and there are no more tears. A feeling of relief takes over.

If the client seems fine and if birth control was not discussed in pre-abortion counseling, post-abortion is the time to bring it up. Most people are highly motivated at this time to prevent another unplanned pregnancy. They are usually eager to receive information and almost always have decided upon which method to use.

Most patients express gratitude for the excellent care they received from all the staff who attended them. It is common for us to receive hugs and handshakes from our patients and from the caring people who came with them. We receive thanks and compliments not only on the day of their procedure but also weeks later on the evaluation forms they send back. It gives us all a lift and replenishes our energy for the next day's work.

POST-ABORTION FOLLOW-UP

Most abortion providers do not call patients back to find out how they're feeling, simply because of patient confidentiality. Many patients live with people whom they have not told and don't want them to find out. We always leave the door open and tell them if they ever need to talk, to call us. We let them know our counseling staff is available to them. The vast majority go on with their lives and never call back. Most abortion clinics report the same experience when they offer post-abortion counseling. Even those clinics that have tried advertising post-abortion support groups have received very little response. As the research shows, most women don't need additional counseling after an abortion. Sometimes a need for counseling occurs much later in the woman's life when other life and death issues are faced, but she is then unlikely to return to the place where the abortion occurred for counseling.

The only routine emotional follow-up we do is through the patient evaluation forms. Before they leave, we give our patients an evaluation form and a self-addressed return envelope to take home. A copy of the form is printed in the Appendix.

Normally we get an 8% rate of return. We have implemented suggestions conveyed to us through these evaluations and distribute the comments to our staff. Responses on their physical and emo-

tional well-being have been fairly consistent through the years. Here are the average results for the years 1988-91:

1. I have felt relieved: 99%

2. I have NOT felt relieved: 1%

3. I have felt guilty: 43%
(80% of those who felt guilty reported five or less on a scale of one to 10, indicating "a little" or "moderate.")

4. I have NOT felt guilty: 57%

5. I have felt sad: 50%
(75% who felt sad reported five or less, indicating "a little" or "moderate.")

6. I have NOT felt sad: 50%

7. I have felt angry: 25%
(57% who felt angry reported five or less and said they felt angry either at self, partner, parents, or "everything.")

8. I have NOT felt angry: 75%

9. I believe I made the best decision: 96%

10. I wish I never had the abortion: 1%

11. I have some doubts: 3%

12. I have someone to talk to: 96%

13. I have no one to talk to: 4%

Follow-Up On Patients We Send Home Without An Abortion

We try to get back in touch with the patients we sent home two months after their initial appointment (See the chapter, How Women Cope After Their Abortion for reasons we send some patients home). If they returned and had an abortion, we still call to ask how they are feeling about their decision. If they haven't returned in a few months, we call and ask what they decided to do. This is done solely to collect data and gain feedback. If they say they are carrying to term, we inquire if they have a doctor and are receiving prenatal care.

In 1992 we were unable to contact one third of the women we had sent home because they had disconnected or changed their phone numbers within two months of their appointment or had given us incorrect phone numbers to begin with. Of the 51 patients we had sent home in 1992 (less than 1% of total number of patients), we were able to contact 33. Data on the 33 cases showed 64% returned and had the abortion. All stated they felt the abortion was the best decision. Two women (6%) went to another clinic for their abortion. Six women (18%) chose to carry to term. One woman returned and was sent home again after she indicated her boyfriend tricked her into coming back to the clinic. She said she didn't know where he was taking her. She chose to carry to term.

One of the most extraordinary "sent home" patients was a middle-aged married woman whose obstetrician repeatedly dismissed her complaints of intense abdominal pain as her pregnancy progressed. By 20 weeks her pain had intensified to the point of disability. She could barely walk, and neither she nor her husband could bear the debilitating psychological effects of her chronic pain. Her physician ran a few tests and told her it was all in her head. He refused to prescribe pain pills for fear the drug would adversely affect the fetus. Due to other known medical conditions, she was considered a high-risk obstetrical case, had no medical insurance, and all other physicians they asked refused to take her as a patient. Since the pregnancy was clearly wanted, and the reason for termination was lack of treatment for intolerable, undiagnosed pain, I asked if they would allow me to take a few days to search for a doctor who would be willing to take her case. They seemed weary of trying, but they agreed. My search ended in success.

I located a physician who was willing to assume her case, and he diagnosed the woman as having a fractured pelvic bone that was getting worse as the fetus grew larger. The patient was given pain medication to help her through the last three months of what would have been excruciating pain. She became completely bed-ridden and unable to walk or sit up. Though she still felt considerable pain, at least she was being humanely treated. She and I stayed in contact through what she called "the longest three months of my life!" At last she had her long-awaited C-section. When I visited her in the hospital, she and her husband looked radiant holding their beautiful baby girl. They were filled with gratitude and joy and quipped, "It took an abortion counselor to help us have our baby!"

Chapter Twenty-Two

Abortion Providers Taking Care Of Their Staffs

HELPING STAFF MANAGE STRESS

The clients you serve will sometimes be sharing intense emotions and tragic life situations with you. Once they have purged themselves, you may find yourself feeling the need to purge in kind. Caregivers tend to take in others' pain and give comfort and strength in return. This process can leave caregivers drained.

Our personal lives are full of sources of stress: our relationship with our partner, children, parents, co-workers, supervisors, and friends; our automobile hassles; the cost of living; our health, weight, or allergies; job performance, education, home chores and bills to pay; having a baby, changing jobs or career, and going back to school. We have a limited amount of time and energy to spend on all these areas of life. If we don't manage our time well and recharge our batteries regularly, we can become emotionally and physically drained, and in great need of revitalization. When we have squeezed dry the last drop of energy and are "running on empty," that's when we are experiencing true "burn-out."

When our energy is depleted by stress factors in one area of our lives, we have less to give to the other areas. If our family problems are consuming our time, we will probably feel drained at work. Likewise, if our conflicts on the job are left unresolved, we may soon find ourselves neglect-

ing our home life. And if we have problems in both or more areas, our need for rejuvenation is increased that much more.

Sometimes the depletion of our energy is so gradual that we overlook the initial warning signs. We must become aware of our own individual symptoms of burn-out and then watch for them to prevent a severe bout. Try to identify some of your symptoms from the following list, and add those that aren't listed.

Burn-out Symptoms

1. Chronically feeling tired when you wake up, draggy during the day, and exhausted when you get home from work. Can't motivate yourself to do anything, continuously procrastinating.

2. Getting sick a lot: getting headaches or abdominal pains, indigestion or breathing difficulties, biting your nails, clenching teeth, sighing a lot, tightening facial and neck muscles, changing eating habits (losing appetite or eating all the time).

3. Increasing dependence on drugs: alcohol, cigarettes, tranquilizers, sleeping pills, caffeine, etc.

4. Complaining a lot.

5. Being more disorganized and forgetful than usual - feeling overwhelmed with chores or duties.

6. Slowing down or speeding up - you're dragging your feet or going so fast you wonder why everyone else is so darn slow!

7. Lacking patience and getting irritable earlier in the day.

8. Driving unsafely; taking more chances in traffic or driving slower or faster than usual. Not wanting to drive at all.

9. Not being able to get to sleep or sleeping more often and longer than usual.

10. Doing nothing but watching TV when you're home.

11. Not being able to concentrate.

12. Denying anything is wrong when someone confronts you with your unusual behavior.

13. Feeling you're not getting anything done.

14. Not wanting to make decisions - "giving in" a lot.

15. Feeling sad and depressed, and you can't put your finger on the cause.

16. Becoming upset at little things that normally don't upset you.

All these symptoms may be telling you something is wrong. To curb the burn-out process, it is essential to recognize your early warning signs. Maybe you start to forget things or chew your fingernails, and as your burn-out progresses, you start losing sleep or gaining weight from nervous munching. You may not know what's wrong, but by talking to a caring, understanding listener, it is likely to come out in the open. DO something about your stress or your behavior will continue to worsen.

Managing Stress

With any source of stress, you can either eliminate it through effective problem solving (for things you CAN control), or get away from the problem mentally if not physically. Give yourself a rest away from the source of stress, even if just for a little time every day.

Listed below are some constructive methods for warding off burn-out before it becomes severe, and for maintaining emotional well-being.

1. Write down the names of your most nurturing friends and family members.

2. Write down the names of friends, neighbors, and family members who are always coming to you with their problems.

3. The nurturing friends are those you want to see more of when you are experiencing your stress symptoms, because you need to be nurtured at this time. You need to avoid problematic friends and family members when you are experiencing your symptoms. They will deplete your energy even more. It is not unkind to avoid these people temporarily; it is necessary for your own emotional health.

4. We all need to develop outside interests - something totally unrelated to our jobs. Write down some activities you really enjoy doing or you would enjoy doing. How often do you do these activities in a week? Is it enough? How do you justify not doing it more often? What would it take to do it more often? Time? Money? A partner? Better planning? What are the obstacles that prevent you from enjoying yourself more often? How can you surmount these obstacles?

Doing nice things for yourself is essential to replenish your supply of emotional and physical energy. However, it takes planning to do those things. You may have to put some money away each paycheck if your activity takes money, plan to make time for it, and schedule the activity. It may take time sitting down with a calendar at the beginning of each week and writing down what you are going to do for yourself that week.

5. Contract with a counselor (not a co-worker) for an hour of his or her time so you can ventilate, problem-solve, or focus on redirecting your energy for yourself. A counselor is sometimes more effective than a friend because he/she has skills that will help you get to the crux of the problem.

6. Keep a journal. Write down your thoughts

at the day's end so at least your problems will be out of your mind and onto a piece of paper.

7. Learn and develop assertiveness to express your needs, validate your rights, and get in touch with your feelings.

8. Spend time alone NOT doing chores, unless the sense of accomplishment will make you feel good. Rather, go someplace that brings peace. Spending time alone allows you to be with yourself rather than expending energy on communicating with another person.

9. Learn "thought-stopping." When you are alone, turn off the worrisome thoughts by purposely thinking about something pleasant. Fantasize, daydream, meditate, or do something like crossword puzzles that forces you to clear your mind and focus on something else. This gives you a rest away from the problem.

10. Ask yourself: How much sleep do you get? Is it enough? Do you feel rested when you wake up? What times of the day are you most alert? Do you maximize that alert time?

11. How much physical exercise do you get? How can you incorporate more into your day? What type of exercise do you enjoy most? What do you need to do it? Work in the helping professions is often sedentary and we need the refreshing balance of physical activity.

12. What kind of food do you eat? How can you change your diet for the better? Plan to get at least one nutritious meal a week, if not per day. Or make it even simpler and eat one nutritious food each day. You cannot afford to mistreat your body since the mental and physical aspects are so intrinsically tied to one another. You need to get proper nourishment, rest, and exercise to be healthy enough to be an effective caregiver. Empathy and problem-solving takes concentrated energy, and it is not unusual for a counselor to feel exhausted after an intense counseling session. You can't give to someone else unless you give to yourself first.

13. Spend some money on yourself. It doesn't have to be extravagant, but something that is all for YOU. Or make yourself something new. Learn something new and fun.

14. Examine how much time you spend on work, education, recreation, friends and family. Which do you spend the most time on, and which do you spend the least? Are the allotted times for each satisfactory? If not, plan how you are going to balance these areas for the coming month.

15. Take a vacation away from it all, even if that means disconnecting the phone and shutting down the TV. Getting away from it all doesn't necessarily mean spending your life savings on a trip to the Caribbean. In fact, don't take a vacation where you run yourself ragged and wind up feeling more exhausted upon returning home than when you left!

16. Periodically ask yourself, "What do I need to be happy? Is my current lifestyle giving me what I need to be satisfied? What do I need to change to improve my morale?"

Management Interventions To Relieve Staff Stress And Burn-out

1. Hire enough people to serve the number of patients you have. Do not overload employees.

2. Reduce patient contact for managers and supervisors.

3. Limit the amount of time an employee spends under high stress conditions or give adequate compensation and time off.

4. Furnish a counselor or crisis team for the employees' utilization when needed.

5. Allow employees to air complaints to someone who is willing and able to deal effectively with conflicts and problems.

6. Allot enough vacation time for an employee to feel refreshed throughout the year.

7. Make employees take their vacation time each year.

8. Allow employees to diversify and grow in their jobs.

9. Allow time and money for employee attendance at workshops and classes to enrich their skills and increase their feeling of achievement.

10. Show appreciation. People can endure hectic work as long as they feel appreciated. Since employees give so much of their energy, they need to receive in order to give. "Receiving" can mean hearing compliments from clients, co-workers, and supervisors. And of course, receiving a pay raise, bonus, or other monetary reward or special privilege is especially uplifting. Everyone needs a pat on the back for his or her efforts from time to time. And when employees feel appreciated, they have more to give to the patients.

Letting Go Of Worry

Hanging on to other people's problems is a source of stress for the helping profession. The "other people" I am referring to may be a client, co-worker, spouse, friend, or family member.

When people "take on" other people's problems, they think about the person and their problem over and over again. These thoughts usually generate feelings of sadness, anger, or fear. For instance, you may fear the person will never be able to solve his or her problem, or that the problem may become worse. You may feel sad for this person's plight, and the more you think about it, the sadder you become. You may feel angry the person has to deal with such terrible hardships and may contemplate the injustice of it all. The more you think about it, the angrier and more frustrated you become because you realize you are unable to do anything about it. The person must take care of it themselves.

There is a continuum of concern we have for people in our lives. On one extreme there is "worry." Worry means continuously stewing over the other person's difficulties. On the other extreme of the continuum is "don't care." Both extremes are unhealthy. In the middle lies "concern."

Worry	Concern	Don't Care

People think if they REALLY care about a person, they'll worry about them. People also believe that if you don't worry about someone, that means you don't really care. We usually learn this distorted thinking from one or both of our parents. The fact is, worrying about someone does NOT mean you care any more or any less

about that person, and it does not help the person you're worrying about! The only effect worrying has is on the worrier. Have you ever heard the expression, "I'm just worried sick!" Worry usually will make you physically and emotionally sick. What good does that do?

The goal is to strike a balance. You want to show the person you are concerned without stewing about them. A healthy concern means letting the person know by what you say and what you do that you care about them. It also means letting go of continual thoughts and feelings about them. Letting go is a skill we can all learn. To understand the letting-go process, we first need to remember that every one of us has a need for kindness, affection, and protection from harm. We need to be gentle with ourselves and to protect ourselves from unnecessary harm. To let go, we need to nurture ourselves.

Self-Nurturing & Self-Talk

When you are worrying about someone, relax and talk to yourself in the following manner: "I know I am a caring person and I want to help people. Taking on my friend's problems doesn't help her, and it only serves to hurt me. I don't need to worry about other people. Worrying does not prove I care about them or that I love them; it does not help solve the problem; what it does is cause me distress. It is not necessary for me to create this stress for myself. By caring for myself I will be able to give that much more to others. I can take joy in helping myself. Worry only depletes the energy I need for more positive action. I am focusing now on positive actions. What can I do for them? Can I send them a card or a treat to let them know I care? Is there anything concrete I can do to help? If not, then I let go and trust they will solve their problem in their own way and in their own time." For those of you who believe in God, you may want to add, "I let go and let God provide them with the strength and guidance needed to solve their problem."

Remember that people solve their own problems and that letting go will help keep you strong.

COPING WITH ANTI-ABORTION TERRORISM

Acts of terrorism directed at abortion clinics have been reported to the National Abortion Federation since 1977 and have included: arson, death threats, stalking of doctors and staff, verbal and physical assault, blockades, clinic invasion, chemical attacks, destruction of property, shootings, kidnapping, and the murder of physicians by "pro-life" activists (Chicago Tribune Wires, 1994; Donovan, 1985; Forrest & Henshaw, 1987; N.A.F., 1992; and St. Louis Post-Dispatch, 1993). These acts of terrorism present an unprecedented epidemic of violence directed at health care providers in the United States (Grimes, Forrest, and Radford, 1991). See N.A.F.'s Incidence of Violence in Appendix.

Many doctors and clinic directors heed the advice of their city police and wear bullet-proof body armor, hire bodyguards and use protection dogs, and vary their daily routine and travel routes. Some providers have resorted to carrying guns (Hewitt, Sider, Campier, Eskind, & Wescott, 1993). Most abortion clinics take maximum security measures to protect property and people and have installed high tech security systems, 24-hour guard service, state-of-the-art fire proofing and fire alarm systems, bullet-proof window glass, video surveillance cameras, and high fences around the building.

None of us in this field of women's health care ever intended to become combat soldiers. Our purpose from the beginning was - and is - to provide care to women who cannot obtain abortion services from their own doctors. Over the years we have realized that while most of our time is spent in caregiving, sometimes we must assume the dual roles of caregiver and freedom fighter.

Examples Of "Pro-Life" Terrorism

Bombing And Arson

In 1982 on a Saturday night in the dead of winter the Hope Clinic burst into flames at 8:40 p.m., just 15 minutes after the cleaning staff had locked up and left for the night. The explosion was heard blocks away, and the fire department was quickly on the scene. In less than an hour the fire had demolished one third of the building.

The next morning as I walked into what was left of the waiting room and saw the dripping wet, charred remnant of my office, I felt myself shaking. Less than 24 hours before, I had been sitting there talking to a patient.

The detectives determined that someone had gained entry to the building minutes after the cleaning staff left, poured and ignited a highly flammable substance onto the floors of the waiting rooms and made a quick exit. Both the police and a private company we hired thought it looked like the work of a professional arsonist. The culprit was never found.

This account is only one of the 119 bombings and arsons of abortion clinics perpetrated by the anti-abortion terrorists from 1977-1993 (National Abortion Federation, 1993). As many as three clinics were firebombed in one day in 1984, the handiwork of people who purport to be "pro-life" and "Christian" (Blanchard & Prewitt, 1993). In addition to actual bombings and arsons, over 200 bomb threats have been reported in the same period (National Abortion Federation, 1993). For these reasons the Federal Department of Alcohol, Tobacco, and Firearms' training sessions on handling bomb threats is common practice for abortion clinic staffs.

Blockades And Protests

From 1977 to 1993 there were 581 incidents of clinic blockades reported to the National Abortion Federation (National Abortion Federation, 1993). Operation Rescue is one of the national, militant organizations led by Fundamentalist Christians whose purpose is to block women from entering abortion clinics and shut clinics down (Faludi, 1989; Shepard, 1991). Other groups include Lambs of God, Rescue America, Missionaries to the Preborn, Life Ministries, and Collegians Activated to Liberate Life (CALL). Their training, lingo, and tactics are highly militaristic and heavily cloaked in the trappings of the Christian religion (Wills, 1989).

In the summer of 1991 hundreds of militant members of Operation Rescue descended upon the clinics in Wichita, Kansas. When they arrived they announced to the media they had secured the first abortion-free zone in the country and would not leave. The next day the police executed a highly effective maneuver that successfully broke through the human blockade obstructing access to the Women's Health Care clinic. In the blink of an eye a police vehicle carrying both staff and patients whisked through the mob with the invaluable help of the mounted police and deposited everyone inside the clinic. When Operation

Rescuers realized they had been foiled, the leaders ordered their troops to march to the next clinic. One of the staff members watched as the mob went berserk, venting their anger at having been defeated. She saw them using pocketknives, cutting the mounted police horses' bellies and legs, grabbing hold of the reins, and bringing the horses to their knees. The police resorted to using tear gas to repel the mob.

One platoon of Operation Rescue followed the doctor to his home and camped across the street for several days and nights. The doctor, his wife, and two teenage daughters feared for their lives. Some of the "pro-life Christians" stormed the house and pounded on the windows and doors in the middle of the night. The next day armed guards were hired to stand at every door of their house. Because of the pro-lifers' treatment of the police horses, the doctor feared he'd find his dogs poisoned, shot, or mutilated. He took them to a kennel and obtained a trained protection dog to keep guard in the backyard.

Stalking

In the first six months of 1993 there were 109 reported stalkings of abortion providers (National Abortion Federation, 1993). For reporting purposes, "stalking" is defined as following, threatening, and harassing a provider or patient away from the clinic site.

During the weeks of Operation Rescue in Wichita, staff members were sometimes followed home and terrorized. One stalker was described as a big man who dressed in black robes and wore chains around his wrists. After clinic hours, he followed an employee home who was a single mother of a teenage son. When she peered out her window one evening after supper she saw this demonic man coming into her front yard. He stood there facing the house, shaking his chains, pulling them taut and growling. She called the police, but by the time the police arrived, he was walking up and down the sidewalk. The police took one look at the guy and told her, "That man is dangerous. Don't do anything foolish." Then the officer left.

The same man tried to follow other staff members home, but they had all been warned to stay alert to cars following them. One employee drove directly to the police station to get him off her trail.

Another drove to a restaurant and called the police.

I have talked to physicians who travel long distances to provide abortions in other states who describe being ambushed and screamed at in airports by stalkers. Both directors and physicians have also described being followed into grocery stores, theaters, and restaurants by stalkers who sometimes point and shriek, "Baby murderer!" The husband of one of the female physicians from a Topeka clinic told a reporter, "I am concerned about how close I can keep her to me so that I can take the bullet for her" (Hollar, 1993).

Chemical Attacks

Clinics have been the target of chemical attacks (butyric acid and mace-like chemicals), sometimes harming staff and patients with noxious fumes as well as destroying property (Hollar, 1993). In Indiana in 1993 a clinic that was heavily picketed by the group, CALL, was destroyed by butyric acid. At the time of CALL's protests, stalking of the clinic director also began.

Death Threats

From 1977 to 1993 there were 144 death threats reported to the National Abortion Federation, with 56 of those threats reported in 1993 (National Abortion Federation, 1993). Doctors, clinic directors, and their families have been the target of death threats. Sometimes the threat is hand-delivered into their mailboxes at their homes, and sometimes they receive threatening phone calls at night. One of the physicians in Dallas, Texas, who has received numerous death threats throughout the years told me, "The usual message is: 'I know where you are; I know your routine; and you're going to die unless you quit killing babies.'"

In 1974 when Hope Clinic opened, our physician **and his two children** received death threats from anti-choice terrorists. In 1994 Dr. John Britton received a written threat left in the door of his Pensacola, Florida home that read, "What would you do if you had five minutes to live?" That same year he was shot and killed by an anti-abortion zealot. (Chicago Tribune Wires, 1994).

Kidnapping

Prior to 1990 a doctor and his wife were kidnapped at gunpoint from their home. They were bound and gagged and taken to a deserted army bunker. There they were kept bound and guarded by one of three armed men who called themselves, "The Army of God." Their purpose, they said, was to make an example of him to the rest of the physicians performing abortions. Every one of the eight days they were held in captivity their kidnappers told them they would be executed. The leader of the Army of God said he heard voices from God telling him to carry out this plan "to save babies." The doctor and his wife spent those eight days mentally preparing themselves to die and periodically wondering how they could escape. On the third day of captivity the leader forced the doctor to make a cassette tape asking that President Ronald Reagan call an end to abortion in exchange for their release. The FBI was called in. On the eighth day of captivity the doctor and his wife were blindfolded and led into the backseat of a vehicle. Thinking they were being taken to their place of execution, they were transported for hours and then miraculously released a few miles from their home. Three months later all three men had been apprehended, and the following year they were tried, sentenced and imprisoned.

Murder

Dr. David Gunn, an unassuming and highly regarded OB-GYN, performed abortions at three clinics in Florida, Georgia, and Alabama due to the shortage of physicians willing to do abortions. Protesters harassed him outside the clinics and sometimes outside his home. Abortion opponents targeted him on their "hit list" by printing his picture and daily routine on a "Wanted" poster. On March 7, 1993 a local pro-lifer prayed aloud for Dr. David Gunn's soul at the Whitfield Assembly of God church. Wednesday, March 10, 1993, protesters from the Assembly of God church picketed outside Women's Medical Services in Pensacola, Florida where Dr. Gunn was due to arrive. When Dr. Gunn got out of his car, the perpetrator walked over to him, pulled out a revolver, and shot the doctor three times in the back. Two hours later Dr. Gunn died at the hospital (Hewitt, Sider, Dampier, Eskind, & Wescott, 1992; Yearwood, 1993).

After Dr. Gunn's murder, an anti-abortion activist organized Defensive Action, a group that publicly condoned murdering physicians who perform abortions. Sixteen months after Dr. Gunn

was shot to death, the leader of Defensive Action shot and killed Dr. John Britton and a clinic escort, James Barrett, outside an abortion clinic in Pensacola. Mr. Barrett's wife, also an escort, suffered a gunshot wound (Chicago Tribune Wires, 1994).

Attempted Murder

Five months after Dr. Gunn was murdered the physician from Women's Health Care in Wichita was shot twice by a protester while leaving the clinic (Bates, 1993; Hollar, 1993). The assailant was apprehended and taken under custody for attempted homicide. According to news reports, she had written numerous letters to the man who murdered Dr. Gunn after he was in custody and hailed him as a hero. She had also been arrested in an Operation Rescue blockade in Atlanta, and edited a Christian anti-abortion newsletter for a fellow terrorist who has been serving prison time for bombing a Cincinnati abortion clinic (Johnson, 1993).

Surmounting The Oppression: How We Keep On Going

1. WE FIND STRENGTH IN EACH OTHER. Attacks from the "pro-lifers" serve to forge stronger bonds between providers, and it strengthens the fighting spirit of the pro-choice community.

When Dr. David Gunn was murdered outside his clinic in Pensacola, Florida, physicians traveled from other cities to keep the clinic open. After Operation Rescue laid siege to clinics in Wichita, Kansas for seven weeks, their next target was Buffalo, New York. However, Buffalo's outraged pro-choice community rose up, surrounded the clinic in a display of strength, and proved a formidable foe. Operation Rescue retreated. Afterwards, Buffalo's organizers shared their successful strategy with the rest of us. In addition, the National Abortion Federation keeps its members informed of terrorist acts and ways to combat them.

2. WE RELY ON LOCAL AND NATIONAL POLITICAL ORGANIZATIONS like the National Abortion and Reproductive Rights Action League, National Coalition of Abortion Providers and National Organization for Women to garner pro-choice support on the federal and state level. In

response to terrorist acts perpetrated on abortion clinics, bills such as the Federal Access to Clinic Entrances Act (1993) and anti-stalking laws have been introduced into the legislature in hopes of providing more protection to clinic staffs and patients. And in October of 1993, Attorney General Janet Reno of the Clinton Administration launched a coordinated national effort to investigate the pattern of terrorism against abortion providers, utilizing the Chief of the Terrorism and Violent Crime Section, the FBI, and the Bureau of Alcohol, Tobacco, and Firearms (NAF, 1993).

3. WE FOLLOW THE MOTTO, "BE PREPARED." Once you have done everything possible to protect patients, staff and property, you are more likely to let go of fear and maintain an appropriate level of vigilance and preparedness.

Being prepared means having regular staff inservices on protocol for clinic invasion, blockades, bomb threats, and fire. It also means "knowing thine enemy." As unpleasant a task as it is, we periodically watch pro-life propaganda films, read their pamphlets and newsletters, keep abreast of their latest terrorist tactics through networking, and know who their leaders are. We don't need to spend a lot of time on this, but having the knowledge helps to keep us one step ahead.

Finally, being prepared means establishing and training a post-trauma debriefing team for staff in times of blockades and other attacks. People who have been subjected to terrorism are likely to experience symptoms of post-trauma stress. Helping staff and their families cope with their symptoms goes a long way toward fortifying their morale, endurance, and human spirit. Once you are in the middle of a fray, time and energy is at a premium, so preparing ahead of time for psychological support will save considerable time and stress.

Hope Clinic's debriefing team is comprised of four hand-picked counselors from the pro-choice community whom I trained in post-trauma debriefing and who are on-call for us. It is important to seek counselors for a debriefing team who are NOT on staff. Every staff member will need to be on the RECEIVING end of the debriefing and support sessions. Essentially the team will assist everyone in the process of healing from a trauma by providing group and individual support and imparting knowledge of post-trauma stress. Just knowing they are there brings a greater sense of security.

To learn how to recruit and train members of your debriefing team, write or call Hope Clinic for Women to purchase the booklet, Survival Kit for Abortion Providers: Emotional Support in Times of Crisis.

4. WE KEEP FOCUSED ON "THE BIG PICTURE." When times get rough, people sometimes ask us, "Why do you stay?" We stay because this issue isn't about abortion, it's about women's lives and fundamental liberty.

Liberty

No woman is truly free unless she has the right to control her own body. Without the freedom to exercise control over if and when she carries a pregnancy, a woman is enslaved by whoever prevents her from exercising that control.

One of the basic human rights that our country was founded upon and that is covered in the Bill of Rights is the freedom of religion. When abortion is legal and accessible, everyone is free to exercise their religious beliefs about abortion. Those who believe it is immoral need not ever have an abortion and thus follow their conscience. Those who believe it is a morally acceptable choice can exercise that option.

Women's Lives

Abortion is and always has been a fact of life. Women all over the world and in every century have practiced abortion to control fertility, prevent birth, and save themselves and their families from a myriad of social, physical, and emotional ills. The question is NOT, "Will it exist?" but "Will it be safe and legal?"

When abortion was not legal, women in the 20th century resorted to drinking turpentine, ammonia, bluing, teas, and other potions in hopes of causing a miscarriage. They have douched with Lysol and other caustic substances and inserted objects into their uteruses such as knitting needles, crochet hooks, hatpins, umbrella ribs, rubber tubing, coat hangers, and T.V. antennae (Gordon, 1976). Submitting to someone else's methods proved just as treacherous, with the added danger of getting raped by the "abortionist" (Fadiman, 1993). Many women died, and those that lived had grisly stories to tell.

Physicians practicing medicine during the days of illegal abortion remember all too well the number of botched abortion cases they saw in the hospitals, the women whose bodies were beyond repair, and those that died. The memory of those wasted young lives motivates many of the doctors who now provide abortion services even under threat to their own safety. Those of us too young to have witnessed the reality of illegal abortion can imagine the desperation women of years past must have felt. We are determined to continue offering compassionate and professional care during a procedure that was once relegated to the back alleys.

WHEN PEOPLE ASK, "WHERE DO YOU WORK?"

Have you ever stopped in your tracks when your new neighbors, dentist, or husband's boss asked "Where do YOU work?" In that instant, a hundred thoughts may be racing through your mind as you try to decide, "Do I want to subject myself to a debate on when life begins? Worse yet, do I want to take the risk of being stalked and picketed at home by a fetus supremacist?" Even though you may encounter occasional hostility, you may very well receive uplifting responses, such as "Good for you! It's a necessary service!" I have received positive remarks from some of the most unlikely people (or so I thought.)

On one occasion a bank teller who spoke with an Italian accent and wore a gold crucifix around her neck scrutinized "The Hope Clinic" name on my paycheck. She surprised me when she said, "I've heard of you." And then she whispered, "I'm glad you're there."

I have come to expect more positive remarks than negative, not only from my past experience, but also because the majority of people in the U.S. are pro-choice. The opinion polls repeatedly demonstrate that fact, year after year. We need to keep in mind it is PROBABLE that we will hear pro-choice comments.

I find it invaluable to share with other staff members the experiences we've had answering the question, "Where do you work?" There are approximately four categories of reactions we receive: positive regard, silence, expressed disapproval, or dark humor. Here are some examples of each reaction and possible responses.

Expressed Disapproval

"I think abortion is just terrible!"
(Our response): "Well, from all my experience working with the many good people who have chosen to end their pregnancy, I see it in a different light."

"I just don't see how anybody can do such a thing!"
(Our response): "Some of the people who have anguished over the decision and chose abortion as the only solution that made sense to them in their situation once professed the same anti-abortion beliefs you have. Sometimes it looks a lot different once you're in the situation."

"Well, I certainly don't believe in abortion!"
(Our response): "That's the beauty of legal abortion - everyone has the right to act upon his or her own beliefs. Some people do not believe that having an abortion is the same thing as killing a baby. The people who don't believe in it never have to use the service. For others, clinics like ours are a godsend!"

"How can anyone kill her own baby?"
(Our response): "Not everyone believes that removing a fetus from a uterus is the same as killing a newborn. You can ask a room full of priests, ministers, biologists and physicians if abortion is killing a baby, and you'll get as many answers as there are people in the room. Everyone has the right to his or her own opinion."

"Those women should put their babies up for adoption!"
(Our response): "Many women say they could never part with their baby once they went through nine months of pregnancy and then gave birth. Could you give up YOUR child for adoption?" (This is especially effective if they have children of their own. They often look at you as though you're crazy to suggest such a thing. In other words, once the shoe is placed on the other foot, the idea doesn't sound so simple after all.) OR "Some of the women I see seeking an abortion have been adopted themselves, and they say they could NEVER do that to someone else because they know what it feels like. And that's even from

197

the women who state they have good adoptive parents! Other women seeking an abortion have placed a baby for adoption in the past and say they could NEVER go through it again! They say that they could cope better emotionally after an abortion than after another adoption experience. Adoption is only a viable alternative for those women who feel they can get through it emotionally."

"Abortion goes against God and nature!"
(Our response): "God and nature have always allowed abortions to occur in the form of spontaneous abortions, or miscarriages."

If someone goes on continuously about the horrors of abortion, and you tire of hearing it, you can state this is an issue theologians and scientists can't agree on, and you'd prefer to put your energy elsewhere.

"Why don't those people use birth control? There's no excuse for abortion nowadays!"
(Our response): "Most of the people we see HAVE used birth control - often they have used several different kinds of contraception in the past. I've seen every type of birth control fail since I've been at Hope Clinic - even vasectomy and tubal sterilization. Then there are people who have not had any education about fertility, and they're using ineffective methods. Some women don't use birth control and get pregnant because their doctors told them they COULDN'T get pregnant. And there is no method of birth control that is 100% effective, 100% available, and 100% side-effect free."

(Another response): "One of the services we offer to every patient is information on contraception. We feel strongly about educating people to help them avoid the sad situation of an unplanned pregnancy."

"I think it's horrible that women use abortion as birth control, as if it's no big deal."
(Our response): "Since I work in an abortion clinic, let me tell you from one who knows: it's a myth that women supposedly use abortion as birth control in this country. I don't know where you get your information, but your idea of abortion patients and the reality are two different things."

"I can see maybe one abortion, but those people

who repeat are just disgusting!"
(Our response): "Some of those people feel just as unhappy about it and place the same judgment on themselves as you have; that they're disgusting because they failed. But I ask you, is there any area of your life you have repeatedly failed to control - like quitting smoking, losing weight, never procrastinating? Their area happens to be fertility; yours may be something else, and mine, something altogether different. We're all human, and we all deserve compassion and help, not condemnation."

"I hear that Planned Parenthood runs the largest chain of abortuaries in the country!"
(Our response): "Oh? How interesting. And did you also know that Planned Parenthood is the one organization that helps to prevent more abortions than any other organization in the world?"

Dark Humor

"I bet your doctor really pulls in the money!"
(Our response): "Any doctor who has the courage to perform abortions in a time when doctors are kidnapped, stalked, and murdered for doing so deserves every penny he or she gets. And quite frankly, they could make a lot more money without any personal danger if they were in another field of medicine."

(Another response):"You must have no idea what medical procedures and surgeries cost these days. An abortion procedure is one of the least expensive surgeries there is! Getting your wisdom teeth removed costs more than an abortion."

"What's it like to kill babies for a living, ha ha!" Or, "I guess you're in charge of the rusty coat hangers!"
(Our response): "You know, because I see so many tragic situations where people have agonized over this decision, it doesn't strike me as funny." The people who make these remarks might be mocking the anti's rhetoric, but there are enough people who think we're cold-blooded, callous humanoids. I don't like to perpetuate these myths by engaging in dark humor with acquaintances.

"How's business? Booming?"
(Our response): "Are you asking how many people are in need of our service?"

Silence

Silence can mean just about anything. They may be a at a loss for words. They may be wondering where they've heard of your clinic. Perhaps they are reflecting on the abortion they've had , or they may be expressing total disapproval.

In that moment of silence, you can make a favorable statement about your work: "I'm lucky to work at a place where at the end of a day I can say I really helped people when they needed understanding the most. It's a good feelng!"

(Another response): "You know, working at The Hope Clinic is really a window to the world. I've talked to people from all walks of life, all religions, all races...and to people who say they would never have dreamed they'd have an abortion."

(Another response): "You know, I'm glad to be a part of an organizaion where people are treated with dignity and respect, and where they can receive excellent patient care."

You can also choose to let the silence stand, go on to talk about something else, or ask them what they believe about abortion (if you want to know).

Positive Regard

"That's wonderful! I believe in your cause!"

"I'm sure your job isn't easy, but I'm glad there are places like yours."

"I know someone who went to your clinic. She just raved about how well she was treated!"

"I admire people who can work in the abortion field, especially when the opposition is so violent and crazy!"

"More power to you! What you're doing is a needed service!"

TAKING PRIDE IN WHAT WE DO

We have every reason to feel proud of working in a field that helps so many people live their lives with dignity and self-determination. While pregnancy can be a beautiful experience of life when it occurs at a GOOD time, a pregnancy can be dev-astating to a woman and her entire family when it occurs at a BAD time.

At a workshop I was conducting for a Planned Parenthood in a conservative Bible Belt town, I asked the participants, "What do you say when someone asks where you work?" One woman recounted a story at which we all laughed and applauded at the tale's end. She said when she first started working for Planned Parenthood, she was reluctant to reveal where she worked because she'd get so angry when her reply was met with snide remarks. "But," she said, "I've changed completely, ever since I witnessed how my ten-year-old daughter, Carla, handled herself one day in Sunday School. I was picking her up one Sunday, and there she was, chatting with Miss Patton, the Sunday school teacher. As I drew closer, I heard Miss Patton ask, 'And, Carla, where does your mother work?' Carla beamed as she proudly announced, 'My Mom works at the Planned Parenthood Federation of America!' At that moment I thought I heard a drum roll as I walked into the room!"

Impact Of Family Planning And Legal Abortion On Society, Families, And Women's Lives

When women lack the means to control their fertility through effective contraceptives and safe abortion, their health often suffers and lifespans are shortened. Repeated childbirth in close succession takes its toll both mentally and physically. For some women with debilitating diseases and health conditions, even one pregnancy can wreak havoc and result in death.

Illegal abortion all too often resulted in major complications and death. In 1942 there were 1,407 **reported** abortion-related deaths, and more that assuredly went unreported. By 1985 the death toll plummeted to only seven (American Medical Association/Council on Scientific Affairs, 1992). The sharp decline in mortality is attributed to the introduction of antibiotics in medical practice in the 1940s and 1950s, the discovery and legalization of contraceptives in the 1960s, and legal abortion in the 1970s.

When these women who died were already mothers, what happened to their children? If the fathers were absent, unwilling, or unable to raise their children, the kids were sent to live with relatives who were not always thrilled to have them, or they were placed in orphan homes.

Infant mortality also declines when women have access to birth control and legal abortion (Gold, 1990). Women at high risk of complicated births, premature delivery, low birth weight babies, fetal abnormality and genetic disease can and often do choose to avoid risky pregnancies. Individuals, families, and society all serve to benefit from these decisions.

When a family's budget is stretched to the breaking point from too many mouths to feed, nerves can fray, relationships break down, and divorces result. Many books and therapists specializing in marriage counseling point to the prominent role of financial problems in the decision to divorce.

The more children a woman has and cannot support, the more trapped she may become in an abusive marriage. The longer she and her children are exposed to and entrenched in abuse, the more mental and physical damage can occur, including long-term depression, post-trauma syndrome, drug and alcohol problems, and physical illness.

With self-regulated fertility control also comes the ability for the female half of the population to be educated and potentially self-supporting. Society stands to benefit when all its people contribute his or her brain power and talents to the whole.

As the planet becomes crowded with too many people, the earth's limited resources diminish, crime and deprivation increases, waste products overflow, animals become extinct, rain forests are destroyed, and the balance of nature is threatened.

When women can choose when they are ready to provide adequately for a child, the entire family reaps the benefits of more resources. More time, attention, and money translates into more opportunity for education, employment, adequate health care, a home in a safe neighborhood, and psychological well-being for both parents and children.

One of my clients brought home this point to me in no uncertain terms. She said, "If I have this baby, neither one of us will have any kind of life. Do you know what poverty is? Let me tell you - I can show you a scar where a rat bit me when I was little. Where we lived, it was called the projects. My mother used to stay up at night sometimes with a baseball bat, watching over us kids, scaring the rats away while we slept on a mattress on the floor. We were on state aid. We had nothing! Sometimes I'd find her crying. She yelled at us a lot. I guess her nerves couldn't take it. I swore to myself I would never be that poor again. That if I ever had a child, it would never have to go through what I went through. If I had this child, I'd have to go on state aid and live that nightmare all over again, and bring another human being down with me. NO way! No way! I'd rather die first!"

For these reasons and many more, everyone who chooses to work in the field of family planning and/or abortion makes a significant contribution to the welfare of society, families, and individuals. We can go home at the end of a day and know we have made a difference in people's lives and in the world as a whole. We help make the dream of reproductive freedom a reality.

Appendix

To help the Hope Clinic staff better serve women's needs, please take a few minutes to fill out this questionnaire.

Name (Optional): _ _ _ _ _ _ _ _ _ _ _ _ _ _ Age: _ _ _ _ _ _ _

Today's Date: _____

Date of Abortion: _____

How Do You Feel?

Have you experienced any of the following as a result of the abortion? (<u>Check all that apply.</u>)

1. _____ Have felt **relieved**.
2. _____ Have not felt relieved
    Circle the number below that describes the degree of relief you have been feeling:

1	2	3	4	5	6	7	8	9	10
not relieved				somewhat relieved				very relieved	

3. _____ I have not felt **guilty**.
4. _____ I have felt guilty.
    If yes, what I felt guilty about was:
    Circle the number below that describes the degree of guilt you have been feeling:

1	2	3	4	5	6	7	8	9	10
strong guilt				moderate				little/no guilt	

5. _____ I have not felt **sad**.
6. _____ I have felt sad.
    If yes, what I felt sad about was:
    Circle the number below that describes the degree of sadness you have been feeling:

1	2	3	4	5	6	7	8	9	10
a deep sense of sadness			a little sad				little/no sadness		

7. _____ I have not felt **angry**.
8. _____ I have felt angry.
    If yes, what I felt angry about was:
    Circle the number below that describes the degree of anger you have been feeling:

1	2	3	4	5	6	7	8	9	10
Very angry				moderate anger				little/no anger	

9. _____ When I think about the abortion, I come to the same conclusion: I made the best decision considering the circumstances.
10. _____ When I think about it, I wish I had never had the abortion, but instead had continued the pregnancy.
11. _____ When I think about it, I have **doubts** whether the abortion was the best decision.
    Circle the number below that describes the degree of doubt you have been feeling:

1	2	3	4	5	6	7	8	9	10
Serious doubts				moderate doubt				little/no doubt	

12 _____ I have someone I can talk to who is supportive to me about the abortion.
13 _____ I have nobody I can talk to who is supportive to me about the abortion.

COMMENTS: _____

_____

Remember: If you would like to talk with a counselor, please don't hesitate to call Hope Clinic.
Toll free: 1/800-844-3130   Local: 1/618-451-5722

INCIDENTS OF VIOLENCE & DISRUPTION AGAINST ABORTION PROVIDERS, 1994[1]

VIOLENCE (# Incidents)	1977–83	1984	1985	1986	1987	1988	1989	1990	1991[2]	1992	1993	1994[1]	TOTAL
Murder	0	0	0	0	0	0	0	0	0	0	1	4	5
Attempted Murder	0	0	0	0	0	0	0	0	0	0	1	8	9
Bombing	8	18	4	2	0	0	2	0	1	1	1	13	40
Arson	13	6	8	7	4	4	6	4	10	16	9	5	92
Attempted Bomb/Arson	5	6	10	5	8	3	2	4	1	13	7	4	68
Invasion	68	34	47	53	14	6	25	19	29	26	24	2	347
Vandalism	35	35	49	43	29	29	24	26	44	116	113	40	583
Assault & Battery	11	7	7	11	5	5	12	6	6	9	9	7	95
Death Threats	4	23	22	7	5	4	5	7	3	8	78	55	221
Kidnapping	2	0	0	0	0	0	0	0	0	0	0	0	2
Burglary	3	2	2	5	7	1	0	2	1	5	3	3	34
Stalking[3]	0	0	0	0	0	0	0	0	0	0	188	16	204
TOTAL	149	131	149	133	72	52	76	68	95	194	434	147	1,700
DISRUPTION													
Hate Mail & Phone Calls	9	17	32	53	32	19	30	21	142	469	628	333	1785
Bomb Threats	9	32	75	51	28	21	21	11	15	12	22	11	308
Picketing	107	160	139	141	77	151	72	45	292	2898	2279	1212	7568
TOTAL	125	209	246	245	137	191	123	77	449	3379	2929	1228	9661
CLINIC BLOCKADES													
No. Incidents	0	0	0	0	2	182	201	34	41	83	66	24	633
No. Arrests[4]	0	0	0	0	290	11732	12358	1363	3885	2580	1236	161	33605

[1] Numbers represent incidents reported to NAF as of 12/31/94; actual incidents are most likely higher. **Please note that final year-end reports of violence have not yet been tabulated. These numbers will increase 1994 totals.**

[2] The sharp increase in incidents for 1991 may be partially attributable to the computerization of NAF's tracking system in mid-1991.

[3] Stalking is defined as the persistent following, threatening, and harassing of an abortion provider, staff member, or patient away from the clinic. Especially severe stalking incidents are noted on NAF's Incidents of Extreme Violence fact sheet. Tabulation of stalking incidents began in 1993.

[4] The "number of arrests" represents the total number of arrests, not the total number of persons arrested. Many blockaders are arrested multiple times.

12/94

References

Adler, N. (1975). Emotional responses of women following therapeutic abortion. <u>American Journal of Orthopsychiatry</u>, **45**, 446-454.

Adler, N. (1979). Abortion: A Social-psychological perspective. <u>Journal of Social Issues</u>, **35**, 100-119.

Adler, N., David, H., Major, B., Roth, S., Russo, N., & Wyatt, G. (1990). Psychological responses after abortion. <u>Science,</u> **248**, 41-44.

Ibid. (1992). Psychological factors in abortion: A review. <u>American Psychologist,</u> **47** (10), 1194-1204.

American Civil Liberties Union/Reproductive Freedom Project (1986). <u>Parental Notice Laws, Their Catastrophic Impact On Teenagers' Right To Abortion</u>, New York: ACLU.

American Civil Liberties Union/Reproductive Freedom Project (1991). <u>Shattering the Dreams of Young Women: The Tragic Consequences of Parental Involvement Laws</u>. New York: Author.

American Health Consultants (1992, August). Changes in OC instructions may cause compliance problems. <u>Contraceptive Technology Update,</u> **13** (8), 117-121.

American Health Consultants (1992, October). There's good news about birth control pills. <u>Women's Health Update: Supplement to Contraceptive Technology Update</u>.

American Medical Association (1992, June 21-25). House of Delegates Proceedings, 141st Annual Meeting, Chicago, IL.

American Medical Association/Council on Scientific Affairs (1992). Induced termination of pregnancy before and after Roe v. Wade: Trends in the mortality and morbidity of women. <u>JAMA</u>, **268**, 3231-3239.

American Psychiatric Association (1987). <u>Diagnostic and Statistical Manual of Mental Disorders, Third Edition, Revised</u>, Washington, D.C.: American Psychiatric Association.

Amon, E. (1988). Limits of fetal viability: Obstetric considerations regarding the management and delivery of the extremely premature baby. Obstetric and Gynecology Clinics of North America, **15** (2), 321-338.

Armsworth, M. (1991). Psychological response to abortion. Journal of Counseling & Development, **69,** 377-379.

Athanasiou, R., Oppel, W., Michaelson, L., Unger, T., & Yaeger, M. (1973). Psychiatric sequelae to term birth and induced early and late abortion: A longitudinal study. Family Planning Perspectives, **5**, 227-231.

Baluk, U., & O'Neill, P. (1980). Health professionals' perceptions of the psychological consequences of abortion. American Journal of Community Psychology, **8**, 67-75.

Bandler, R., & Grinder, J. (1979). Frogs Into Princes. Moab, Utah: Real People Press.

Bass, E., & Davis, L. (1988). The Courage to Heal. NY: Harper and Row.

Bates, M. (1993, August 20). Wichita abortion doctor wounded. The Topeka Capitol-Journal, pp. 1-A, 2-A.

Bennett, M. (1989). Personhood from a neuroscientific perspective. In E. Doerr & J. Prescott (Eds.), Abortion Rights and Fetal 'Personhood.' (pp. 83-85). Long Beach, CA: Centerline Press.

Beresford, T. (1977). Short-Term Relationship Counseling. Baltimore, MD: Planned Parenthood of Maryland.

Berger, L. (1978). Abortions in America: The effects of restrictive funding. The New England Journal of Medicine, **298**, 1474-1477.

Blanchard, D. & Prewitt, T. (1993). Religious Violence and Abortion: The Gideon Project. University Press of Florida.

Blumberg, B., Golbus, M., & Hansen, K. (1975). The psychological sequelae of abortion performed for a genetic indication. American Journal of Obstetrics and Gynecology, **122**, 799-808.

Blumenthal, S. J. (1991). An overview of research findings. In: Stotland, N. L., ed. Psychiatric Aspects of Abortion. Washington, D.C.: American Psychiatric Press.

Bongar, B. (Ed.), (1992). Suicide: Guidelines for Assessment, Management, and Treatment. New York: Oxford University Press.

Borysenko, J. (1990). Guilt Is The Teacher, Love Is The Lesson. New York: Warner Books, Inc.

Bracken, M.B., Klerman, L., & Braken, M. (1978). Coping with pregnancy resolution among never-married women. American Journal of Orthopsychiatry, **48**, 20-334.

Bracken, M.B., Phil, M., Hackamovitch, M., & Grossman, G. (1974). The decision to abort and psychological sequelae. The Journal of Nervous and Mental Disease, **158**, 154-162.

Bracken, M., Hellenbrand, K., Holford, T., Bryce-Buchanan, C. (1986). Low birthweight in pregnancies following induced abortion: no evidence for an association. American Journal of Epidemiology, **123**, 604-613.

REFERENCES

Brown, S. (1993). Aggressive management of LBW infants: Survival at what cost? <u>Ob. Gyn. News</u>, **28** (3), 5.

Campbell, N., Franco, K. & Jurs, S. (1988). Abortion in adolescence. <u>Adolescence</u>, **23**, 813-823.

Chicago Tribune Wires (July 30, 1994). Doctor, aide slain at abortion clinic. <u>Chicago Tribune</u>, pp. 1, 6.

Cohen, L., & Roth, S. (1984). Coping with abortion. <u>Journal of Human Stress</u>, **10**, 140-145.

Cvejic, H., Lipper, I., Kinch, R., & Benjamin, P. (1977). Follow-up of fifty adolescent girls two years after abortion. <u>Canadian Medical Association Journal</u>, **116**, 44-46.

Dagg, P. (1991). The psychological sequelae of therapeutic abortion: Denied and completed. <u>American Journal of Human Stress</u>, **148,** 578-585.

David, H., Friedman, H., Vandertak, J.,& Sevilla, M. (Eds.), (1978). <u>Abortion in Psychosocial Perspective: Trends In Transnational Research</u>. New York: Springer.

David, H., Dytrych, Z., Matejcek, Z., & Schuller, V. (1988). <u>Born Unwanted: Developmental Effects of Denied Abortion</u>, New York: Springer Publishing Co.

David, H. Rasmussen, N., & Holst, E. (1981). Postpartum and postabortion psychotic reactions. <u>Family Planning Perspectives</u>, **13**, 88-93.

Diamond, S. (1993, September/October). Watch on the Right: No place to hide. <u>The Humanist</u>, pp. 39-41.

Doerr, E., & Prescott, J., eds. (1989). <u>Abortion Rights and Fetal 'Personhood.'</u> Long Beach, CA: Centerline Press.

Donnai, D., Charles, N., & Harris, R. (1981). Attitude of patients after genetic termination of pregnancy. <u>British Medical Journal</u>, **282**, 621-622.

Donovan, P. (1983). Judging teenagers: How minors fare when they seek court authorized abortions. <u>Family Planning Perspectives</u>, **15**, 259.

Donovan, P. (1985). The holy war. <u>Family Planning Perspectives</u>, **17** (1), 5-9.

Doyle, J. (1984). The unborn as person. <u>Restoring the Right To Life/The Human Life Amendment</u>, Salt Lake City, UT: Brigham Young University Press.

Droegemueller, M.D., W. & London,M.D., R. (1990). Patient compliance. <u>Clinical Consensus in Obstetrics & Gynecology</u>, Berlex Laboratories, Inc.

Egan, G. (1990). <u>The Skilled Helper</u>. Pacific Grove, CA: Brooks/Cole Publishing Co.

Ewing, J., & Rouse, B. (1973). Therapeutic abortion and a prior psychiatric history. <u>American Journal of Psychiatry</u>, **130**, 37-40.

Faludi, S. (November, 1989). Where did Randy go wrong?, <u>Mother Jones</u>.

Fertel, P., Holowinsky, S., Iams, P., Winterstein, M., Gatlin, S., & Scribner, S. (1988). <u>Difficult Decisions</u>, Omaha, NE: Centering Corporation.

Fingerer, M. (1973). Psychological sequelae of abortion: Anxiety and depression. Journal of Community Psychology, **1,** 221-225.

Flower, M. (1989). Neuromaturation and the moral status of human fetal life. In E. Doerr & J. Prescott (Eds.), Abortion Rights and Fetal 'Personhood.' (pp. 71-82). Long Beach, CA: Centerline Press.

Forrest, J., & Henshaw, S. (1987). The harassment of U.S. abortion providers. Family Planning Perspectives, **19** (1), 9-13.

Forward, S., & Torres, J.(1986). Men Who Hate Women and The Women Who Love Them, New York: Bantam Books, Inc.

Francoeur, R. (1989). Summing up the linchpin question: When does a human become a person, and why? In E. Doerr & J. Prescott (Eds.), Abortion Rights and Fetal 'Personhood.' (117-122). Long Beach, CA: Centerline Press.

Franz, W., & Reardon, D. (1992). Differential impact of abortion on adolescents and adults. Adolescence, **27,** 105.

Freeman, E. (1978). The Ambivalence of Abortion. New York: Random House.

Furuhjelm, M., Ingelman-Sundberg, A., and Wirsen, C. (1976). A Child Is Born. New York: Dell Publishing Co., Inc.

Gold, R. (1990). Abortion and Women's Health: A Turning Point for America? New York and Washington, D.C.: The Alan Guttmacher Institute, pp. 35-36.

Gordon, L. (1976). Woman's Body, Woman's Right. New York: Grossman Publishers.

Gordon, T. (1977). Leader Effectiveness Training, L.E.T. New York: Bantam Books.

Grimes, M.D., D. (1984). Second trimester abortion in the United States. Family Planning Perspectives, **16,** 260-266.

Grimes, M.D., D. (1987, Summer). The safety of mid-trimester abortion. Medical Digest, pp.1-3.

Grimes, M.D., D., Forrest, J., Kirkman,A., & Radford, B. (1991). An epidemic of antiabortion violence in the United States. American Journal of Obstetrics and Gynecology, **165** (5), 1263-1268.

Grimes, D., Schulz, K., & Cates, W. Jr. (1979). Local versus general anesthesia: Which is safer for performing suction abortions? American Journal of Obstetrics and Gynecology, **135,** 1030.

Grobstein, C. (1988). Science and the Unborn, NY: Basic Books.

Grobstein, C. (1989, September). When does life begin? Psychology Today, pp. 43-46.

Handy, J. (1982). Psychological and social aspects of induced abortion. British Journal of Clinical Psychology, **21,** 29-41.

Hatcher, R., Stewart, F., Trussell, J., Kowal, D., Guest, F., Steward., G. Cates, W. (1990-1992). Contraceptive Technology, NY: Irvington Publishers, Inc.

Heisterberg, L. & Kringlebach, M. (1987). Early complications after induced first trimester abortion. Acta Obstetrica Et Gynecologica Scandinavica, **66,** 201-204.

Henshaw, S. (1986). Induced abortion: A worldwide perspective. <u>Family Planning Perspectives</u>, **18**, 250-254.

Henshaw, S. (1990). Induced abortion: a world review. <u>Family Planning Perspectives</u>, **22**, 76-90.

Henshaw, S., Forrest, J. & Van Vort, J. (1987). Abortion services in the United States. <u>Family Planning Perspectives</u>, **19**, 63.

Henshaw, S., & Kost, K. (1992). Parental involvement in minors' abortion decisions. <u>Family Planning Perspectives</u>, **24** (5), 196-213.

Henshaw, S., & Silverman, J. (1988). The characteristics and prior contraception use of U.S. abortion patients. <u>Family Planning Perspectives</u>, **20**, 158-168.

Hern, M.D., H. (1990). <u>Abortion Practice</u>. Philadelphia: J.B. Lippincott, Co.

Hewitt, B., Sider, D., Dampier, C., Eskind, A., & Wescott, G. (1993, March 29). In life's name. <u>People</u>, pp. 44-46.

Hollar, M. (1993, August 22). Perilous practice. <u>The Topeka Capitol-Journal</u>, pp. 1-D, 7-D.

Hovick, T., Vintzileos, A., Campbell, W., Rodis, J., & Nochimson, D. (1989). Neonatal survival rates based on estimated fetal weights in extremely premature infants. <u>American Journal of Perinatology</u>, **6** (3), 329-330.

Iles, S. (1989). The loss of early pregnancy. <u>Bailliere's Clinical Obstetrics and Gynacology</u>, **3** (4), 769-790.

Illinois Caucus on Teenage Pregnancy/Reproductive Choice Project (1991). <u>The Right To Choose: Teen Access to Reproductive Services in Illinois</u>, Chicago: Author.

Jaworski, P. (1989). Thinking about **The Silent Scream**. In E. Doerr & J. Prescott (Eds.), <u>Abortion Rights and Fetal 'Personhood.'</u> (pp.61-70). Long Beach, CA: Centerline Press.

Johnson, D. (1993, August 28). Abortions, Bibles and bullets and the making of a militant. <u>New York Times</u>, pp. 1, 8.

Jones, O., Penn, N., Shuchter, S., Stafford, C., Richards, T., Kernahan, C., Gutierrez,J., & Cherkin, P. (1984). Parental response to mid-trimester therapeutic abortion following amniocentesis. <u>Prenatal Diagnosis</u>, **4**, 249-256.

Kalmar, R. (1977). <u>Abortion: The Emotional Implications.</u> Dubuque: Kendall/Hunt.

Kantrowitz, B., & Crandall, R. (1990, Aug. 20). A vital aid for preemies. <u>Newsweek</u>, p. 70.

Kilbride, H., Daily, D., Claflin, K., Hall, R., Maulik, D., & Grundy, H. (1990). Improved survival and neurodevelopmental outcome for infants less than 801 grams birthweight. <u>American Journal of Perinatology</u>, **7** (2),160-165.

Knight, J., & Callahan, J. (1989). Elective abortion: The moral debate. <u>Preventing Birth: Contemporary Methods and Related Moral Controversies</u>, Salt Lake City, UT: University of Utah Press.

Kummer, J. (1963). Post-abortion psychiatric illness - a myth? <u>American Journal of Psychiatry</u>, **119**, 980-983.

LeBolt, S., Grimes, D., & Cates, W., Jr. (1982). Mortality from abortion and childbirth: Are the populations comparable? JAMA, 248 (2),188-191.

Lister, M., & Lovell, S. (1991). Healing Together: For Couples Whose Baby Dies, Omaha, NE: Centering Corporation.

Luker, K. (1976). Taking Chances: Abortion and the Decision Not To Contracept, Berkeley, CA: University of California Press.

Lloyd, J., & Laurence, K. (1985). Sequelae and support after termination of pregnancy for fetal malformation. British Medical Journal, 290, 907-909.

Lumley, J. (1986). Very low birthweight (l,500 g) and previous induced abortion: Victoria 1982-1983. Australia and New Zealand Journal of Obstetrics and Gynecology, 26, 268-272.

Magyari, P., Wedehase, B., Ifft, R., & Callanan, N. (1988). A supportive intervention protocol for couples terminating a pregnancy for genetic reasons. Birth Defects, 23 (6), 76-83.

Major, B., & Cozzarelli, C. (1992). Psychosocial predictors of adjustment to abortion. Journal of Social Issues, 48 (3), 121-142.

Major, B., Cozzarelli, C., Sciacchitano, A., Cooper, M., Testa, M., & Mueller, P. (1990). Perceived social support, self-efficacy, and adjustment to abortion. Journal of Personality and Social Psychology, 59, 452-463.

Major, B., Cozzarelli, C., & Testa, M. (1992). Male partners' appraisals of undesired pregnancy and abortion: Implications for women's adjustment to abortion. Journal of Applied Social Psychology, 22, 599-614.

Major, B., Mueller, P., & Hildebrandt, K. (1985). Attributions, expectations, and coping with abortion. Journal of Personality and Social Psychology, 48, 585-599.

Margolis, A., Davison, L., Hanson, K., Loos, S., & Mikkelsen, C. (1971). Therapeutic abortion: Follow-up study. American Journal of Obstetrics and Gynecology, 110, 243.

Maris, R. (Ed.), (1992). Assessment and Prediction of Suicide. New York: Guilford Press.

Mayer, A. (1993). Incest: A Treatment Manual for Therapy With Victims, Spouses and Offenders. Holmes Beach: Learning Publications, Inc.

Melton, G. (1986). Adolescent Abortion: Psychological and Legal Issues. Lincoln: University of Nebraska Press.

Mendelson, M., Maden, C., & Daling, J. (1992). Low birthweight in relation to multiple induced abortions. American Journal of Public Health, 82 (3), 391-394.

Minnick, M., Delp, K., & Ciotti, M. (1991). A Time to Decide, A Time to Heal. East Lansing, MI: Pineapple Press.

Moore, K. (1989). Before We Are Born: Basic Embryology and Birth Defects. Philadelphia: W.B. Saunders Co.

Mosley, D., Follingstad, D., Harley, H., & Heckel, R. (1981). Psychological factors that predict reaction to abortion. Journal of Clinical Psychology, 37, 276-279.

Mueller, P., & Major, B. (1989). Self-blame, self-efficacy, and adjustment to abortion. Journal of Personality and Social Psychology, **57** (6), 1059-1068.

National Abortion Federation (1990). Women who have abortions fact sheet. Washington, D.C.: National Abortion Federation.

National Abortion Federation (1993). Incidents of violence and disruption against abortion providers fact sheet. Washington, D.C.: National Abortion Federation.

National Abortion Federation (1993, October 29). News Release. (Available from National Abortion Federation, 1436 U Street, N.W., Washington, D.C. 20009).

Niswander, K., & Porto, M. (1986). Abortion practices in the United States: A medical viewpoint. In J.D. Butler & D.F. Walbert (Eds.), Abortion, Medicine, and the Law (pp. 248-265). New York: Facts on File Publications.

Osofsky, H., Osofsky, J., & Rajan, R. (1973). Psychological effects of abortion. In H. Osofsky & J. Osofsky (Eds.), The Abortion Experience (pp.188-205). New York: Harper & Row.

Pacter, J., & Nelson, F. (1974). Factors in the unprecedented decline in infant mortality in New York City. Bulletin of the New York Academy of Medicine, **50**, 839-868.

Payne, E., Kravitz, A., Notman, M., & Anderson, J. (1976). Outcome following therapeutic abortion. Archives of General Psychiatry, **33**, 725-733.

Peck, A., & Marcus, J. (1966). Psychiatric sequelae of therapeutic interruption of pregnancy. Journal of Nervous and Mental Diseases, **143**, 417-425.

Perez-Reyes, M., & Falk, R. (1973). Follow-up after therapeutic abortion in early adolescence. Archives of General Psychiatry, **28**, 120-126.

Plutzer, E., & Ryan, B. (1985). Individual reasons and the social influences on women's decision to tell or not tell the co-conceiver about the pregnancy: A study of abortion clients. Unpublished research, The Hope Clinic for Women, Ltd.

Rando, T. (1988). How To Go On Living When Someone You Love Dies. New York: Bantam Books.

Richardson, J. (1987). The Magic of Rapport. Cupertino, CA: Meta Publications.

Rizzardo, R., Novarin, S., Forza, G., & Cosentino, M. (1991). Personality and psychological distress in legal abortion, threatened miscarriage and normal pregnancy. Psychotherapy Psychosomatics, **56**, 227-234.

Robbins, J., & DeLamater, J. (1985). Support from significant others and loneliness following induced abortion. Social Psychiatry, **20**, 92-99.

Romans-Clarkson, S. (1989). Psychological sequelae of induced abortion. Australian and New Zealand Journal of Psychiatry, **23** (4), 555-565.

Rosenthal, M., & Rothchild, E. (1975). Some psychological considerations in adolescent pregnancy and abortion. Advances in Planned Parenthood, **9** (3), 60-69.

Rubin, A. (1992, March 22). The other abortion case. Washington Post.

Russo, N., & Zierk, K. (1992). Abortion, childbearing, and women's well-being. Professional Psychology: Research and Practice, **23,** 269.

Seidman, D., Ever-Hadani, P., Slater, P., Harlap, S., Stevenson, D., Gale, R. (1988). Childbearing after induced abortion: Reassessment of risk. Epidemiological Community Health, **42,** 294-298.

Shannon, D. (1990). Guide for Pro-Choice Catholics. Catholics for Free Choice.

Sharpe, R. (1990, July/August). She died because of a law. Ms. p. 80.

Shepard, C. (1991, November 24). Operation rescue's mission to save itself. The Washington Post.

Simmons, P.(1990). Personhood, The Bible,and the Abortion Debate. Washington, D.C.: The Religious Coalition for Abortion Rights Educational Fund, Inc.

Simon, N., & Senturia, A. (1976). Psychological sequelae of abortion: Review of the literature, 1935-64. Archives of General Psychiatry, **16,** 378-392.

Smith, E. (1973). A follow-up study of women who request abortion. American Journal of Orthopsychiatry, **43,** 574-585.

Speckhard, A. (1987). The Psycho-Social Aspects of Stress Following Abortion. Kansas City, MO: Sheed & Ward.

Stewart, G., Goldstein, P. (1971). Therapeutic abortion in California: Effects on septic abortion and maternal mortality. Obstetrics and Gynecology, **37,** 510-514.

Stotland, M.D., N. (1992). The myth of the abortion trauma syndrome. JAMA, **268** (15), 2078-2079.

Stubblefield, M.D., P. (1989). Control of pain for women undergoing abortion. International Journal of Gynecology and Obstetricians, **3,** 131-140.

Suprato, K., & Reed, S. (1984). Naproxen Sodium for pain relief in first trimester abortion. American Journal Obstetrics and Gynecology. **150,** 1000.

Thoren, H. (1993). Physicians urged to encourage use of ocs in perimenopausal women. Ob. Gyn. News, **28** (8),1.

Tietze, C., & Henshaw, S. (1986). Induced abortion: A world review. New York: The Alan Guttmacher Institute.

Tietze, C., & Lewit, S. (1977). Legal abortion. Scientific American, **236,** 21-28.

Wade, R. (1978). For Men About Abortion (available from Roger C. Wade, P.O. Box 4748, Boulder, CO 80306).

Wallerstein, J., Kurtz, P., & Bar-Din, M. (1972). Psychological sequelae of therapeutic abortion in young unmarried women. Archives of General Psychiatry, **27,** 828-927.

Wells, N. (1989). Management of pain during an abortion. Journal of Advanced Nursing, **14,** 56-62.

Wells, N. (1992). Reducing distress during abortion: A test of sensory information. Journal of Advanced Nursing, **17,** 1050-1056.

Williams-Deane, M., & Potter, L. (1992). Current oral contraceptive use instructions: An analysis of patient package inserts. Family Planning Perspectives, **24** (3), 111-115.

Wills, G. (1989, May 1). Save the babies. Time.

Yearwood, L. (1993, March 22). Protester guns down clinic doctor. St. Louis Post-Dispatch, pp. 1, 11.

Zabin, L., Hirsch, M., & Emerson, M. (1989). When urban adolescents choose abortion: Effects on education, psychological status and subsequent pregnancy. Family Planning Perspectives, **21**, 248-255.

Zimmerman, M. (1977). Passage Through Abortion: The Personal and Social Reality of Women's Experiences. New York: Praeger.

Index

A

Abnormalities, fetal: Anencephaly, 132; Cystic Fibrosis, 132; Down's Syndrome, 132; Huntington's Disease (Chorea), 132; Hydrocephalus, 132; Klinefelter's Syndrome, 133; Niemann-Pick Disease, 132; Spina Bifida, 132; Tay-Sachs Disease, 132; Turner's Syndrome, 132; tests to determine, 133; amniocentesis, 133; chorionic villus sampling, 133; fetoscopy, 133; ultrasound, 133

Abortion: after, first trimester, 104, second trimester, 172-73; client's coping after an abortion, 69-74; emotional reactions on the day of the abortion and during counseling, 52, 57-64; complications of, first trimester, 104-106, second trimester, 173-76; counseling, 53-55, 64-77, 93-101, 103, 104, 107-112, 113-161, 176-179, 180-184; counselor's attitudes toward, 11-12; history of, 5, 196; illegal, 5, 196, 199; impact on society, families, and women's lives, 199-200; number of, in the United States, 50; procedure, first trimester, 103-104, second trimester, 172-175; profile of women choosing, 49; reasons for choosing, 50-52, 200, in the second trimester, 169-172; safety of, 175-176, 199; saline, 174-175; second trimester, 169-187; steps to obtaining, 49. See also Counseling, repeat abortion, second trimester abortion

Abstinence: adolescents, post-abortion and, 161, 166; discussing the reality of, in post-abortion counseling, 166-167; discussion of, in self-help booklet, 161, 167

Abuse: by male partner, 94, 115-117, long-term effects, 200, risks of post-abortion complications, 177; by parents, 73, 100, 149; long-term effects, 200; by significant others, and effects on client's post-abortion coping, 71, 73, 100, 115, 117; history of, and potential for poor coping post-abortion, 71, 73, 87; of abortion clinic staff by anti-abortion clients, 141-142; by anti-abortion terrorists, 192-195; statements made by clients revealing the probability of, by male partner, 115-116

Adolescents: abuse by parents and effects on post-abortion coping, 73, 100-101; abuse by parents and parental involvement laws, 149-150; anger toward parents, 89-90, 154, 155; baby fantasies, 42, 177; financial dilemmas, 37, 39; in the pre-abortion counseling session, 158-160; mistrust of the counselor, 158; reactions to a pregnancy, 146; reality testing for parenthood, 37; reasons for abortion, 42, 51, 170; risk-taking, 15-16; second trimester abortion, 170, 171, 177, 179-180; sexuality, 12-13; using denial about the pregnancy, 170, 177; who are too far in the pregnancy for an abortion, 183; who don't tell their parents about their pregnancy, 150; who tell their parents about their pregnancy, 150. See also Men, adolescent

Adoption: as atonement for previous abortion, 143; attitudes toward, 12; laws, questions about, 47-48; reasons for choosing, 45-47, 183; reasons for rejecting, 45-47, 51-52, 197; by incest survi-

About the Author

Anne Baker is the Director of Counseling at The Hope Clinic for Women, an abortion provider in Granite City, Illinois. She holds a Master of Arts in Counseling Psychology from Lindenwood College in St. Louis, Missouri. Ms. Baker has counseled over 15,000 women before their abortions and has conducted research on post-abortion emotions and how women cope. She has conducted counselor training workshops across the United States and Canada on pregnancy options and abortion counseling.

Anne Baker is the author of <u>The Complete Book of Problem Pregnancy Counseling</u>, <u>Survival Kit for Abortion Providers: Emotional Support in Times of Crisis</u>, and the self-help booklets, <u>How To Cope Successfully After An Abortion</u>, <u>How To Cope With Guilt</u>, <u>After Her Abortion: For Parents, Male Partners, and Friends</u>, and <u>I'll Never Have Sex Again</u>. Ms. Baker received the 1993 C. Lalor Burdick Award from the National Abortion Federation for her contribution to the field of abortion and reproductive health.

NOTES